UNDERSTANDING KIDNEY DISEASES

A SIMPLIFIED APPROACH

Authored by leading nephrologists and physicians. Simplifies nephrology for non-nephrologists.
Includes one page illustrated infographic with each chapter.

Dr Priti Meena | Dr Garima Aggarwal | Dr Urmila Anandh
Dr Narinder Pal Singh | Dr Anupam Prakash

Section Editors: Dr Edwin M. Fernando, Dr Vinant Bhargava

notionpress.com

INDIA • SINGAPORE • MALAYSIA

ISBN

Hardcase 979-8-89673-452-9
Paperback 979-8-89066-888-2

CONTENTS

SECTION 1
Introduction to Kidney Diseases

SECTION 2
Glomerular Diseases

SECTION 3
Acute Kidney Injury

SECTION 4

Chronic Kidney Disease

SECTION 5

Kidney Disorders In Systemic Diseases

SECTION 6
Renal Replacement Therapy

SECTION 7
Miscellaneous

SECTION 8
Electrolyte Disorders

ABOUT THE EDITORS

1. Dr. Priti Meena, a nephrologist, FASN, MD in General Medicine from Maulana Azad Medical College and MBBS from LHMC, New Delhi. Currently, she holds the position of Assistant Professor at AIIMS Bhubaneswar. She has published her research in numerous peer-reviewed national and international journals. Dr. Meena is an Editorial Fellow at the prestigious kidney journal NDT and Associate Editor of the Indian Journal of Nephrology. She is also an editor of the book Textbook of Kidney Transplantation. She is a council member of the Indian Hemodialysis Society and a Visual Abstract Editor for Kidney International, Kidney 360, and IJN.
2. Dr. Garima Aggarwal is a consultant Nephrologist and Transplant specialist at Manipal Hospital, Varthur Road, Bangalore. She has a stellar academic background, earning a gold medal in MD Medicine and securing top rank in DM Nephrology training. Recognized by the Indian Medical Association for Academic Excellence in Kidney Care, she is actively engaged in promoting kidney disease education. She is a sought-after speaker, faculty member, and active participant in national and international nephrology and medicine conferences.

3. Dr. Urmila Anandh is a senior nephrologist currently working at Amrita Hospitals, Faridabad. She had her early training in AIIMS (New Delhi) and CMC Vellore. She has more than 25 years of experience as a nephrologist and is part of various committees of International Society of Nephrology. Education is her area of interest and she has mentored students from all over the world. She has many publications from both international and national journals. She is the founder president of Women In Nephrology India.
4. Dr. (Prof.) Narinder Pal Singh possesses over 30 years of extensive experience in Internal Medicine and Nephrology. He currently serves as the Professor and Dean of Research at Eternal University in Baru Sahib, Himachal Pradesh. Previously, Dr. Singh held prestigious positions including Medical Director and Senior Director of Medicine at Max Super Speciality Hospital in Vaishali, Ghaziabad, and Director Professor of Medicine and Head of Nephrology at MAMC in New Delhi. With over three decades of teaching experience, he now coordinates NBE academic activities for DNB (General Medicine) and trains medical professionals for MRCPUK. His contributions have earned him numerous awards, and he has authored numerous publications, chapters, and edited books in the field of medicine.
5. Dr. Anupam Prakash did his MBBS from UCMS, Delhi and MD (Medicine) from Maulana Azad Medical College, Delhi. He is presently the Director Professor of Medicine at Lady Hardinge Medical College, New Delhi. He has been a medical Teacher for 23 years with over 250 publications in journals and texts, and has authored eight books/monographs. He is Editor-in-Chief of Indian Journal of Medical Specialities, and is on the Editorial Board of Journal of Association of Physicians of India, API. He is the President of Indian Society for Atherosclerosis Research and Delhi Diabetic Forum and is a Governing Body Member of API. He is a recipient of several orations and awards.

ACKNOWLEDGMENT

As the editors of "Understanding Kidney Diseases: A Simplified Approach", we stand on the shoulders of giants, and it is with deep gratitude that we acknowledge those who have contributed to the creation of this book.

First and foremost, we extend our heartfelt thanks to our seniors and mentors in the field of nephrology and medicine. Your guidance, wisdom, and unwavering support have been instrumental in shaping our understanding of kidney diseases. Your dedication to patient care and teaching have inspired us continuously, and we are honored to carry forward your legacy.

We are immensely grateful to our authors, whose expertise and passion have enriched the chapters of this book. Your commitment to sharing knowledge and advancing the field of medicine is commendable.

A special mention and thanks to our graphic designer, Suguna Ganesh, who helped us design and beautify the infographics submitted by the authors.

At the heart of every meaningful endeavor lies inspiration, often sparked by a need, a gap, or a challenge. We want to thank the myriad of clinicians and non-nephrology colleagues who expressed the pressing demand for a resource like this.

Our patients have played a vital role in our journey. Their resilience, stories, and experiences have served as a constant reminder of the real-world impact of kidney diseases. We thank them for entrusting us with their care and for being a crucial part of our teaching and learning process.

Finally, we extend our heartfelt gratitude to our family members. Your unwavering support, understanding, and encouragement have been our rock throughout this endeavor.

This book would not have been possible without the collective contribution and support of all these individuals. Thank you for helping us make "Understanding Kidney Diseases: A Simplified Approach" a reality.

FOREWORD

The book, "Understanding Kidney Diseases" is a blue rose. The painstaking effort of the editors has bestowed a rare distinction and flavor to this book. It is simple and straightforward; in a reader-friendly lexicon and style. Keeping in mind that practitioners and specialists are reading it to solve day-to-day, real world, and real time challenges, this book provides hands-on information. To blend depth in brevity is an art. For me, it was non-put-downable.

I trust the editors have achieved their goal of helping clinicians and caregivers in early identification and better management of kidney diseases. Thoughtfully crafted, this book presents practical insights into common kidney ailments encountered in everyday clinical practice. It serves as an indispensable resource for doctors, navigating the dynamic landscape of modern medicine.

The authors celebrate the kidneys as masters of the internal milieu. Simple statements like 'Urine is liquid gold' and 'Examining the urine is poor man's kidney biopsy' capture the necessary import. Tables similar to the one depicting CKD by GFR and albuminuria categories are a delight to understand and could be put to use straight away. Obstetricians can delve into the chapter "Pregnancy and kidneys" as a ready reference.

In a nation as diverse as India, empowering our clinicians with knowledge is the only way to reach quality care out to people. The authors have bridged the gap between specialized expertise and primary care. I express my gratitude for this act of nation-building and extend my appreciation towards the passionate team who have left their footprints in the sands of time. This book has enriched the clinicians' choices in understanding the diseases of the kidneys.

– Dr RV ASOKAN
National President,
Indian Medical Association,
PUNALUR, Kerala, India.

FOREWORD

It is my distinct privilege as the President of the Indian Society of Nephrology to introduce this collaborative effort on kidney diseases, authored by eminent nephrologists. Hans Hofmann, an abstract painter artist, said it so succinctly, "The ability to simplify means to eliminate the unnecessary so that the necessary may speak." This book addresses a critical imperative in a simplified way for the intended readers—general practitioners, physicians, and non-nephrologists—with the knowledge and tools necessary for the early detection and effective management of common kidney cases in clinical settings.

Kidney diseases pose a significant health challenge, and timely intervention is paramount in mitigating their impact. This book, a testament to the collective expertise of our nephrological community, simplifies the complexities of renal disorders into a resource accessible to medical professionals across disciplines. The aim is to empower practitioners at the frontline of patient care by providing practical insights, diagnostic approaches, and management strategies.

I extend my heartfelt appreciation to the dedicated nephrologists whose contributions make this book a beacon of knowledge. May it serve as a catalyst for heightened awareness, early detection, and ultimately, improved outcomes for individuals suffering from kidney diseases.

To our colleagues embracing the challenges of diverse medical landscapes, your commitment to advancing healthcare is commendable. Together, let us champion a holistic approach to kidney care, ensuring that every practitioner, regardless of specialization, is equipped to contribute meaningfully to the well-being of our patients.

With sincere regards,

– Harbir Singh Kohli
President,
Indian Society of Nephrology,
PGIMER, Chandigarh, India.

FOREWORD

It is my pleasure to endorse a remarkable book that is poised to make a significant impact on our collective approach to kidney health. Nephrology, with its intricate concepts and involvement of basic sciences, can often appear daunting to non-specialists, general practitioners, and physicians in clinics. This book, a product of the expertise and dedication of its authors, seeks to demystify these complexities. By breaking down intricate concepts, it aspires to empower clinicians, making the diagnosis and treatment of kidney diseases more accessible.

What sets this book apart is its commitment to keeping practitioners informed about the latest advancements in kidney therapeutics. In an ever-evolving field, staying current with the latest knowledge is paramount. The authors have succeeded in presenting not only a guide to understanding common kidney conditions but also an invaluable resource on the most recent developments in treatment modalities. I especially appreciate the illustrated summaries at the end of each chapter.

I extend my sincere appreciation to the editors for their tireless efforts in creating this invaluable nephrology resource. To all practitioners, I urge you to explore the pages of this book, confident that it will enrich your understanding and practice in the realm of kidney diseases.

Wishing you a rewarding journey through the insights and practical wisdom presented within these pages.

Sincerely,

– Dr Milind Y Nadkar
Past-president,
Association of Physicians of India (API),
Seth G S Medical College &
KEM Hospital, Mumbai, India.

LIST OF CONTRIBUTORS

1. Dr Ajay Kher
   Co-founder and Director,
   Epitome- Kidney Urology Institute and Lions Hospital,
   New Friends Colony, Delhi, India.

2. Dr Alpana Raizada
   Professor, Dept of Medicine, UCMS and GTB Hospital, Delhi, India.

3. Dr Amit Roy
   Senior Resident, Department of Nephrology, Gauhati Medical College and Hospital, Guwahati, Assam, India.

4. Dr Anirban Ganguli
   Staff Nephrologist and Research Associate, Kidney Disease Branch,
   National Institutes of Digestive, Diabetic and Kidney Diseases,
   National Institutes of Health, Bethesda, MD, USA.

5. Dr Anish Garg
   Senior Resident, Department of Nephrology, AIIMS Bhubaneswar, Odisha, India.

6. Dr Anish Kumar Gupta
   Consultant (Research and Development),
   Faculty of Medicine and Health Sciences,
   SGT Medical College Hospital and Research Institute,
   SGT University Gurugram, Haryana, India.

7. Dr Anupam Prakash
   Director Professor, Dept of Medicine, LHMC and SSK Hospital, Delhi, India.

8. Dr Arpita Roy Choudhary
   Professor, Dept of Nephrology, IPGMER & SSKM Hospitals, Kolkata, West Bengal, India.

9. Dr Arvind Kumar Verma
   Resident, Department of Medicine, KGMU, Lucknow, India.

10. Dr Avinash Kumar
    Resident, Department of Medicine,
    KGMU, Lucknow, Uttar Pradesh, India.

11. Dr Balbir Singh Kohli
    Consulting Critical Care Physician at Jupiter Hospital, Thane, Maharashtra, India.
    Consulting Critical Care Physician at Fortis Hospital Mulund, Mumbai, Maharashtra, India.
    Head Department of Critical Care & Emergency at Hira Mongi Navneet Hospital,
    Mulund, Mumbai, Maharashtra, India.

12. Dr Dinesh Khullar
    Chairman, Department of Nephrology and Renal Transplant Medicine at Max Super Speciality Hospital, Saket, New Delhi, India.

13. Dr Divya Bajpai
    Professor (Addl), Department of Nephrology; Seth G.S.M.C and K.E.M. Hospital, Mumbai, Maharashtra, India.

14. Dr Gireesh Reddy
Consultant Interventional Nephrologist and Transplant Physician,
Institute of NephroUrology, Victoria Hospital Campus, Bangalore, Karnataka, India.

15. Dr Gurleen Kaur
Assistant Professor, Department of Nephrology,
George Washington University, NW, Washington, USA.

16. Dr Jithu Kuiren
Assistant Professor, Department of Nephrology
Pushpagiri Medical College, Thiruvalla, Kerala, India.

17. Dr Kamal Kumar Sawlani
Professor, Department of Medicine, KGMU, Lucknow, Uttar Pradesh, India.

18. Dr Karthik Ganesh
Consultant Nephrologist, VPS Lakeshore Hospital, Kochi, Kerala, India.

19. Dr Kirti Singh
Senior Resident, Department of Urology and Renal Transplant, AIIMS, Bhubaneswar, Odisha, India.

20. Dr Kulwant Singh,
Consultant Nephrologist, Department of Nephrology,
Ivy Hospital, Mohali, Punjab, Mohali 160071, Punjab, India.

21. Dr Manisha Dassi
Principal Consultant, Department of Nephrology and Renal Transplant
Max Super Speciality Hospital, Vaishali, Ghaziabad, India.

22. Dr Manisha Sahay
Professor and Head, Department of Nephrology,
Osmania Medical College & Osmania General Hospital, Hyderabad, Telangana, India.

23. Dr Manjuri Sharma
Professor and Head of Department of Nephrology, Guwahati Medical College and Hospital, Guwahati, Assam, India.

24. Dr Manjusha Yadla
Professor and Head, Department of Nephrology,
Gandhi Medical College,
Hyderabad, Telangana, India.

25. Dr Manoj Das
Department of Urology and Renal Transplant, AIIMS, Bhubaneswar, Odisha, India.

26. Dr M Edwin Fernando
Head of Department, Professor,
Stanley Medical College, Chennai, Tamil Nadu, India.

27. Dr M Subashri
Assistant Professor, Department of Nephrology,
Government Thoothukudi Medical College & Hospital, Thoothukudi, Tamil Nadu, India.

28. Dr Narayan Prasad
Professor and Head, Department of Nephrology;
Sanjay Gandhi Postgraduate Institute of Medical Sciences, Lucknow, Uttar Pradesh, India.

29. Dr Narinder Pal Singh
Dean Research, Eternal University, Baru Sahib, Himachal Pradesh, India.
Advisor Research (Medical Sciences), Shree Guru Gobind Singh Tricentenary University, Gurugram, Haryana, India.
Consultant – Academic Programs in Nephrology, Max Super Speciality Hospital,
Saket, Delhi, India.

30. Dr. Natarajan Gopalakrishnan
Director, Institute of Nephrology, Madras Medical College, Chennai, Tamil Nadu, India.

31. Dr Padmini Sirkanungo
Assistant Professor, Department of Nephrology, MGM Medical College & Superspeciality Hospitals, Indore, Madhya Pradesh, India.

32. Dr Pallavi Prasad
Assistant Professor, Department of Nephrology, Vardhman Mahavir Medical College and Safdarjung Hospital, New Delhi, India.

33. Dr Paromita Das
Senior Resident, Department of Nephrology, AIIMS, Bhubaneswar, Odisha, India.

34. Dr Priti Meena
Assistant Professor, Department of Nephrology,
All India Institute of Medical Sciences, Bhubaneswar, Odisha, India.

35. Dr Raja Ramachandran
Associate Professor, Department of Nephrology,
PGIMER, Chandigarh, India.

36. Dr Sandip Panda
Associate Professor, Department of Nephrology
All India Institute of Medical Sciences, Bhubaneswar, Odisha, India.

37. Dr Santosh Varughese
Professor, Department of Nephrology, Christian Medical College, Vellore, Tamil Nadu, India.

38. Dr Saurabh Nayak
Associate Professor, Department of Nephrology,
AIIMS, Bathinda, Punjab, India.

39. Dr Sayali Thakare
Assistant Professor, Department of Nephrology,
Seth G.S.M.C and K.E.M. Hospital, Mumbai, Maharashtra, India.

40. Dr Shambhavi Sinha
Junior Resident, Department of Medicine, KGMU, Lucknow, Uttar Pradesh, India.

41. Dr Sharmas Valli
Senior Consultant, Department of Nephrology,
AINU, Dilsukhnagar, Hyderabad, Telangana, India.

42. Dr Shyam Chand Chaudhary
Professor, Department of Medicine, KGMU, Lucknow, Uttar Pradesh, India.

43. Dr Smriti Sinha
Consultant, Department of Nephrology,
Marengo Asia Hospita, Faridabad, Delhi NCR, India.

44. Dr Sreejith Parameswaran
Professor, Department of Nephrology,
Jawaharlal Institute of Postgraduate Medical Education and Research (JIPMER),
Pondicherry, India.

45. Suguna Ganesh
Graphic Designer, sugunaganesh1995@gmail.com

46. Dr Sujit Suren
Assistant Professor, Stanley Medical College, Chennai, Tamil Nadu, India.

47. Dr Swarnalatha Guditi
Professor and Head, Department of Nephrology,
NIMS Hospital, Hyderabad, Telangana, India.

48. Dr Swarnendu Mandal
Dept of Urology, AIIMS,
Bhubaneswar, Odisha, India.

49. Dr Swati Pal
Senior Resident, Department of Medicine, VMMC and Safdarjung Hospital, Delhi, India.

50. Dr Tanuj Moses Lamech
Assistant Professor, Institute of Nephrology, Madras Medical College, Chennai, Tamil Nadu, India.

51. Dr Urmila Anandh
Senior Consultant and Head, Department of Nephrology, Amrita Hospitals, Faridabad, Delhi NCR, India.

52. Dr Vijay Kher
Chairman, Nephrology and Kidney Transplant,
Epitome- Kidney Urology Institute and Lions Hospital,
New Friends Colony, Delhi, India.

53. Dr Vinant Bhargava
Senior Consultant Nephrologist, Sir Ganga Ram Hospital, New Delhi, India.

54. Dr Vineet Behara
Consultant Nephrologist, Professor of Medicine,
INHS Kalyani, Visakhapatnam, Andhra Pradesh, India.

55. Dr Vishwanath Siddini
Professor and Head, Department of Nephrology,
Manipal Hospital, Old Airport Road, Bengaluru, Karnataka, India.

56. Dr (Prof) V Narayanan Unni – MD, DM, FRCP, FASN, FISN
Lead Senior Consultant Nephrologist,
Aster Medcity, Kochi, Kerala, India.

SECTION 1

Introduction to Kidney Diseases

01

INTRODUCTION TO KIDNEY DISEASES (WHEN TO SUSPECT, HOW TO SCREEN)

M Subashri, M Edwin Fernando

Introduction:

Superficially, it might be said that the function of the kidneys is to make urine; but in a more considered view, one can say that the kidneys make the stuff of philosophy itself.

– Homer Smith 'The Evolution of the Kidney', Lectures on the Kidney (1943).

Kidneys are the masters of the 'internal milieu'. They are responsible for a wide range of functions, which include the maintenance of acid-base and electrolyte balance, production of erythropoietin, maintenance of bone mineral metabolism, and regulation of blood pressure along with excretion of nitrogenous wastes and urine. Hence, the diseases of the kidneys can manifest as an abnormality in any of the above. Also, the optimal functioning of the kidneys involves its crosstalk between multiple other organs, and hence, the diseases of the kidneys can occur in isolation or as part of a systemic illness. Thus, suspecting and diagnosing a kidney disease at the earliest requires thorough history taking, complete physical examination, and a structured investigative approach.

- **Referral of Asymptomatic Patients with Suspected Renal Disease:**

The referral usually occurs after a clinical or laboratory test reveals an abnormality that is not causing symptoms. These come up during routine medical exams at school, for employment, life insurance, immigration, major surgery, potential live kidney donation, as a part of the health screening in at-risk individuals with systemic diseases, at booking for pregnancy care, or while evaluating infertility.

- **Signs and Symptoms Indicative of Renal Disease:**

Patients with kidney disease present with one or many of the following features. These include:

  - Abnormal blood laboratory values (e.g., elevated blood urea nitrogen and serum creatinine, decreased estimated glomerular filtration rate, or abnormal serum electrolyte values).
  - Abnormalities in urine composition (e.g., microalbuminuria, microscopic hematuria, proteinuria).
  - Changes in urine volume (anuria, oliguria, polyuria).
  - Changes in voiding (hesitancy, intermittency, double stream, dribbling of urine, and straining), or storage (altered bladder sensation, increased daytime frequency, nocturia, urgency or stress incontinence).
  - New-onset hypertension or hypertension in the young.
  - Worsening edema in dependent areas such as ankle or periorbital puffiness.
  - Pain originating along the urinary tract (renal colic, ureteric colic, pyelonephritis, and loin pain-hematuria syndrome).

- Anatomical abnormalities in the kidney and urinary tract (incidentally discovered on imaging studies or clinical presentation, e.g., horseshoe kidney, congenitally absent or ptotic kidney, asymmetric kidneys, angiomyolipoma, renal mass, polycystic kidneys, pelviureteric junction obstruction, and ectopic ureter).
- Manifestations of uremia (e.g., nausea, vomiting, intractable hiccups, pruritus, easy fatigability, breathlessness, unexplained anemia, altered mentation, seizures, asterixis, and decreased libido) (Figure 1.1).
- Other nonspecific signs and symptoms (neurological weakness in hypokalemia, seizures, or gait abnormalities in hyponatremia, abdominal pain, or psychiatric manifestations in hypercalcemia).
- Failure to thrive, bony abnormalities such as bow legs or windshield deformities, renal stones (in renal tubular acidosis, especially in children).
- Symptoms associated with underlying systemic illness (arthralgia, rash due to vasculitic conditions such as systemic lupus erythematosus, anti-neutrophil cytoplasmic antibody syndrome, multiple spontaneous abortions in antiphospholipid antibody syndrome, and arthritis due to gout).

- **Renal Disease Screening in Special Populations:**

The most common cause of chronic kidney disease worldwide is diabetes mellitus, followed by hypertension. Hence, periodic follow-up of these patients has to be done on a regular basis to identify the disease early during its course. To curb the growth of chronic kidney diseases as a global pandemic, screening programs should be considered to identify places that are similar to 'hot spots' of chronic kidney diseases of unknown etiology, such as Uddanam, Tondaimandalam, Canacona, Marthwada, etc.

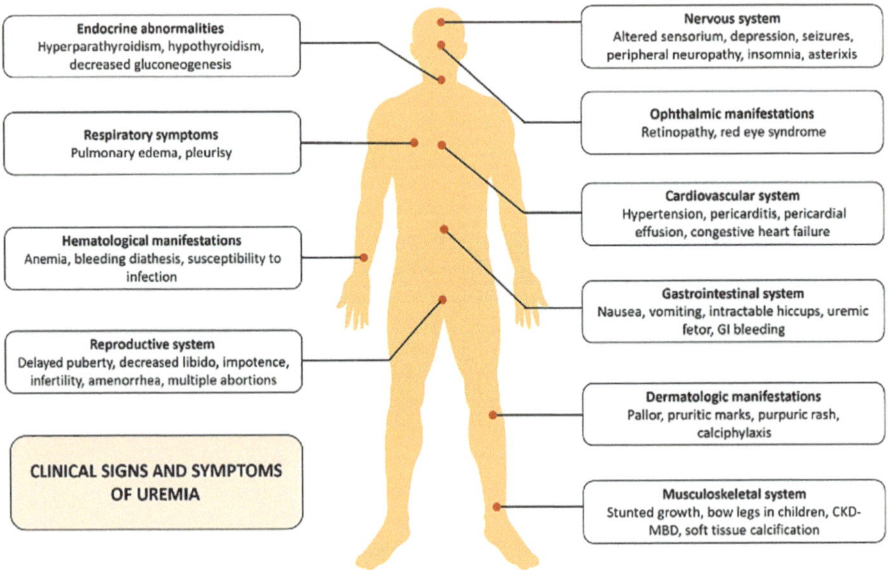

Figure 1.1: Clinical Manifestations of Uremia

Abbreviations: CKD-MBD, Chronic kidney disease-mineral bone disease; GI, Gastrointestinal.

- **How to Screen for Kidney Disease:**

1.1 Urinalysis:

Urine is liquid gold. It is a fundamental step in diagnosing renal disease and is considered an extension of clinical examination. Freshly voided morning urine is preferred. Three characteristics should be observed: physical, biochemical, and microscopic. In clinical practice, direct examination and dipstick testing are usually sufficient.

1.1.1 Physical Properties:

i. **Color** – The most important color change to observe is a red-through-brown discoloration, which occurs in hematuria, hemoglobinuria, myoglobinuria, bilirubinuria, ingestion of food dyes (beetroot, blackberries, vegetable dyes), or drugs (rifampicin, phenazopyridine, chloroquine, nitrofurantoin, doxorubicin), and the presence of metabolites (porphyrin, melanin, homogentisic acid).

ii. **Turbidity** – Pyuria, chyluria, or excessive salt (urate, phosphate, oxalate).

iii. **Frothiness** – Proteinuria.

iv. **Specific Gravity (SG)** – Urine SG, defined as the weight of the urine compared with that of an equal volume of pure water, reflects the solute load. In general: fixed SG 1.010 (isosothenuria) is suggestive of chronic kidney disease.

1.1.2 Biochemical Properties:

- Commercially available urine Multistix strips can yield semiquantitative detection of albumin, blood, glucose, nitrites, leukocytes, ketone, and pH.
- Microalbuminuria can be detected using a specialized dipstick, which usually yields a semiquantitative estimation of urine albumin to creatinine ratio.
- Urine protein can also be checked by adding 5% sulphosalyclic acid and graded according to flocculation.
- 24-hour protein estimation is done to quantify proteinuria (Normal < 150 mg/day). Nephrotic proteinuria is when it exceeds 3.5 gm/24hrs/1.73m^2. The ratio of urine protein to creatinine can be a simple and practical substitute for 24-hour urine protein for outpatient care.

1.1.3 Microscopy:

- Microscopy allows the identification of abnormal cells, casts, crystals, and even microorganisms.
- Examination of the urine is akin to a poor man's kidney biopsy.
- Dysmorphic red blood cells (RBC) of glomerular origin can be distinguished from non-glomerular RBCs.

- The absence of RBCs together with dipstick-positive hematuria is a classic sign of myoglobinuria in acute rhabdomyolysis.
- The presence of white blood cells may signify a urinary tract infection (the significant range of pus cells in males and females suggestive of UTI is different)). Sometimes, bacteria may also be seen.
- Epithelial cells lining the urinary tract at any level sloughing into the urine are generally of little diagnostic utility.
- Commonly observed urinary crystals in association with renal stones include calcium oxalate, uric acid, and magnesium ammonium phosphate.

1.2 Interpretation of Laboratory Tests:

1.2.1 Assessment of Renal Function Using Plasma Creatinine

The standard measure of renal function is the glomerular filtration rate (GFR). The GFR is equal to the sum of the filtration rates in all of the functioning nephrons. The filtering units of the kidney – the glomeruli – filter approximately 180 liters of plasma per day (125 mL/min). The normal value for GFR depends upon age, sex, and body size, and is approximately 140 to 173 liters per day/1.73 m^2 (90 to 120 mL/min/1.73 m^2), with considerable variation even among healthy individuals. In clinical practice, creatinine clearance (CrCl) is often used to reflect the GFR. CrCl is calculated using either a timed urine collection or Serum Creatinine values (SCr), given by

$$[UCr \times V] \div PCr;$$

where UCr – urine creatinine concentration, V – urine volume, and PCr – plasma creatinine concentration, or accepted equations.

Commonly used estimation equations include:

a. **The CKD-EPI equation 2021**, expressed as a single equation, is:
GFR = 141 * min(Scr/κ,1)α * max(Scr/κ, 1)-1.209 * 0.993Age * 1.018 [if female] * 1.159 [if black]
Scr is serum creatinine (mg/dL), κ is 0.7 for females and 0.9 for males, α is -0.329 for females and -0.411 for males, min indicates the minimum of Scr/κ or 1, and max indicates the maximum of Scr/κ or 1.

b. **The abbreviated 4-variable MDRD** (Modification of Diet in Renal Disease study) equation: GFR (mL/min/1.73 m^2)= 175 x $SerumCr^{-1.154}$ x $age^{-0.203}$ x 1.212 (if the patient is black) x 0.742 (if female), where PCr (plasma creatinine concentration) is in mg/dL. It is most accurate in subjects with moderate chronic kidney disease (CKD) and less accurate at the extremes of GFR, underestimating at high GFR but overestimating with advanced CKD. All these equations can be used in Android applications and the calculators are available online.

1.2.2 Assessment of Renal Function Using Plasma Cystatin C

Cystatin C is a small, 13-kDa basic protein produced by all nucleated cells at a constant rate and eliminated exclusively by GFR. Plasma cystatin C level increases earlier than PCr as GFR decreases, and hence, is useful in detecting early renal function impairment. Plasma cystatin C level starts to rise at a GFR of around 90 mL/min/1.73 m^2. Cystatin C measurement is more expensive than PCr assay and is not routinely performed.

1.3 Renal Biopsy:

Percutaneous renal biopsy under real-time ultrasound guidance using spring-loaded automated 16G to 18G core needles is the favored approach. Indications are diagnosis of renal parenchymal disease (proteinuria, abnormal sediments, or impaired function), diagnosis of renal allograft rejection, and recurrent or de novo disease in allograft.

1.4 Other Ancillary Investigations:

Anemia is one of the cardinal manifestations of CKD and a peripheral smear showing normocytic normochromic anemia is diagnostic. Blood urea, electrolytes including calcium, phosphorus, uric acid, 25-hydroxy Vitamin D, and parathormone levels help in the diagnosis of kidney disease in many ways as the case may be.

1.5 Imaging:

An x-ray of the abdomen is useful to locate mid-ureteric and renal calculi. Ultrasonogram is an essential part of the workup for kidney disease. Besides showing the location and size of the kidneys, it can show calculi, mass, or scars, which help in the diagnosis. Computerized axial tomograms aid in diagnosis and radiocontrast study aids in understanding the anatomy and physiology of the kidney. 99mTc-DTPA(diethylenetriaminepentaacetic acid) is used in the evaluation of glomerular filtration. DTPA is cleared by the renal glomeruli, and measurement of its excretion can provide an accurate estimate of the GFR. Renal artery doppler is useful in the diagnosis of renal artery stenosis.

1.6 Immunological Tests:

Many autoimmune diseases affect the kidneys. Tests like an antinuclear antibody, anticytoplasmic neutrophilic antibody, and serum complement levels may help in the diagnosis of various glomerulonephritis.

References:

1. Zoccali, C. et al. The systemic nature of CKD. Nat. Rev. Nephrol. **13**, 344–358 (2017).

2. Chen TK, Knicely DH, Grams ME. Chronic Kidney Disease Diagnosis and Management: A Review. JAMA. 2019 Oct 1;322(13):1294-1304. doi: 10.1001/jama.2019.14745. PMID: 31573641; PMCID: PMC7015670.
3. Stevens PE, Levin A; Kidney Disease: Improving Global Outcomes Chronic Kidney Disease Guideline Development Work Group Members. Evaluation and management of chronic kidney disease: Synopsis of the kidney disease: improving global outcomes 2012 clinical practice guideline. Ann Intern Med. 2013 Jun 4;158(11):825-30. doi: 10.7326/0003-4819-158-11-201306040-00007.
4. Almutary H, Bonner A, Douglas C. Symptom burden in chronic kidney disease: A review of recent literature. J Ren Care. 2013 Sep;39(3):140-50. doi: 10.1111/j.1755-6686.2013.12022.x.

KIDNEY DISEASE

1 CLINICAL PRESENTATION

- Asymptomatic patient with abnormal laboratory values
- Renal disease presenting in isolation
- Renal manifestation of systemic disease

2 SIGNS AND SYMPTOMS

- New onset HTN, in young
- Edema
- Pain along the urinary tract
- Uremic manifestation: nausea, vomiting, fatigue, seizures, loss of appetite
- Abnormalities in urine, volume composition, voiding & storage symptoms
- Tubular defects: failure to thrive, renal stones, neurological weakness, increase in urinary frequency
- Systemic illness: vasculitic rash, arthralgia, arthritis

3 CLINICAL SYNDROME

- Acute nephritic syndrome
- Nephrotic syndrome
- AKI
- Asymptomatic urinary abnormalities
- CKD
- Urinary tract obstruction
- Nephrolithiasis
- HTN
- Renal tubular defects

4 SCREENING TOOLS

- Blood pressure monitoring
- Monitoring of blood glucose
- Urinalysis
- CBC
- Blood urea, serum creatinine
- USG KUB
- When warranted: serum complements, viral serology, anti dsDNA antibodies, anti-neutrophil cytoplasmic antibodies

AKI : Acute Kidney Injury, ***CBC :*** Complete blood count, ***CKD :*** Chronic Kidney Disease, ***HTN :*** Hypertension, ***KUB :*** Kidney ureter bladder, ***USG :*** Ultrasound/ Sonography

02

URINE ANALYSIS

Alpana Raizada, Swati Pal, Anupam Prakash

> The simplest things give me great ideas
>
> – Joan Miro

Sometimes, the simplest of things, like a small amount of urine voided by the human body, can provide great insight into renal pathologies. Urine analysis is a very informative diagnostic tool that is easily accessible and simple to perform. Over the past years, it has helped us in establishing early diagnosis of various acute and chronic kidney diseases and guided us through the need for renal biopsy. This chapter aims to highlight various aspects of urine analysis and its significance for a physician.

Specimen Collection:

A midstream "clean catch" urine specimen has to be collected in a clean and dry container. The first 200 mL of early morning urine should be discarded. Women should clean the external genitalia (from front to back) before collection to avoid contamination. In catheterized patients, a sample should be obtained directly from the catheter tubing, rather than the drainage bag to avoid contamination by debris in the collection bag.

Indications for urine analysis

1. **Suspected urinary tract infection.**
2. **Suspected renal diseases like glomerulonephritis, tubulo-interstitial disease, pyelonephritis, nephrotic syndrome.**
3. **Evaluation of kidney dysfunction / azotemia.**
4. **Diabetes and its complications: diabetic nephropathy, diabetic ketoacidosis.**
5. **Detection of plasma cell dyscrasias.**
6. **Screening for pregnancy, beta HCG secreting tumours and urological malignancies.**

Box 2.1: Indications for Urine Analysis

Specimen Processing:

The specimen should ideally be examined at room temperature within 30–60 minutes of voiding. If not possible, it should be refrigerated at 2–8°C and then warmed again to room temperature prior to assessment.

Components of Urine Analysis:

- **Gross Assessment**

Normal urine is clear and light yellow in color with a faint ammoniacal odor.

Color: Figure 2.1 describes the causes of abnormal urine color.

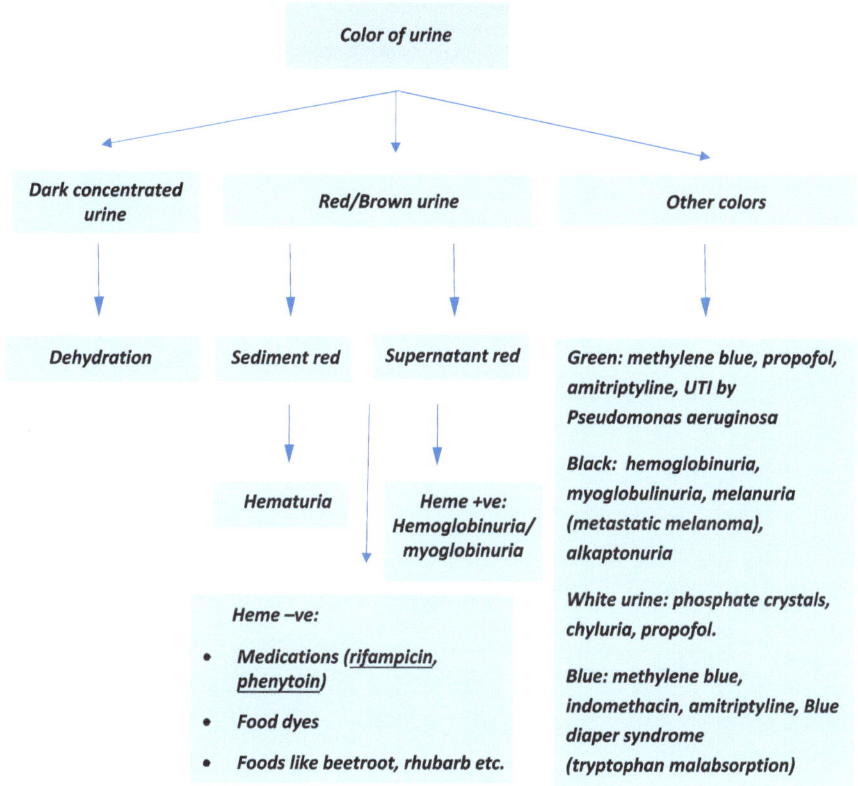

Figure 2.1: Causes for Abnormal Urine Color

Turbidity:

Depends on substances in the urine, like cells, casts, crystals, bacteria, and proteins. Vaginal discharge, sperm, and prostatic secretions also alter the clarity.

Odor:

An abnormal pungent odor is mostly caused by the production of ammonia by bacteria. Other disorders with specific odors are:

- Ketonuria – sweet fruity smell
- Maple syrup urine disease – maple syrup odor
- Phenylketonuria – musty or mousy odor
- Isovaleric academia – sweaty feet odor
- Hypermethioninemia – rancid butter or fishy odor

Urine Dipstick Analysis

Urine dipstick renders a semi-quantitative assessment of the urinary characteristics on a series of colorimetric pads embedded on a test strip. It may lack the 100% accuracy of quantitative tests but provides rapid insight into the possible renal pathology.

Following are the components of urine dipstick:

- **Specific Gravity:** It is a measure of urine osmolality and represents the ability of the kidney to concentrate urine. It generally varies with the osmolality, rising by approximately 0.001 for every 35 to 40 mOsmol/kg increase in urine osmolality. It is often reflective of hydration and the status of the patient.
- **pH**: Hydrogen ion concentration in urine is expressed as the pH and reflects the degree of acidification of urine. The physiologic urine pH ranges from 4.5 to 8, depending upon the acid-base balance in the body. A higher value suggests the presence of renal tubular acidosis. Infection with pathogens that produce urease like Proteus mirabilis, can result in urine pH above 8.
- **Protein**: The urine dipstick test for protein is most sensitive to albumin and insensitive to non-albumin proteins, most notably immunoglobulin light chains. The semi-quantitative categories of albuminuria that are reported (trace, 1+, 2+, and 3+) may be misleading. A dilute urine might underestimate the degree of albuminuria. By contrast, concentrated urine may register as 3+ but may not have high-grade albuminuria.

Recent exposure to iodinated radiocontrast agents can induce transient albuminuria.

Confirm reagent strip positive albuminuria by quantitative laboratory measurement and express as a ratio to creatinine (rather than the concentrations alone) in a random untimed sample, preferably followed by a confirmation on an early morning timed sample. The term microalbuminuria should no longer be used.

Measurements for initial testing of proteinuria (in descending order of preference):

1. Urine albumin-to-creatinine ratio (ACR)
2. Urine protein-to-creatinine ratio (PCR)
3. Reagent strip urinalysis for total protein with automated reading
4. Reagent strip urinalysis for total protein with manual reading

Sulfosalicylic Acid (SSA) Test: SSA detects all proteins in urine and is useful in patients with acute kidney injury of unclear etiology and a urine dipstick that is negative for protein. A

Box 2.2 defines the important terminologies used in the evaluation of proteinuria.

Proteins in urine

1. **Normal = up to 150 mg/ 24 hrs**
2. **Significant proteinuria in pregnancy = >300mg/ 24 hrs**
3. **Nephrotic proteinuria = >3.5g/ 24 hrs**
4. **Normal urinary albumin excretion <30mg/24hrs (ACR<30mg/g)**
5. **Severely increased albuminuria = >300mg/24 hrs (ACR >300mg/g)**
6. **Nephrotic albuminuria = >2200mg/24 hrs (ACR >2200mg/g)**
7. **Overflow proteinuria = proteinuria other than albumin (e.g. Light chains)**

Box 2.2: Important Definitions of Proteinuria

positive SSA test in conjunction with a negative dipstick usually indicates the presence of non-albumin proteins in the urine, most often immunoglobulin light chains.

- **Glucose**: Glycosuria can be due to either the inability of the proximal convoluted tubule to reabsorb glucose despite normal plasma glucose or an overflow related to high plasma glucose. In patients with normal kidney function, significant glycosuria does not generally occur until the plasma glucose exceeds 180 mg/dL. Causes of glycosuria with normal plasma blood glucose include:
    - Intake of SGLT-2 inhibitors.
    - Fanconi syndrome (phosphaturia, uricosuria, renal tubular acidosis, and aminoaciduria) is caused by multiple myeloma, heavy metal exposure, and drugs like tenofovir, lamivudine, cisplatin, etc.
- **Heme:** It may be positive in the presence of urinary RBC and free hemoglobin/free myoglobin. May be falsely positive if there is semen present in the urine.
- **Leukocyte Esterase**: It is released by lysed neutrophils and macrophages and is a marker for the presence of WBCs.
- **Nitrite**: Many Enterobacteriaceae species produce the enzyme nitrate reductase, which converts urinary nitrate to nitrite. Thus, nitrite-positive urine may indicate bacteriuria. Whereas, UTI with enterococci species, which express low levels of nitrate reductase, may test negative for nitrites.

- **Microscopic Examination**
    - **Red Blood Cells:** Hematuria may be gross or microscopic. Microscopic hematuria is defined as the presence of 3 or more RBCs/hpf in a spun urine

sediment. Transient hematuria is seen following exercise, sexual intercourse, menstruation, and UTIs. Persistent hematuria should always be evaluated. The more common pathologic causes include kidney stones, malignancy, and glomerular disease.

Distinguishing between glomerular and non-glomerular causes is the first step in an evaluation. Isomorphic RBCs with normal appearance can be seen with any cause of hematuria. Whereas, dysmorphic RBCs (altered morphology) are suggestive of glomerular disease. Figure 2.2 demonstrates the hallmarks of glomerular hematuria.

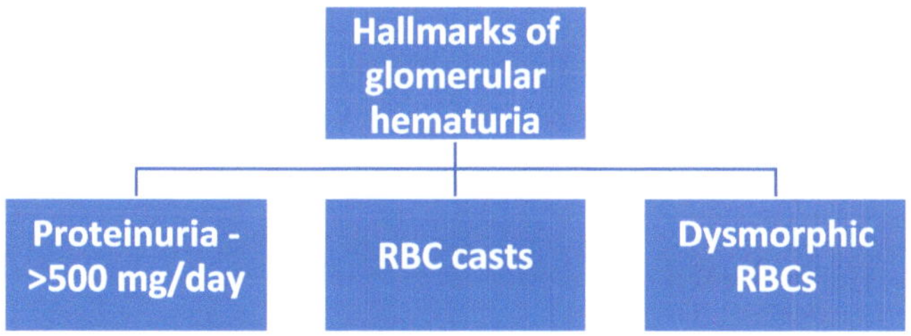

Figure 2.2: Hallmarks of Glomerular Hematuria

- **White Blood Cells:** The number of WBCs considered normal in urine is typically 2–5 WBCs/hpf or less. Neutrophils and eosinophils are cell types of the greatest significance. Neutrophils are commonly associated with bacteriuria. However, if the urine culture is negative, other possibilities include interstitial nephritis, renal tuberculosis, and nephrolithiasis.
  The presence of eosinophiluria has traditionally been considered a marker of acute interstitial nephritis.
- **Casts:** These are cylindrical structures formed in the tubular lumen. All casts have a matrix composed of

Tamm-Horsfall protein. They are defined by the cells or other elements that are embedded in the cast matrix. Table 2.1 shows the various types of casts that are seen on urine microscopy and the associated pathology.

Table 2.1: Types of Casts on Urine Microscopy

a. RBC casts	**Proliferative glomerulonephritis**
b. WBC casts	**Interstitial nephritis, less commonly glomerular inflammation, pyelonephritis**
c. Renal tubular epithelial cell casts	**Desquamation of tubular epithelium including acute tubular necrosis (ATN), acute interstitial nephritis, and glomerulonephritis**
d. Granular casts	**Deeply pigmented granular "Muddy-brown" casts in ATN**
e. Hyaline casts	**Healthy individuals, small volumes of concentrated urine, diuretic therapy**

- **Crystals**: Solid forms of a particular dissolved substance in the urine.
    - Calcium oxalate or calcium phosphate crystals.
    - Magnesium ammonium phosphate crystals(struvite): Occur only when ammonia is increased and urine is alkaline, which decreases the solubility of phosphate. Both these things occur only in the setting of a UTI with urease-producing organisms like Proteus or Klebsiella.
    - Uric acid crystals: Tumour lysis syndrome, hyperuricemia.
    - Cystine crystals: Cystinuria.
    - Drug-induced crystals by drugs like acyclovir, sulphonamides, and methotrexate.

- **Microorganisms**: Bacteria are often seen in the urine, although the clinical significance of bacteriuria is dependent on patient symptoms. Patients without UTI symptoms have to be managed according to the algorithm for the management of asymptomatic bacteriuria as demonstrated in Figure 2.3. Fungi (yeast) are not normally found in the urine specimen. The most common yeast that we come across is the Candida species, which may colonize the vagina, urethra, or bladder. Yeast cells may signify true infection or contamination.

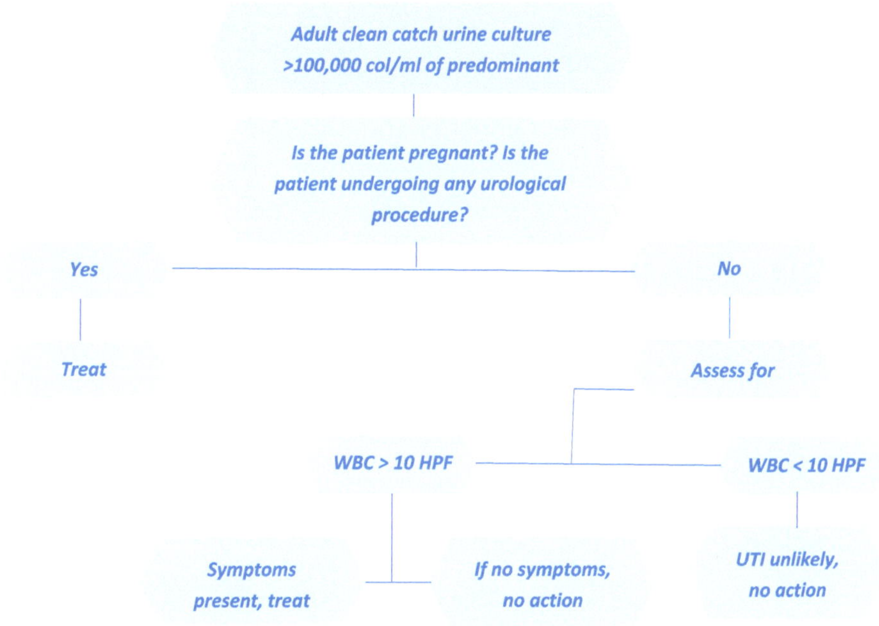

Figure 2.3: Algorithm for the Management of Asymptomatic Bacteriuria

- **Urinary lipids:** Commonly seen in patients with nephrotic syndrome. They show the typical "Maltese cross" appearance on polarized microscopy.

The Extra Edge on Urine Analysis:

1. **Urine Proteomics**

   Proteomics in the simplest words means the large-scale study of proteomes, which is a set of proteins produced in an organism. Urine is a very relevant bio-fluid in proteomics because of its stability and non-invasive retrieval in large quantities and is studied using various methods, namely mass spectrometry, 2D gel electrophoresis coupled to mass spectrometry (2DE-MS), surface-enhanced laser desorption/ionization with spectrometry (SELDI-MS), and liquid chromatography coupled to mass spectrometry (LC-MS), to name a few.

Its application has been studied up till now as a biomarker for various diseases, including diabetic nephropathy, glomerulonephritis, acute kidney injury, and renal allograft rejection.

2. **Urinary Biomarkers**

   There has been a discovery of promising biomarkers that report on kidney and tubule functions, detect an early tubular injury, and distinguish pre-renal AKI from ATN as well as ATN from CKD.

   The major types of urinary biomarkers fall into three classes:

   1. Inflammatory – Neutrophil gelatinase-associated lipocalin, IL-18.
   2. Renal tubular proteins that are excreted into the urine after injury – Kidney Injury Molecule-1, Na^+/H^+ Exchanger Isoform 3.
   3. Surrogate markers of tubular injury – Cystatin C, α-1 microglobulin, and retinol-binding protein.

References:

1. KDIGO 2012 Clinical Practice Guideline for the Evaluation and Management of Chronic Kidney Disease
2. https://kdigo.org/wp-content/uploads/2017/02/KDIGO_2012_CKD_GL.pdf
3. Hitchins, M., Bouchard, J., Ingram, C., & Orvin, A. (2023). Implementation of an asymptomatic bacteriuria assessment protocol for patients discharged from the emergency department. Antimicrobial Stewardship & Healthcare Epidemiology, 3(1), E37. doi:10.1017/ash.2023.117.
4. Stéphane Decramer, Anne Gonzalez de Peredo, Benjamin Breuil, Harald Mischak, Bernard Monsarrat, Jean-Loup Bascands, Joost P. Schanstra, Urine in Clinical Proteomics, Molecular & Cellular Proteomics, Volume 7, Issue 10,2008, Pages 1850-1862, ISSN 1535-9476 https://doi.org/10.1074/mcp.R800001-MCP200.
5. Wu J, Chen YD, Gu W. Urinary proteomics as a novel tool for biomarker discovery in kidney diseases. J Zhejiang Univ Sci B. 2010 Apr;11(4):227-37. doi: 10.1631/jzus.B0900327. PMID: 20349519; PMCID: PMC2852539.
6. Coca, Steven G.; Parikh, Chirag R.. Urinary Biomarkers for Acute Kidney Injury: Perspectives on Translation. Clinical Journal of the American Society of Nephrology 3(2):p 481-490, March 2008. | DOI: 10.2215/CJN.03520807.

URINE ANALYSIS

EXAMINE WITHIN 30-60 MINS, ELSE REFRIGERATE AT 2-6° C

MID STREAM CLEAN CATCH SPECIMEN AFTER VOIDING FIRST 200ML

Gross Examination

- Color
- Turbidity
- Odor

Dipstick

- Specific gravity, Ph
- Protein
- Glucose
- Sulfosalicylic acid
- Nitrite
- Leuocyte esterase
- Heme

Microscopy

- RBC
- WBC
- Casts
- Crystals
- Micro Organisms
- Lipid

GLOMERULONEPHRITIS

- PROTEINURIA >500MG/DAY
- DYSMORHIC RBC
- RBC CASTS

PROTEINURIA GRADING

Negative	0 mg/dL
Trace	15-30 mg/dL
1+	30-100 mg/dL
2+	100-300 mg/dL
3+	300-1000 mg/dL
4+	>1000 mg/dL

- *TRANSIENT PROTEINURIA:* UTI, Fever, Pregnancy, Excerise, Stress, Postural, CHF
- *PERSISTENT PROTEINURIA:* Glomerular/Tubulointerstitial Disease

GLYCOSURIA

- SGLT-2 INHIBITORS
- HYPERCLYCEMIA (>180MG/DL) CAUSING OVERFLOW AT PCT
- FANCONI SYNDROME
- DRUGS LIKE TENOFOVIR, LAMIVUDINE, VALPROATE

CRYSTALS WITH MICROSCOPY

Uric Acid | Ca Phosphate | Ca Oxalate | Triple Phosphate

- Use of as biomarker for diabetic nephropathy, IgA nephropathy, lupus nephritis, AKI etc
- Urinary biomarkers for AKI like NGAL, 1L-18, KIM 1, cystatin C, retinol binding protein

CASTS	CAUSES
RBC	Glomerulonephritis
WBC	Interstitial Nephritis
Renal Tubular Epithelial cell	ATN, acute interstitial nephritis,and glomerulonephritis
Granular	"Muddy-brown"casts in ATN
Hyaline	Healthy individuals small volumes of concentrated urine diuretic therapy

AKI : Acute Kidney Injury, ***ATN :*** Acute tubular necrosis, ***CA :*** Calcium ***CHF :*** Congestive heart failure, ***DL :*** Deciliter, ***IgA :*** Immunoglobulin A, ***IL :*** Interleukin, ***KIM :*** Kidney Injury Molecule, ***NGAL :*** Neutrophil gelatinase-associated lipocalin, ***RBC :*** Red Blood Cell, ***PCT :*** Proximal convulated tubule, ***UTI :*** Urinary Tract Infection, ***WBC :*** White Blood Cell

03

APPROACH TO PROTEINURIA

Saurabh Nayak, Raja Ramachandran

Introduction:

Proteinuria is a common laboratory abnormality that often leads to nephrologist referrals. Urine protein appearance often portends kidney disease but may sometimes be unassuming. Proteinuria that persists beyond a single measurement warrants attention. An increase in the permeability of glomerular capillaries or reduced tubular resorption of filtered proteins results in proteinuria. Proteinuria is often the first sign of kidney disease. Proteinuria plays a crucial role in the pathogenesis of progressive kidney damage. Irrespective of the etiology, progressive nephron loss exaggerates glomerular pressure and loss of selectivity to the filtered protein, leading to non-selective proteinuria. Assessment of proteinuria is a cornerstone for the identification, evaluation, and management of patients with kidney disease. Proteinuria is vital in risk assessment and therapeutic decision-making for various kidney diseases.

Physiological Proteinuria:

The average urinary protein excretion per day is normally 150 mg. Albumin and other plasma proteins (immunoglobulins, beta-2-microglobulin) constitute 15% and Tamm Horsfall (tubular) protein comprises 85% in a healthy person.

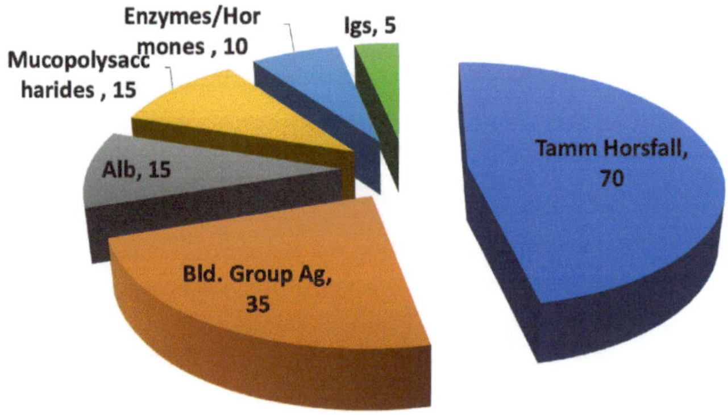

Figure 3.1: Normal Constituents of Urinary Protein (< 150 mg/day) (Igs- Immunoglobulins, Alb- Albumin, Bld group Ag- Blood group antigens)

Proteinuria beyond 500 mg/day is pathological. Occasionally, proteinuria can be isolated and transient (e.g., orthostatic). Benign isolated proteinuria is primarily because of erroneous dipstick testing during routine health checkups. Such 'isolated proteinuria' having normal kidney functions and bland urinary sediments (less than three erythrocytes per high-power field) are not concerning.

Various Causes of Transient/Physiological Proteinuria:

1. Dehydration
2. Hypotension
3. Fever
4. Exercise
5. Kidney Stone
6. Urinary Tract Infection
7. Prolonged Cold Exposure
8. Orthostatic Proteinuria

Pathological Proteinuria:

Urinary excretion of abnormal quantities of protein persisting beyond three months constitutes CKD. Proteinuria is an independent risk factor for cardiovascular disease, end-stage renal disease, stroke, and death in the general population and patients with chronic kidney disease. The presence of proteinuria is associated with higher mortality in critically ill patients. The degree of proteinuria post-renal transplantation is predictive of allograft and patient survival.

Most ominous proteinuria is glomerular in origin, which tends to be highly selective (albuminuria) and portends multiple complications owing to lipiduria, hypoalbuminemia, and the progressive loss of kidney function. Proteinuria because of glomerulosclerosis (resulting from the aftermath of the primary disease process) may not be that catastrophic owing to the loss of non-albumin proteins (non-selective). Tubular proteinuria is usually limited to 1–2 g per day.

Table 3.1: Various Causes of Pathological Proteinuria

Pathological Proteinuria			
Glomerular	**Tubular**	**Overflow**	**Post-renal**
From damaged glomerulus	From damaged tubules	Massive glomerular excretion or overwhelmed tubular resorption of proteins	From urinary tract stones, tumors, or infections

Overflow Proteinuria

Increased excretion of low-molecular-weight proteins can occur with marked overproduction of a particular protein, leading to increased glomerular filtration and excretion. The aforementioned is almost always due to immunoglobulin light chains in multiple myeloma. However, it may also be due to lysozyme (in acute myelomonocytic leukemia), myoglobin (in rhabdomyolysis), or free hemoglobin (in intravascular hemolysis) that is not bound to haptoglobin.

Proteinuria vs Albuminuria:

In a healthy person, a small amount of albumin is excreted from the intact glomerulus and reclaimed by proximal tubular cells. Albumin excretion of up to 10–20 mg per day is normal. Persistent albumin excretion between 30 and 300 mg per day is called moderately increased albuminuria (formerly called "microalbuminuria"). Albumin excretion above 300 mg daily is overt proteinuria or severely increased albuminuria (formerly called "macroalbuminuria"). Albuminuria is more ominous and accurate than proteinuria in predicting CKD progression. It is well-validated for chronic kidney disease progression and cardiovascular events. Proteinuria is a poor prognostic sign in all stages of CKD.

Microalbuminuria is misleading and thus an abandoned term. Kidney Disease Improving Global Outcomes (KDIGO 2012) classified the risk of CKD progression based on albuminuria categories defined as (Figure 3.2):

1. A1 – Normal to mildly increased albuminuria; < 30 mg/g or < 3 mg/mmol
2. A2 – Moderately increased albuminuria; 30–300 mg/g or 3–30 mg/mmol
3. A3 – Severely increased albuminuria; > 300 mg/g; > 30 mg/mmol.

Standard Dipstick (dye-based) is more sensitive to detecting albumin than other urine proteins. In contrast, the direct measurement of albumin (immunology-based detection) still needs to be standardized and is often inaccurate with large inter-laboratory variabilities. High-performance liquid chromatography-based tests may undoubtedly be more helpful but are underway with standardization. Albuminuria specifies selectivity, acute and active glomerular injury, and steroid responsiveness (in patients with glomerular disease). In contrast, non-selective proteinuria signifies previous damage and irreversibility.

Prognosis of CKD by GFR and albuminuria categories: KDIGO 2012			Persistent albuminuria categories Description and range		
			A1	A2	A3
			Normal to mildly increased	Moderately increased	Severely increased
GFR categories (ml/min/1.73 m²) Description and range			< 30 mg/g < 3 mg/mmol	30–300 mg/g 3–30 mg/mmol	> 300 mg/g > 30 mg/mmol
G1	Normal or high	≥ 90	low risk	increased risk	high risk
G2	Mildly decreased	60–89	low risk	increased risk	high risk
G3a	Mildly to moderately decreased	45–59	increased risk	high risk	very high risk
G3b	Moderately to severely decreased	30–44	high risk	very high risk	very high risk
G4	Severely decreased	15–29	very high risk	very high risk	very high risk
G5	Kidney failure	< 15	very high risk	very high risk	very high risk

Figure 3.2: Prognosis of CKD by GFR and Albuminuria Category, KDIGO 2012

Testing for Proteinuria

Testing for proteinuria is done by the following methods:

Semi-quantitative Methods

1. Dipstick
2. Sulfosalicylic acid (SSA)

Quantitative Methods

1. 24-hour urine protein quantification – this is the gold standard.
2. Urine albumin creatinine ratio (UACR)
3. Urine protein creatinine ratio (UPCR)

Urine albumin creatinine ratio (UACR) and Urine protein creatinine ratio (UPCR), if available, may be considered as surrogates for 24-hour urine protein. However, the dipstick is the least preferred test, as per KDIGO 2009 guidelines, for monitoring treatment response.

Dipstick grading (negative to 4+, based upon the increasing intensity of color changes) and SSA grading (negative to 4+, based upon increasing turbidity and precipitated flocculent) are highly dependent upon urine concentration. Very concentrated urine, alkaline urine, pus, vaginal secretions, or semen can give false-positive results, and a dilute one can give a false-negative result.

Table 3.2: Urine Dipstick Protein Grading and Its Correlation with Urine Protein Excretion

Dipstick protein	Protein excretion gm/24 hour	Protein excretion mg/dl	Albuminuria category
Negative	< 0.1	< 10	A1
Trace	0.1–0.2	15	A1/A2
1+	0.2–0.5	30	A2
2+	0.5–1.5	100	A3
3+	2.0–5.0	300	A3
4+	>5.0	> 1000	A3

Table 3.3: False Positive for Proteinuria Results Seen in Various Conditions

Dipstick method	SSA method
Chlorhexidine, Benzalkonium-based antiseptics use	Penicillin, Sulfisoxazole-based antibiotics use
Within 24 hours of Radio-iodine contrast use	Within 24 hours of Radio-iodine contrast use
Urine Ph >8	-
Gross hematuria, Pyuria	Gross hematuria

Urine lysozyme	Urine lysozyme
Semen	-

Quantitative Urine Protein Calculation (24-hour protein)

24-hour timed urine protein calculation is the gold-standard test recommended for assessing persistent proteinuria. It is cumbersome and often ends up with incorrect collections. One way to counter this is to simultaneously ask for creatinine excretion from the same sample. For an adult female, 15–20 mg per kg and 20–25 mg per kg for an adult male is the appropriate urinary creatinine excretion per day. Since creatinine excretion drops by 50% after 50 years, appropriate age-based correction is necessary.

Spot urine protein creatinine ratio (UPCR) of the early morning first urine is a good correlate of daily protein excretion on a population level. Nevertheless, due to increased individual variability, especially in those losing or gaining muscle mass, it is only recommended when timed urine collection is not feasible. There can be wide variability in 24-hour protein excretion at a given total protein-to-creatinine ratio. Therefore, UPCR or UACR values do not find a place while defining treatment response in nephrotic syndrome. Following are the challenges faced with spot versus timed protein estimation:

1. It depends highly on the denominator (urinary creatinine excretion). It overestimates proteinuria in cachectic people and underestimates it in overweight cases.
2. It does not correlate well with 24-hour urine protein excretion, especially in patients with lower protein excretion.
3. Urine protein excretion varies throughout the day and on a day-to-day basis, which makes the timed collection more accurate. Protein excretion is approximately 50% higher during the middle of the day than during sleep.

Suggested Approach to Quantification:

Initial proteinuria quantification must be performed on a timed urinary sample – a complete 24-hour urine collection is desirable. Subsequent proteinuria assessments may be reliably done using a spot urinary sample (for ease).

Approach to a Patient with Proteinuria

After detecting proteinuria, the foremost is to know the clinical and historical perspective leading to the conducting of the test. The next step must include a urine microscopic examination for erythrocytes, leucocytes, casts, and lipiduria. A patient with isolated proteinuria may have normal urine sediment and glomerular filtration rate, with no apparent etiology identified by the history and physical examination. If so, the next step should be to detect transient and orthostatic proteinuria by repeating the test in an early morning sample. Once transient and orthostatic proteinuria has been ruled out, a patient is said to have isolated persistent proteinuria, for which a nephrologist referral is deemed necessary for further evaluation.

Transient and orthostatic proteinuria is less than 1 g per day, but orthostatic proteinuria may sometimes exceed 3.5 g per day in selected patients. It is unclear what level of persistent isolated non-nephrotic proteinuria should be subjected to a kidney biopsy. In response to a questionnaire, many practicing nephrologists consider conducting a kidney biopsy when proteinuria is greater than 1 g per day.

Conclusion:

Proteinuria assessment should include both dipstick testing (qualitative) as well as quantification, using 24-hour urine collection (quantitative). Spot urine protein creatinine ratio may be utilized for follow-ups. It is essential to keep in mind the daily and day-to-day variation of protein excretion and its relation to various physiological activities. Interpretation of urine protein may be misleading without the clinical context.

References:

1. Rose BD. Pathophysiology of Renal Disease, 2nd edition, McGraw-Hill, New York 1987. P.11
2. Dickson LE, Wagner MC, Sandoval RM, Molitoris BA. The Proximal tubule and albuminuria: really! J Am Soc Nephrol. 2014 Mar;25(3):443-53.
3. Ginsberg JM, Chang BS, Matarese RA, Garella S. Use of single voided urine samples to estimate quantitative proteinuria. N Engl J Med. 1983;309(25):1543.
4. Schwab SJ, Christensen RL, Dougherty K, Klahr S. Quantitation of proteinuria by the use of protein-to-creatinine ratios in single urine samples. Arch Intern Med. 1987;147(5):943.

APPROACH TO PROTEINURIA

History, Physical Exam, Urine Sediment analysis

NORMAL FINDINGS

Recheck Proteinuria
Early morning sample or Overnight sample

- NEGATIVE
  - **Transient Proteinuria**: Exercise; Fever; UTI
  - **Orthostatic Proteinuria**: Exercise; Tall Adolescents
- POSITIVE → Persistant Proteinuria → Quantify Proteinuria

ABNORMAL FINDINGS

Quantify Proteinuria
24hrs Urine protein (gold standard)
Urine Albumin creatinine ratio
Urine protein creatinine ratio

- <3.5gm/day Proteinuria → Dipstick Analysis
  - Dipstick negative → **Work up for Multiple Myeloma**
    - SPEP
    - UPEP
    - Serum & urine light chains (kappa lambda)
    - Monoclonal Protein → **Overflow Proteinuria**: Multiple Myeloma; MGRS
    - Negative Workup → Tubular Proteinuria → **Poor Resorption**: Fanconi's Syndrome; RTA; Drugs
  - Mostly Albumin → KIDNEY BIOPSY
- >3.5gm/day Proteinuria → Nephrotic Range Proteinuria → KIDNEY BIOPSY

Glomerular Proteinuria

With active urine sediment	With bland sediment, Nephrotic Proteinuria
IgA nephropathy	Minimal change disease
Membranoproliferative GN	FSGS
ANCA associated vasculitis	Membranous Nephropathy
SLE	Diabetic kidney disease
Anti GBM Disease	Protein deposition (eg Amyloidosis, light chain deposition disease)
Post Infectious GN	
HSP	

Tests for proteinuria

- Urine Dipstick
- SSA
- 24-hour UP
- UPCR
- UACR

Common Symptoms

- Bilateral pitting edema or anasarca
- Frothy/ foamy urine
- Breathlessness on exertion/at rest
- High Blood Pressure

Special Tests

- ANA, Anti ds DNA
- Complements
- ANCA MPO & PR3, Anti GBM level
- HIV
- Hepatitis serology
- Serum protein electrophoresis
- Serum Anti-phospholipase A2 receptor antibody

URINE DIPSTICK PROTEIN GRADING AND ITS CORELATION WITH URINE PROTEIN EXCRETION

Dipstick Protein	Protein excretion gm/24hour	Protein excretion mg/dl	>Albuminuria Staging	Interpretation
Negative	<0.1	<10	A1	
Trace	0.1-0.2	15	A1/A2	Microalbumin Uria +/-
1+	0.2-0.5	30	A2	
2+	0.5-1.5	100	A3	Macroalbumin uria
3+	2.0-5.0	300	A3	Nephrotic range proteinuria
4+	>5.0	>1000	A3	

ANA: Antinuclear antibody, ***ANCA:*** Antineutrophilic cytoplasmic antibody, ***FSGS:*** Focal segmental glomerulosclerosis, ***GBM:*** Glomerular basement membrane, ***GN:*** Glomerulonephritis, ***GPA:*** Granulomatosis with polyangiitis, ***HIV :*** Human immunodeficiency virus, ***HSP :*** Henoch-Schonlein purpura, MGRS: Monoclonal Gammopathy of renal signicance, ***MPA:*** Microscopic polyangiitis, ***MPO :***Myeloperoxidase, ***PR3 :*** Proteinase-3, ***RTA:*** Renal tubular acidosis, ***SLE:*** Systemic lupus erthematosus, ***SSA :*** Sulfosalicylic acid, ***SPEP:*** Serum protein electrophoresis, ***UACR :*** Urine albumin creatinine ratio, ***UPCR:*** Spot urine protein creatinine ratio, ***UP :*** Urine Protein, ***UPEP :*** Urine Protein electrophoresis, ***UTI :*** Urinary Tract infection,

04

APPROACH TO HEMATURIA

Sayali Thakare, Santosh Varughese

Introduction:

Hematuria is the passage of blood through the urinary tract. Hematuria may be gross (visible to the naked eye) or microscopic (discovered on urine microscopy). It is one of the most common urological presentations, likely accounting for over 20% of urological evaluations. Hematuria may be symptomatic or asymptomatic. Similarly, it may be an incidental finding with no immediate consequences, or on the other hand, be a harbinger of a serious underlying pathology of the urinary tract. By definition, hematuria is defined as the presence of ≥ 3 red blood cells (RBCs) per high power field (HPF) in a spun urine sediment.

Etiology of Hematuria – Where is the Blood Coming From?

Red blood cells in the urine may arise from anywhere along the urinary tract, starting from the glomerulus to the urethral meatus. While evaluating, it is useful to separate glomerular causes from non-glomerular causes of hematuria. So, while glomerular hematuria needs attention from a nephrologist, non-glomerular hematuria, arising from structural or other pathologic conditions, warrants referral to a urologist. Some patients may have spurious hematuria due to the presence of colorigenic substances from dietary sources (beets, blackberries, food dyes) or medications (phenazopyridine, rifampicin).

Initial Evaluation of Hematuria:

A careful history and physical examination are the initial steps when evaluating any patient with hematuria. The onset, duration, history of gross hematuria, and other associated symptoms can give valuable directions toward planning further investigations. Medical history of systemic or local urological disease, concomitant medications, especially anticoagulants, surgical procedures, and history of smoking should be specifically asked for. A family history of renal failure (hereditary nephritis) or cystic kidney disease should be sought. When carefully elicited, symptoms such as pain can point towards the etiology of hematuria, e.g., unilateral flank pain radiating to the groin may suggest a blood clot or calculus. Physical examination in a woman should include a urethral and vaginal examination to rule out any local cause of hematuria.

After a thorough clinical review, a comprehensive urine examination is the important next step. Urine dipstick testing has a sensitivity of 95% and specificity of 75% for detecting microscopic hematuria. However, dipstick testing can be misleading since it cannot distinguish red blood cells from hemoglobin or myoglobin in the urine. A follow-up urine microscopy is needed to confirm the presence of red blood cells. The clean-catch, mid-stream, first-morning void urine, which preserves red blood cells best due to higher pH and osmolality, is the ideal sample. If a clean-catch specimen is difficult to obtain (vaginal contamination, obesity, phimosis in a male), urethral catheterization may be performed for collecting the same.

Patients having macroscopic hematuria/gross (Figure 4.1) may have an immediate plausible cause for hematuria (urinary tract infection [UTI], injury to the urinary tract, vigorous exercise, menstruation, or offending medications). If a repeat urine analysis—48 hours after the inciting event—remains abnormal, then further workup can be pursued. Infections, trauma, and any urological or gynecological causes must be treated appropriately and the urinalysis repeated. If a follow-up urinalysis, 6 weeks after completion of therapy of UTI, reveals resolution of hematuria, usually no further investigations are mandated.

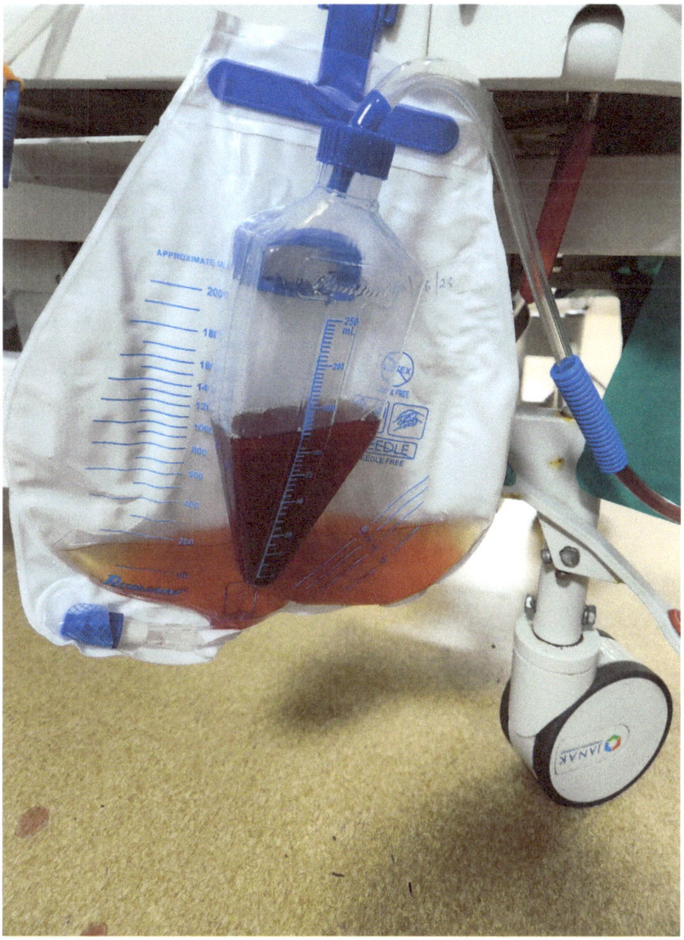

Figure 4.1: Hematuria in an ICU Patient.

Specialized Tests for Hematuria:

The next step is determining whether it is a glomerular or non-glomerular cause of hematuria. The presence of concomitant new-onset hypertension, proteinuria, raised creatinine levels, RBC casts, or dysmorphic RBCs are clues towards the presence of glomerular disease and should be referred to a specialist for further work-up, including a kidney biopsy. Similarly, hypertension and renal insufficiency are red flags for suspecting a glomerular etiology. Several glomerulonephritis initially present with only microscopic hematuria and hence most nephrologists would perform a kidney biopsy if it appears glomerular in origin.

If a glomerular etiology is reasonably ruled out, patients with microscopic hematuria should undergo systematic radiographic assessment of the upper and lower urinary tracts and urine cytology studies. A risk-based approach to the evaluation of hematuria has been suggested by the American Urological Association (AUA) in order to give a reasonable algorithm for planning tests or observations.Microscopic hematuria may indicate urological malignancy in up to 10% of the patients. Urothelial cancers are the most commonly detected malignancies in patients with microscopic hematuria. The choice of tests depends upon the risk of developing urinary tract malignancy in a given individual. Imaging studies are used to evaluate upper urinary tract disease and direct endoscopy is preferred for lower urinary tract. Renal ultrasound has adequate sensitivity and specificity for renal cortical tumors. However, it is a poor modality for upper tract urothelial carcinoma. Intravenous pyelography (IVP) in 3 phases gives a better resolution of the urothelial tumors of the upper urinary tract. Urine cytology is a useful adjunct for cystoscopy in cases with irritative bladder symptoms, especially in those with high risk from transitional cell carcinoma or carcinoma in situ. Sensitivity of urine cytology for the detection of bladder cancer is 40%–76% and is higher for the invasively obtained bladder wash cytology. However, cystoscopy with 98% sensitivity for the detection of bladder tumors is the investigation of choice. Referral to a urologist for specialized procedures like cystoscopy is mandatory for early detection and management of urological malignancies, especially in patients who are at high risk. Factors constituting an increased risk are:

1. Age > 40 years
2. Smokers
3. Males
4. Family history of urothelial cancers
5. Occupational exposure
6. Past irritative voiding symptoms
7. Analgesic abuse
8. Pelvic irradiation
9. Cyclophosphamide use

Deciding how aggressively to evaluate hematuria is based on tradeoffs; e.g., the risk of missing important diagnoses of malignancy versus risks of imaging and invasive cystoscopy. Also, imaging and invasive diagnostics have substantial adverse event implications and cost considerations. Studies suggest that cystoscopy as a diagnostic test is under-utilized. However, cystoscopy may be deferred in low-risk patients at the discretion of a urologist. A large population-based study showed that the incidence of renal cell carcinoma or urothelial carcinoma in microhematuria was low, and hence, an intensive workup was unnecessary. Similarly, asymptomatic microscopic hematuria in women is less likely to be associated with malignancy, and a rigorous evaluation may lead to potentially more harm than benefit. Screening asymptomatic patients for microscopic hematuria in the general population is not recommended. About 8%–10% of patients with unexplained hematuria may harbor an underlying glomerular disease or metabolic derangements like hypercalciuria or hyperuricosuria, indicating a tendency for stone formation. Further clinical probing and repeat periodic urinalysis may uncover the etiology at a later date in such cases.

Approximately 1% of patients with a negative initial examination will develop urinary tract malignancy in 3–4 years. Periodic urine cytology is hence indicated for high-risk patients. Imaging may also need to be repeated at intervals in such patients. The AUA guidelines recommend a similar evaluation for hematuria for patients on anticoagulation since anticoagulation by itself is not expected to cause de novo hematuria. The frequency of macroscopic hematuria in patients on anticoagulants varies between 2% to 24% in the reported literature. Studies have shown that up to a quarter of patients having gross hematuria on aspirin or anticoagulant therapy have an underlying malignancy.

Conclusion:

Hematuria may thus result from minor causes that may be transient and non-recurring, with minimal consequences for future health, but could also include others that may be serious, requiring urgent medical attention, and may occasionally even be life-threatening. Because the incidence of these etiologies varies in different populations, it is difficult to establish uniform algorithms for the evaluation of hematuria. Such decisions can be highly nuanced and require shared decision-making between patients, primary practitioners, and specialists. Knowledge of the causes and their relative frequencies in the region of practice is important for avoiding unnecessary investigations, follow-ups, and patient anxiety while being cognizant of conditions that mandate medical intervention.

Table 4.1. Causes of Hematuria

1.	Glomerular causes: Immunoglobulin A nephropathy Lupus nephritis Membrano-proliferative glomerulonephritis Mesangio-proliferative glomerulonephritis Post-infectious glomerulonephritis ANCA-associated vasculitis Anti-GBM antibody disease Hemolytic uremic syndrome Genetic disorders – Alport's syndrome, Fabry's disease, Nail-patella syndrome, Thin basement membrane disease
2.	Upper urinary tract disease (kidney and ureter): Solitary renal cyst Cystic kidney disease – Polycystic kidney disease, Multi-cystic kidney disease, Medullary cystic kidney disease Interstitial nephritis – Drug-induced (penicillins, cephalosporins, diuretics, non-steroidal anti-inflammatory drugs, cyclophosphamide, chlorpromazine, anti-convulsants) Metabolic – Hypercalciuria, Hyperuricosuria, Renal calculus disease Urinary tract infection – Pyelonephritis, Ureteritis Other infections – Syphilis, CMV, EBV, Toxoplasmosis, Mycobacterial Urinary tract obstruction – Ureteropelvic junction obstruction, Ureteral strictures Malignancy Systemic disease – Sjogren's syndrome, Sarcoidosis, Lymphoma Acute tubular necrosis
3.	Lower urinary tract disease (bladder and urethra): Obstruction – Benign prostatic hyperplasia, Posterior urethral valves, Urethral strictures, Meatal stenosis Urinary tract infection (cystitis, trigonitis, prostatitis, urethritis, epididymitis)

	Congenital anomalies of the kidney and urinary tract (CAKUT) – Vesico-ureteral reflux, Neurogenic bladder, Cystocele, Ureterocele, Pelvic kidney Calculus disease – Bladder, Prostate Malignancy Radiation cystitis Trauma Others – Bladder polyps, Telangiectasias, Diverticuli
4.	Vascular disease: Arterio-venous malformations, Malignant hypertension, Renal artery/vein thrombosis, Sickle cell disease

References:

1. Grossfeld GD, Litwin MS, Wolf JS, et al. Evaluation of asymptomatic microscopic hematuria in adults: the American Urological Association best practice policy – part I: definition, detection, prevalence, and etiology. Urology. 2001;57(4):599-603. doi:10.1016/s0090-4295(01)00919-0.
2. Grossfeld GD, Litwin MS, Wolf JS Jr, et al. Evaluation of asymptomatic microscopic hematuria in adults: the American Urological Association best practice policy – part II: patient evaluation, cytology, voided markers, imaging, cystoscopy, nephrology evaluation, and follow-up. Urology. 2001;57(4):604-610. doi:10.1016/s0090-4295(01)00920-7.
3. Barocas DA, Boorjian SA, Alvarez RD, et al. Microhematuria: AUA/SUFU Guideline. J Urol. 2020;204(4):778-786. doi:10.1097/JU.0000000000001297.
4. Takeuchi M, McDonald JS, Takahashi N, et al. Cancer Prevalence and Risk Stratification in Adults Presenting With Hematuria: A Population-Based Cohort Study. Mayo Clin Proc Innov Qual Outcomes. 2021;5(2):308-319. Published 2021 Jan 21. doi:10.1016/j.mayocpiqo.2020.12.001.
5. Committee Opinion No.703: Asymptomatic Microscopic Hematuria in Women. Obstet Gynecol. 2017;129(6):e168-e172. doi:10.1097/AOG.0000000000002059.

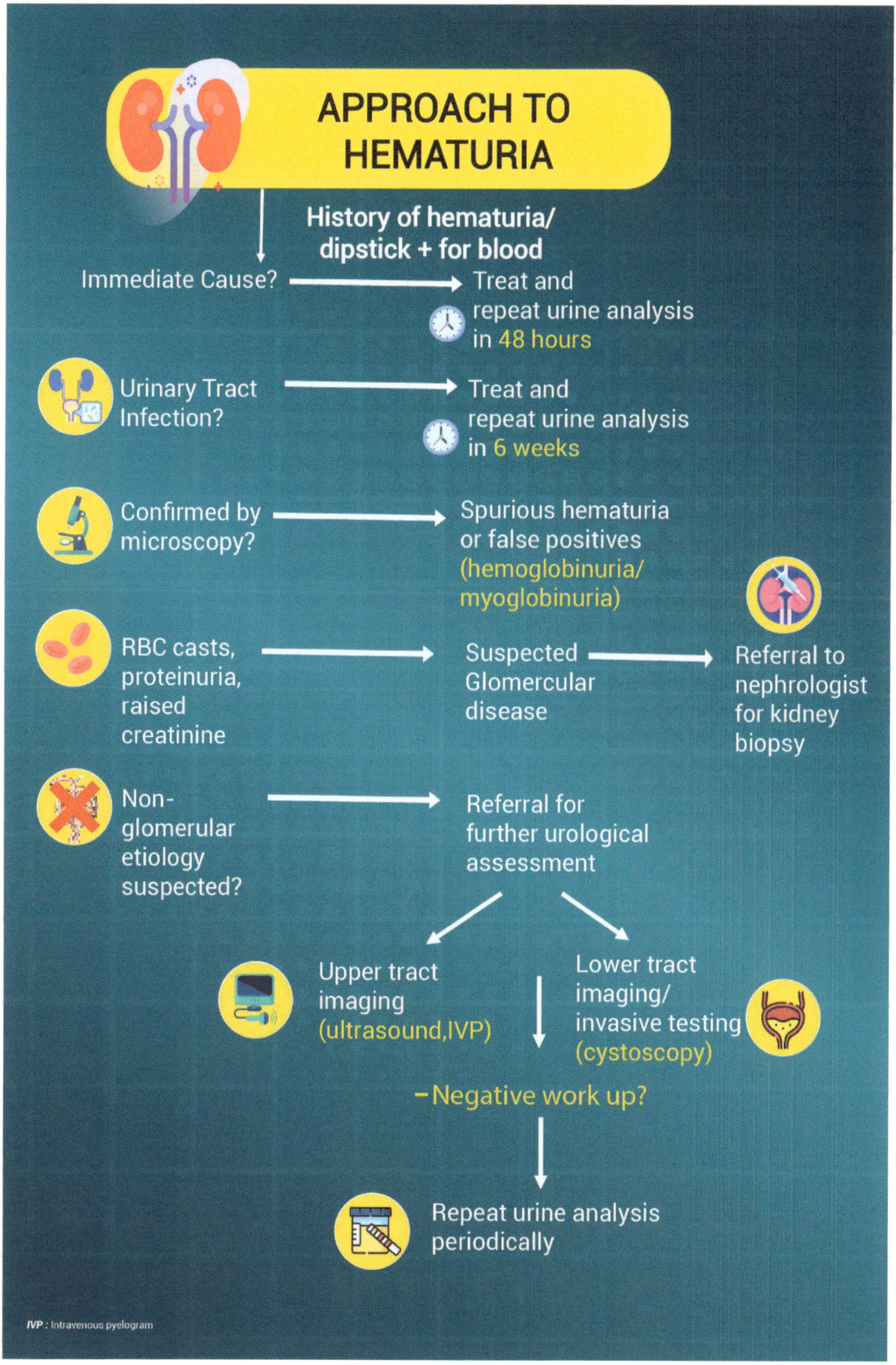
APPROACH TO HEMATURIA
History of hematuria/ dipstick + for blood
Immediate Cause?
Treat and repeat urine analysis in 48 hours
Urinary Tract Infection?
Treat and repeat urine analysis in 6 weeks
Confirmed by microscopy?
Spurious hematuria or false positives (hemoglobinuria/ myoglobinuria)
RBC casts, proteinuria, raised creatinine
Suspected Glomercular disease
Referral to nephrologist for kidney biopsy
Non-glomerular etiology suspected?
Referral for further urological assessment
Upper tract imaging (ultrasound,IVP)
Lower tract imaging/ invasive testing (cystoscopy)
Negative work up?
Repeat urine analysis periodically
IVP : Intravenous pyelogram

05

RENAL BIOPSY

Balbir Singh Kohli, Priti Meena

Introduction:

Renal biopsy is a gold-standard, invasive diagnostic procedure that involves removing a tiny piece of kidney tissue and examining it under a microscope with relevant stains. This aids in the identification of underlying diseases impacting kidney function.

A renal biopsy was first performed in 1951 by Brun and Iversen, using a suction needle and intravenous urography, but the results were not favorable. Later, in 1954, Kark and Muehrcke used a Vim-Silverman needle to perform a kidney biopsy in the prone position. The process for performing a renal biopsy hasn't changed much since then. The biopsy pistol is an automatic spring-loaded device. Furthermore, the location of the kidney and the positioning of the biopsy needle become more precise with the use of ultrasonography, or sometimes, computerized tomography.

Indications for Renal Biopsy: For all practical purposes, following are the broad indications for a renal biopsy:

1. Nephrotic syndrome

2. Unexplained acute kidney injury
3. Evaluation of renal dysfunction
4. Glomerulonephritis
5. Rapidly proliferative renal failure
6. Systemic disease with renal involvement for example lupus nephritis, ANCA associated Vasculitis
7. Diabetes with atypical features
8. Renal allograft dysfunction
9. Significant proteinuria or microscopic hematuria that cannot be explained by any other etiology

Note: Renal biopsy may not be required if clinical and laboratory investigations are suggestive of a histological pattern.

Contraindications for Renal Biopsy:

Absolute

1. Small kidneys
2. Bleeding diathesis
3. Uncontrolled severe hypertension
4. Patient's refusal

Relative contraindications

1. Solitary kidney
2. Multiple bilateral cysts
3. Horseshoe-shape kidney
4. Skin infection over the site of needle insertion
5. Unable to lie in prone position

Pre-biopsy Work Up:

Prior to the procedure, the patients' and their families' informed consent should be sought.

Recommendations:

- CBC, kidney function tests, PT-INR, APTT, bleeding and clotting time, urine examination, and kidney ultrasound.

- Discontinue aspirin/clopidogrel, prasugrel, ticagrelor/warfarin for patients at low risk of cardiovascular events 5 to 7 days before biopsy.
- Discontinue direct thrombin inhibitors (dabigatran) and factor Xa inhibitors (Apixaban, Rivaroxaban) 48–72 hours before the biopsy.
- Unfractionated heparin 6–8 hours and low-molecular weight heparin 24 hours before biopsy to be stopped.
- The platelet counts should be > 50,000/µL and APTT, PT-INR within normal limits.

Renal Biopsy technique:

Position of the Patient:

For Native Kidney: Prone position (In some cases, a wedge is placed under the abdomen to eliminate lumbar lordosis).

Supine anterolateral position (SLAP) position in an obese or pregnant patient with breathing difficulty.

Site: The lower pole of the left kidney is usually preferred to reduce the risk of inadvertent injury to major vessels.

For Transplant Kidney: Supine position

Biopsy Instrument

The era of biopsy instruments has evolved from the Vim-Silverman needle to a manually operated sheathed needle (Tru-Cut), and now recommended are automatic spring-loaded biopsy guns using 14-, 16-, or 18-gauze needles, as they are associated with fewer complications and provide adequate tissue samples.

Percutaneous Renal Biopsy (PRB)

It is currently considered as the standard of care to do real time ultrasound guided kidney biopsy. After proper positioning, the kidneys' size and position are assessed and localized using an ultrasound machine/CT scan in difficult cases (obesity/ complicated anatomies, etc.). Once the biopsy site is found, the skin is marked and cleaned with an antiseptic, where the biopsy needle is to be inserted. A local anesthetic medication is injected using a syringe with a needle at the site of entry to numb the area. Using the ultrasound probe as a guide, a biopsy needle is inserted at an angle of 70^0 to the skin and the patient is asked to hold his breath until the lower pole of the kidney rests just under the biopsy needle while collecting the sample and a pop or sharp clicking sound is heard. The biopsy needle may be inserted a few times to get an adequate sample.

Kidney biopsy tissue is immediately preserved in Formalin solution for light microscopy examination, normal saline for immunofluorescence examination and in glutaraldehyde for Electron microscopy examination (if needed)

Laparoscopic Renal Biopsy/Open biopsy

It is safe and reliable, allowing direct visualization of the kidney tissue and hemostasis is better achieved under direct view, using a fulgurated argon beam coagulator, and thereupon a sheet of oxidized cellulose can be applied.

The possible indications include:

1. Failed percutaneous biopsy
2. Bleeding diathesis
3. Morbid obesity
4. Solitary kidney or multiple bilateral kidney cysts
5. Kidney artery aneurysm

The advantages of laparoscopy biopsy as against open biopsy are as follows:

1. Less wound infection as compared to that in an open biopsy
2. Adequate hemostasis achieved

3. Reliable and safe; if needed, prompt conversion to open can be made

Disadvantages:

1. Requires general anesthesia and is costly
2. More invasive than a closed percutaneous biopsy

Transjugular Renal Biopsy

The biopsy needle is directed via the veins into the kidney after being punctured in the internal jugular vein. The advantage of a transjugular biopsy is that it is safer because the needle is passed into a vein and away from the main vessels.

The disadvantage is the risk of an arterio-calyceal bleed.

Post-renal Biopsy Care

Immediately after the biopsy, the site is compressed and the patient is instructed to lie flat on the bed for 6–8 hours.

Symptoms such as pain abdomen, hematuria, and vitals are monitored.

The common practice is to observe the patient for up to 18–24 hours in the hospital. Hemoglobin and hematocrit are to be monitored after 6 hours.

The patient is also advised to abstain from heavy physical exercise for 1–2 weeks.

Complications of Kidney Biopsy

Kidney biopsies are typically performed by skilled medical professionals who take efforts to reduce risks and maintain patient safety. The healthcare professional should, however, address the potential hazards of a kidney biopsy, which include bleeding (3–10%), hematoma, bleeding that may require blood transfusion and intervention, perirenal soft tissue infection, arteriovenous fistula, pneumothorax, page kidney after allograft kidney biopsy, and allergic response to the local anesthetic used during the kidney biopsy.

Adequacy of Tissue Sampling

A sample size of two cylinders with a minimal length of 1cm & diameter of 1.2mm is needed.

Biopsy adequacy: Biopsy tissue should ideally contain more than 7 glomeruli.

Sectioning and Fixation

After that, the biopsy tissue is examined using a light microscope (LM), an electron microscope (EM), and immunofluorescence (IF).

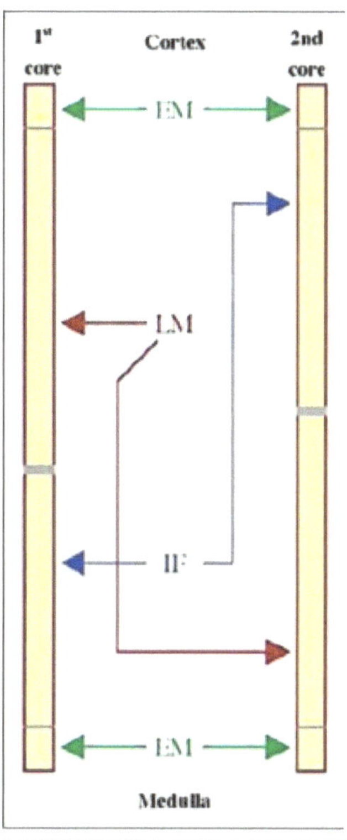

- EM – 1mm cubes from ends of both cores
- Remaining tissues are cut in half by cross-sectioning
- LM – larger 2 pieces
- IF – smaller 2 pieces

Figure 5.1: Diagram to Illustrate the Division of the Kidney Core

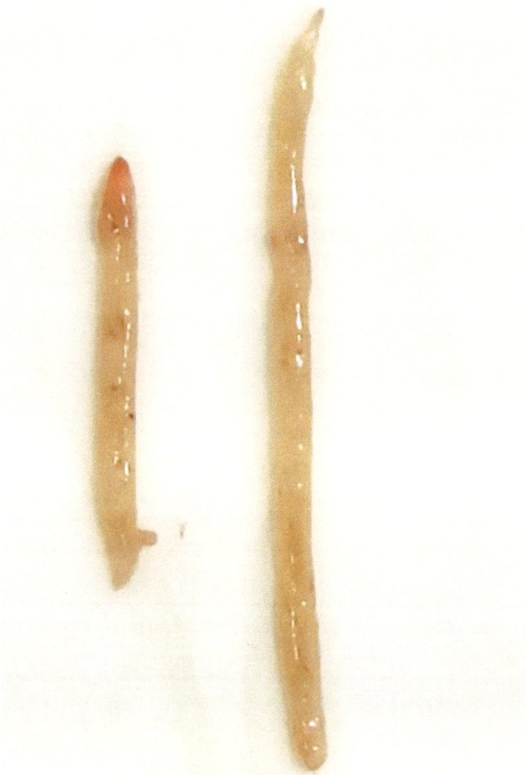

Figure 5.1: The figure shows the sample of a renal biopsy obtained via an 18G renal biopsy gun

Staining and Light Microscopy:

To better understand the glomerular lesion and its cellularity in LM, thin sections of 2–3 mm are produced and stained with the various histochemical stains listed in the table below.

Table 5.1: Various Histochemical Stains and Their Utility in Light Microscopy

Stain	Utility
Hematoxylin & eosin stain(H&E)	General evaluation, cellular characteristic type inflammation
Periodic acid-schiff stain	Glomerular cell number, basement membrane, mesangium, hyaline (red color)
Silver Methanamine (Jones)	Basement details (black color)
Congo red	Amyloid
Masson's tricome	Extracellular glomerular matrix & TBM (blue or green)
Acid fuschin-orange G	Protein deposition (immune complex)
Sirus red	Fibrosis

Immunofluorescence:

In addition to being utilized in conjunction with EM and histology to accurately diagnose renal disease, it aids in the resolution of the differential diagnosis in patients with glomerulonephritis. Sections are fixed with acetone and mostly stained with fluorescein-tagged antibodies against IgG, IgA, IgM, complement pathway components C3 and C1q and/or C4 (classical pathway), κ and λ light chain, fibrinogen, and albumin.

Electron Microscopy:

For glomerular and some tubulointerstitial diseases, this method helps to localize extremely small deposits and document the alteration of a cellular or basement membrane structure. It is mostly useful in:Hereditary nephropathies such as Alport's syndrome, hereditary onychodysplasia (Nail-patella syndrome) and collagenofibrotic glomerulopathy, thin glomerular basement membrane disease, Fabry's disease and other lipidosis, fibrillary and immunotactoid nephropathies and other nephropathies with organized deposits. EM is also helpful in detection of immunoglobulin light and heavy chain deposition diseases and amyloidosis.

Immunohistochemistry (IHC)

IHC detects specific proteins by mono or polyclonal antibodies raised against that protein in biopsy.

Tissue Examination and Interpretation: Microscopic examination is carried out first using low-powered light microscopy followed by high-resolution examination.

A. Localization: Glomerular/tubulointerstitial /vascular.
B. Site of lesion:
    - Diffuse change: Changes occurring in all the glomeruli
    - Focal change: Changes occurring in few glomeruli only
    - Global changes: Whole glomerulus is involved
    - Segmental changes: Some part of glomerulus is involved.
C. Category of lesion:

Table 5.2: Characteristics of Lesions on Light Microscopy

Active Lesion	Chronic Lesion
Proliferation	Glomerulosclerosis
Cellular crescent	Fibrous crescent
Necrosis	Tubular atrophy/ interstitial fibrosis
Inflammation (e.g., Glomerulitis tubulitis, vasculitis)	Vascular sclerosis

Finally, the nature and pathogenesis of the lesion are interpreted by the context of history, LM, IF, and EM. Thus, kidney biopsy is a key tool; if appropriately processed and interpreted, it will yield a correct clinicopathological diagnosis, leading to an appropriate therapeutic strategy.

References:

1. MacGinley R, Champion De Crespigny PJ, Gutman T, Lopez-Vargas P, Manera K, Menahem S, et al. KHA-CARI Guideline recommendations for renal biopsy. Nephrology (Carlton). 2019 Dec;24(12):1205-1213.
2. Agarwal SK, Sethi S, Dinda AK. Basics of kidney biopsy: A nephrologist's perspective. Indian J Nephrol. 2013 Jul;23(4):243-52.
3. Fogo AB. Approach to renal biopsy. Am J Kidney Dis. 2003 Oct;42(4):826-36.
4. Amann K, Haas CS. What you should know about the work-up of a renal biopsy. Nephrol Dial Transplant. 2006 May;21(5):1157-61.
5. Moutzouris DA, Herlitz L, Appel GB, Markowitz GS, Freudenthal B, Radhakrishnan J, D'Agati VD. Renal biopsy in the very elderly. Clin J Am Soc Nephrol. 2009 Jun;4(6):1073-82.
6. Hull KL, Adenwalla SF, Topham P, Graham-Brown MP. Indications and considerations for kidney biopsy: an overview of clinical considerations for the non-specialist. Clin Med (Lond). 2022 Jan;22(1):34-40.

KIDNEY BIOPSY

EXAMINATION

1. Light microscopy
2. Immunofluorescence
3. Electron microscopy

INDICATIONS

1. Nephrotic syndrome
2. Acute nephritic syndrome
3. Unexplained Acute Kidney Injury
4. Graft dysfunction
5. Evaluation of renal dysfunction, proteinuria and active urinary sediments

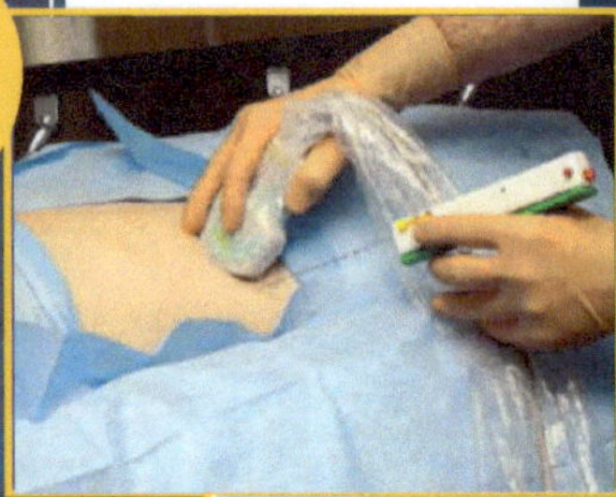

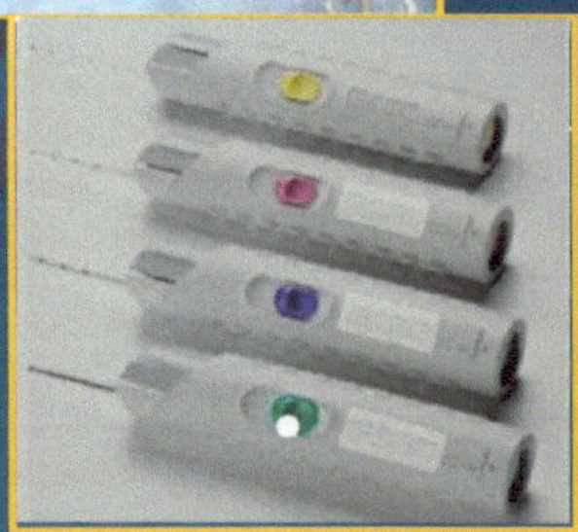

COMPLICATIONS

1. Pain at biopsy site
2. Hematuria
3. Perinephric hematoma
4. Requirement for Blood transfusion or intervention for bleeding
5. AV Fistula (Very rare)
6. Page Kidney
7. Rarely, puncture of liver, pancreas, spleen

CONTRAINDICATION

Absolute

- Small Kidneys or ESKD
- Bleeding diathesis
- Uncontrolled severe hypertension
- Patients' refusal

Relative

- Solitary Kidney
- Uncooperative patient
- Unable to lie flat on bed
- Multiple bilateral Cysts
- Hydronephrosis
- Horseshoe shape kidney
- Hemostasis-altering drugs
- Severe Thrombocytopenia
- Skin infection over the site of needle insertion
- Pyelonephritis or perirenal abscess
- Obesity

AVF : Arteriovenous Fistula, ***ESKD :*** End Stage Kidney Disease

SECTION 2

Glomerular Diseases

06

NEPHROTIC SYNDROME

Urmila Anandh, Jithu Kurien

Introduction:

Nephrotic syndrome is a constellation of signs and symptoms that is characterized by:

1. Proteinuria > 3.5 grams day OR > 40 mg/hour/m^2
2. Serum albumin < 3.5 gm/dl
3. Edema
4. Hyperlipidemia
5. Lipiduria

It is caused by the alteration in the structure of the filtering unit of the kidney. The etiology could vary from a disease intrinsic to the kidneys (primary nephrotic syndrome) to those that are caused because of a systemic disease affecting the kidneys (secondary nephrotic syndrome).

Primary Nephrotic Syndrome:

Primary nephrotic syndrome is characterized by the classical description of nephrotic syndrome and is associated with edema, hypoalbuminemia, and hyperlipidemia. The etiology of the primary nephrotic syndrome varies from children to adults and also varies in different age groups of patients in adulthood. The common pathologies of primary nephrotic syndrome are given in Table 6.1.

Table 6.1: Pathology of Primary Nephrotic Syndrome

Children	Young Adults	Older adults
Minimal change disease	Focal segmental glomerulosclerosis (FSGS)	Membranous nephropathy
FSGS	Minimal change disease	Minimal change disease
Inherited mutation	Membranous nephropathy	Amyloidosis

Secondary Nephrotic Syndrome:

Proteinuria in secondary nephrotic syndrome is caused either due to a systemic disease or because of hyper filtration of the existing glomeruli, resulting in excessive protein loss. This is mostly characterized by nephrotic/non-nephrotic range proteinuria, minimal edema, and normo-albuminemia. The common causes of secondary nephrotic syndrome are given in Table 6.2.

Clinical Features and Complications:

Hypoalbuminemia

The loss of protein in the urine results in hypoalbuminemia.

Edema

Hypoalbuminemia results in a decrease in plasma oncotic pressure and extravasation of fluid into the interstitial space leading to edema. Central to the pathophysiology of nephrotic syndrome is sodium retention. Two theories are postulated for the sodium retention noted in nephrotic syndrome.

Table 6.2: Causes of Secondary Nephrotic Syndrome

Causes of Secondary Nephrotic Syndrome
Infections
Hepatitis B, C
Human Immunodeficiency Virus
Malaria
Toxoplasmosis
Syphilis
Leprosy
COVID-19 infection
Drugs
Gold
Lithium
Non-steroidal anti-inflammatory drugs
Pamidronate
Interferon alpha
Heroin
Lithium
Malignancies
Lymphoma
Leukemia
Solid tumors – breast, lung, gastric cancers
Familial/Genetics
Nephrin mutations (NPHS1/2)
Podocin mutations
Maladaptive Phenomenon
Sickle Cell nephropathy
Congenital heart disease
Obesity
Miscellaneous
Diabetic nephropathy
Systemic lupus erythematosus
Amyloidosis
Paraproteinemias

a. **Underfilling Theory:** The underfilling of the vascular compartment due to fluid extravasation causes renin activation and sodium retention. This also causes an increase in vasopressin, resulting in water retention.

b. **The Overfilling Theory:** This occurs due to the activation of the ENaC channel in the distal tubules by the filtered proteins, resulting in sodium absorption and resultant water retention.

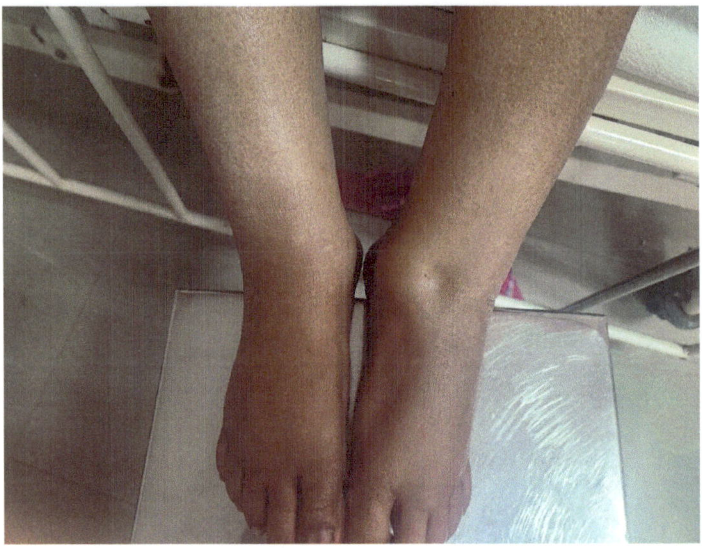

Figure 6.1: Showing Pitting Pedal Oedema in a Patient with Nephrotic Syndrome

Hyperlipidemia

Characterized by an increase in cholesterol and triglycerides. There is an increased synthesis of VLDL, IDL, LDL and a decrease in peripheral lipoprotein lipase activity.

Lipiduria

This is characterized by lipid accumulation in the casts and cellular debris of the urine.

Hyper Coagulability

This is characterized by an increase in the levels of certain procoagulant factors associated with an increase in platelet aggregation. The hemo-concentration and hyperlipidemia might contribute towards hypercoagulability. The clinical correlate for this is an increased risk of thrombosis in nephrotic syndrome.

a. Venous thrombosis is more common than arterial thrombosis.
b. The risk of thrombosis also varies as per the cause of nephrotic syndrome. Thrombotic events are more common in membranous nephropathy.
c. Serum albumin level is used as a surrogate marker for the risk of thrombosis. A serum albumin of less than 2 g/dl is associated with increased risk.

Acute Kidney Injury (AKI)

Causes of AKI in nephrotic syndrome include:

a. Pre-renal failure secondary to volume depletion
b. Acute tubular necrosis
c. Renal vein thrombosis
d. Transformation of the underlying glomerular disease to a crescentic GN
e. Acute interstitial nephritis
f. Intrarenal edema

Evaluation:

Patients suspected of nephrotic syndrome should be evaluated with the following investigations.

Investigation to establish the diagnosis of nephrotic syndrome:

- Urinary spot protein:creatinine ratio (PCR)
- 24-hour urinary protein excretion (gold standard)
- Serum albumin

- Fasting lipid profile
- Urine routine microscopy for urinary activity

Basic evaluation of any underlying etiology responsible for the nephrotic syndrome

Clinical Evaluation:

- Medication/toxin exposure
- Risk factors for HIV and viral hepatitis
- History of diabetes/ SLE/other systemic illnesses
- Pregnancy

Laboratory Evaluation:

- Viral markers – Hepatitis B, Hepatitis C, HIV
- Anti Nuclear Antibody
- Anti Phospholipase A2 receptor Antibodies (Anti PLA2R Ab)
- Complement levels (C3, C4)
- Cryoglobulins
- Serum immunofixation electrophoresis, serum-free light chains
- Renal biopsy to find out the histopathology is indicated in most adults with nephrotic syndrome and in children in certain clinical situations.

Management:

The management of nephrotic syndrome can be divided into:

1. Managing the underlying glomerular diseases in primary nephrotic syndrome
2. Managing the systemic disease/underlying etiology in case of a secondary glomerular disease
3. Managing the proteinuria
4. Managing oedema
5. Management of hypercoagulability
6. Managing dyslipidemia

Managing underlying glomerular diseases:

The primary glomerular diseases causing nephrotic syndrome are diagnosed based on the clinical/laboratory features and/or renal biopsy. They are often treated with immunosuppressive medications. It is usually managed by nephrologists. The preferred immunosuppression and the duration vary with the type of primary glomerular disease.

Managing the systemic disease:

The secondary glomerular diseases are due to an underlying systemic disorder like diabetes, obesity, infections, etc. The management of the underlying systemic disorder is of prime importance, with which the nephrotic syndrome usually improves.

Managing the proteinuria:

In addition to the treatment of nephrotic syndrome with immunosuppression for primary glomerular disease and treatment of underlying systemic diseases in nephrotic syndrome due to secondary glomerular disorders, all efforts should be taken to reduce proteinuria with anti-proteinuric therapy. ACE inhibitors/ARB blockers should be used to do the same and the dose of the drugs should be slowly escalated. Monitoring of creatinine and serum potassium after 3 weeks of initiation and escalation of dosage is very important. A rise in creatinine levels up to 30% after initiation of ACE inhibitors or ARB blockade is acceptable. Newer medications like sodium glucose transporter 2, inhibitors (SGLT2i) like dapagliflozin, empagliflozin, etc., and mineralocorticoid receptor antagonist (finrenone) have revolutionized the therapy of proteinuric kidney disease.

The definitions of remission and relapse of proteinuria are different for adults and pediatric patients and are as follows:

Table 6.3: Definitions and Response to Treatment in Proteinuria

	Adult	Pediatric
Nephrotic syndrome	Proteinuria > 3.5 gram/day + hypoalbuminemia < 2.5 g/dl	Urine PCR > 2000 mg/g and hypoalbuminemia < 2.5 g/dl
Complete remission	Reduction of proteinuria < 0.2 g day and serum albumin > 3.5 g/dl	Urine PCR < 200 mg/g for 3 consecutive days
Partial remission	Reduction of proteinuria to between 0.2 to 3.4 g/day or decrease in proteinuria of > 50% from baseline	Proteinuria reduction > 50% or greater from the baseline value and absolute urine PCR between 200 and 2000 mg/g
No remission	Failure to reduce urine protein excretion by 50% or persistent uPCR > 2000 mg/g	
Relapse	Proteinuria > 3.5 gm/day after attaining complete remission for a month	Urine PCR > 2000 mg/g or 3 + protein on urine dipstick for 3 consecutive days

UPCR: Urinary spot protein: creatinine ratio (PCR)

Management of edema:

Mainstay of the treatment of edema is diuretic therapy with salt restriction. There is a considerable amount of diuretic resistance during a nephrotic relapse due to decreased delivery of the diuretic to the site of action of the drug and due to the decreased binding of the diuretic to albumin within the tubular lumen due to hypoalbuminemia, hence, preventing its action.

Daily weight loss with diuresis should not be more than 2 kg per day.

The order and preference of diuretics are as follows:

1. Oral loop diuretic > furosemide 40 mg BID/Bumetanide 1 mg BID.
2. Double the dose of loop diuretics until diuresis or ceiling dose is reached (Furosemide 240mg, Bumetanide 5mg daily).
3. If no response, add on oral thiazide diuretics: Hydrochlorothiazide 25–50 mg daily/Metolazone 2.5–5mg daily.
4. If poor response, then change loop diuretic to IV bolus or infusion (oral absorption of diuretic can be inhibited by gut edema).
5. If no response, then consider albumin infusion (20%, 100 ml) with IV bolus diuretics.
6. If no response, then consider ultrafiltration.

The clinical use of diuretics doses in the pediatric population is as follows:

1. Assess for hypovolemia.
2. If the weight gain < 7% then dietary salt restriction should be suffice.
3. If weight gain > 7% then this is considered to be moderate weight gain and diuretics need to be used.

The choice of diuretics is as follows:

1. Oral furosemide (1–4 mg/kg/day).
2. Add spironolactone (2–3 mg/kg/day).
3. If refractory > to consider adding thiazide diuretics > Metolazone (0.2–0.4 mg/kg day) or Hydrochlorothiazide (1–2 mg/kg/day).
4. If the edema continues to be refractory, furosemide 1–2 mg/kg IV bolus repeat Q 12 hourly, followed by infusion 0.1–0.4 mg/kg/hour.

5. If refractory, consider albumin (20%) 1g/kg over 4 hours followed by IV furosemide 1–2 mg/kg at the end of infusion.
6. If the edema continues to be refractory, consider ultrafiltration.

Management of hypercoagulability:

Nephrotic syndrome is a prothrombotic state and can be associated with arterial and venous thrombosis. The risk increases with decreasing albumin levels. KDIGO guidelines suggest prophylactic anticoagulation for patients with albumin levels less than 2.5 gm/dl. The prophylactic anticoagulation can be done with low molecular weight heparins, warfarin, and other direct-acting oral anticoagulants. Full-dose anticoagulation is recommended if a venous or arterial thrombosis is documented.

Management of hyperlipidemia

Hyperlipidemia often resolves with the remission of nephrotic syndrome. Statins are mostly reserved for special situations in adults (high risk of cardiovascular events, diabetic kidney disease, etc.).

Conclusion:

Nephrotic syndrome is a diagnosis encapsulating nephrotic range proteinuria and its attendant clinical and laboratory features. In children, it is primary, whereas in adults, diabetic kidney disease is the commonest etiology. Treatment requires a thorough evaluation and treatment of the cause. Often immunosuppression is used in primary nephrotic syndrome and nephrotic syndrome secondary to auto-immune diseases.

References:

1. Rodriguez-Ballestas E, Reid-Adam J. Nephrotic Syndrome. Pediatr Rev. 2022 Feb 1;43(2):87-99. doi: 10.1542/pir.2020-001230. PMID: 35102405.
2. KitsouK,AskitiV,MitsioniA,SpoulouV.Theimmunopathogenesis of idiopathic nephrotic syndrome: a narrative review of the literature. Eur J Pediatr. 2022 Apr;181(4):1395-1404. doi: 10.1007/s00431-021-04357-9. Epub 2022 Jan 31. PMID: 35098401.
3. Noone DG, Iijima K, Parekh R. Idiopathic nephrotic syndrome in children. Lancet. 2018 Jul 7;392(10141):61-74. doi: 10.1016/S0140-6736(18)30536-1. Epub 2018 Jun 14.
4. de Seigneux S, Martin PY. Management of patients with nephrotic syndrome. Swiss Med Wkly. 2009 Jul 25;139(29-30):416-22. doi: 10.4414/smw.2009.12477.
5. Rovin BH, Adler SG, Barratt J, Bridoux F, Burdge KA, Chan TM, Cook HT, Fervenza FC, Gibson KL, Glassock RJ, Jayne DRW, Jha V, Liew A, Liu ZH, Mejía-Vilet JM, Nester CM, Radhakrishnan J, Rave EM, Reich HN, Ronco P, Sanders JF, Sethi S, Suzuki Y, Tang SCW, Tesar V, Vivarelli M, Wetzels JFM, Lytvyn L, Craig JC, Tunnicliffe DJ, Howell M, Tonelli MA, Cheung M, Earley A, Floege J. Executive summary of the KDIGO 2021 Guideline for the Management of Glomerular Diseases. Kidney Int. 2021 Oct;100(4):753-779. doi: 10.1016/j.kint.2021.05.015.

NEPHROTIC SYNDROME

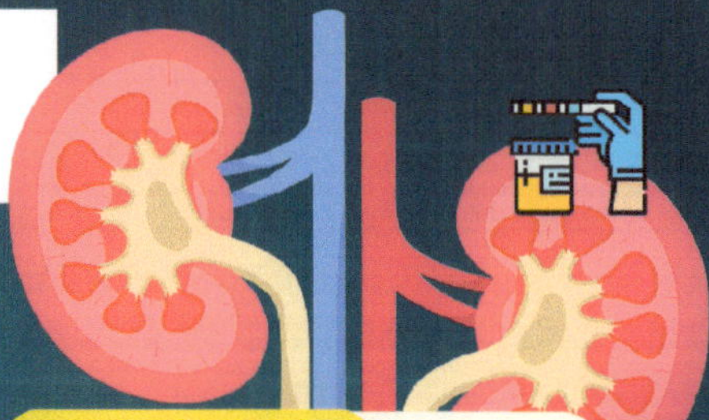

DEFINITION

Constellation of findings including: Proteinuria (nephrotic range), hypoalbuminemia, hyperlipidemia & edema caused by a variety of renal glomerular disease

PRIMARY CAUSES

- Minimal Change Disease
- Focal Segmental Glomerulosclerosis (FSGS)
- Membranous Nephropathy (MN)
- Membranoproliferative Glomerulonephritis (MPGN)
- IgA nephropathy
- Hereditary (Finish-type, Denys-Drash, Frasier)

SECONDARY CAUSES

- Systemic disease (diabetes, lupus)
- Infection (HIV, hepatitis B, hepatitis C)
- Pre-eclampsia
- Certain drugs and toxins
- Congenital due to intrauterine infections

COMPLICATIONS

- FLUID OVERLOAD
- INFECTIONS
- THROMBOEM-BOLISM
- AKI
- DRUG RELATED
- HYPOVOLEMIC CRISIS

INVESTIGATIONS

- Urine r/m
- Urinary protein quantification
- Serum: Basic metabolic panel to assess cbc, renal function serum albumin & lipids
- To rule out secondary causes (HbA1C, Autoimmune markers, viral serologies, work up for multiple myeloma)
- USG abdomen
- Imaging for suspicious thromboembolism
- Renal biopsy

TREATMENT

1 GENERAL MANAGEMENT:

- Diuretics for edema
- Sodium restriction
- Antibiotics for infection
- Anticoagulation for thrombosis

2 TREAT FOR ETIOLOGY

Immunosuppression: Corticosteroids, cyclosporine, MMF, Cyclophosphamide, rituximab

AKI : Acute Kidney Injuyry, ***CBC :*** Complete Blood Count, ***HIV :*** Human immunodeficiency virus, ***MMF :*** Mycophenolate Mofetyl , ***R/m :*** Routine and microscopy, ***USG :*** Ultasonography

07

GLOMERULONEPHRITIS

Karthik Ganesh, V Narayanan Unni

The glomerulus or renal corpuscle is the filtering unit of the nephron. The glomerulus is essentially a collection of capillaries held together by connective tissue called the mesangium in an outpouching of the renal tubular epithelium called the Bowman's capsule. The capillary bed is supported by foot processes of specialized cells called podocytes; movement of water and solutes from the blood in these capillaries occur across the capillary membrane to produce urine. This glomerular ultrafiltrate is then passed into the anatomically contiguous renal tubule.

The glomerular filtration barrier is a highly specialized semipermeable membrane that prevents leakage of blood and proteins into the urine. This barrier is comprised of fenestrated capillary endothelium, the glomerular basement membrane, and the podocytes. It has size and charge selectivity (does not allow passage of solutes bigger than a particular size and those that are negatively charged). Damage to these components results in the leakage of blood and protein into the urine.

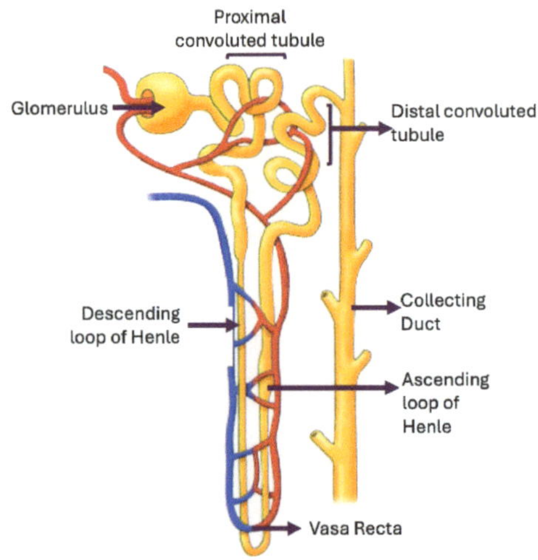

Figure 7.1: Labelled Diagram of a Nephron

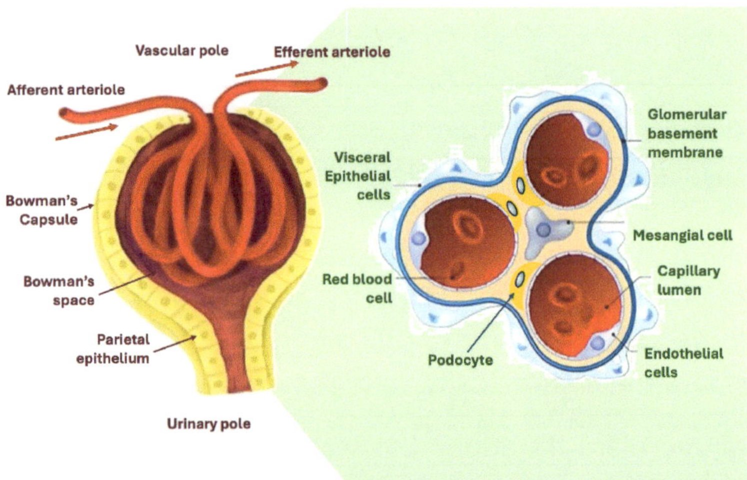

Figure 7.2: Labelled Diagram of the Glomerulus

The term 'glomerulonephritis' comprises a set of diseases that affect the glomerulus. Broadly, these can be classified as proliferative and non-proliferative diseases. Proliferative glomerulonephritis causes inflammation of the glomerular tissue, predominantly via immune mechanisms. The inflammation may lead to the proliferation of the cells of the glomerulus. Etiopathogenetic mechanisms are varied and are summarized in Table 7.1. Frequently, as in the case of genetic mutations in complement factors, a 'second hit' may cause manifestation of the disease. Infiltration of the glomerular apparatus by inflammatory cells induced by one or more of the above mechanisms results in the leakage of protein or blood in the urine. Left unchecked, the inflammatory process involves other segments of the kidney, ultimately resulting in irreversible fibrosis of the interstitium and tubular atrophy resulting in kidney failure.

Classification:

Glomerulonephritis may be classified in multiple ways. Traditional classification systems are based on histopathology (given below). A classification system based on pathogenesis is useful in understanding the disease mechanisms and planning treatment (Table 7.2). Classification according to clinical presentation is another useful way to help the clinician (Table 7.3).

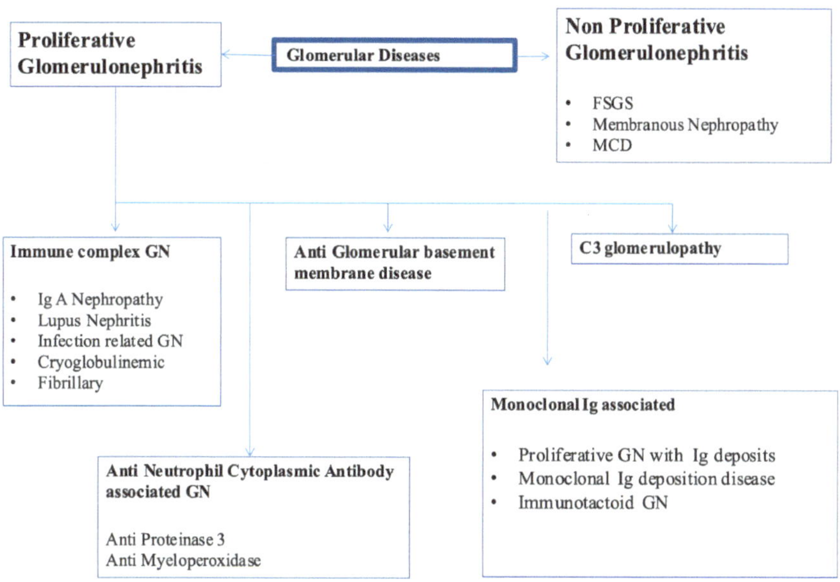

Classification of Glomerulonephritis- based on histology

Figure 7.3: Classification of Glomerulonephritis
FSGS: Focal segmental glomerular sclerosis, Minimal change disease, GN: Glomerulonephritis

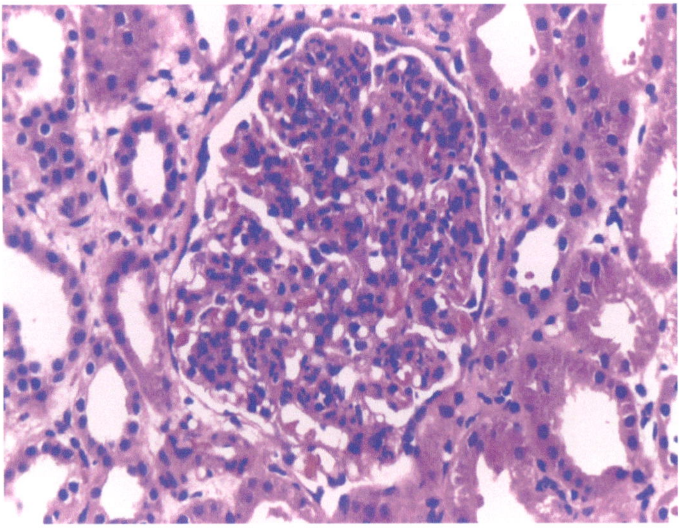

Figure 7.4: Hematoxylin and Eosin (H&E) Stain 40x: Proliferative Glomerulonephritis with Cellular Crescent.

(Images courtesy Dr Renu M Thomas, VPS Lakeshore Hospital, Kochi)

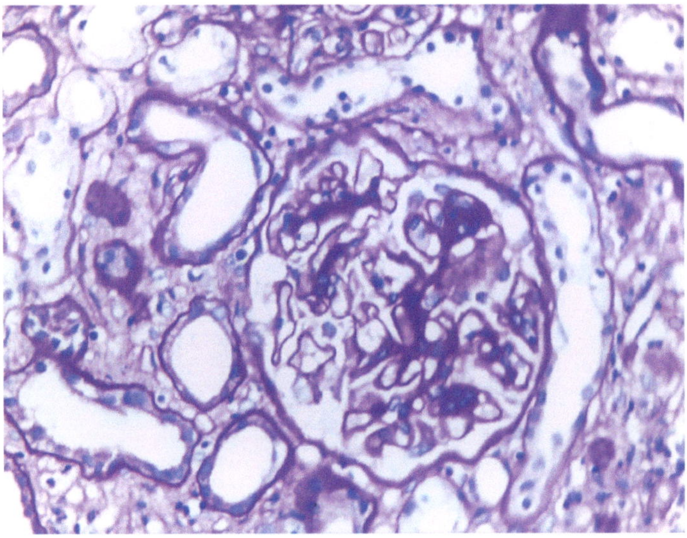

Figure 7.5 Periodic Acid-Schiff (PAS) Stain 40x: Non-proliferative Glomerulonephritis (no cells) Membranous Nephropathy.

(Images courtesy Dr Renu M Thomas, VPS Lakeshore Hospital, Kochi)

Table 7.1: Pathogenic Mechanisms of Glomerulonephritis

Pathogenic Mechanism	Examples
Genetic	Focal segmental glomerulosclerosis, Atypical hemolytic uremic syndrome
Antibody mediated	Anti GBM disease, ANCA vasculitis, Lupus nephritis
Immune complex mediated	IgA Nephropathy, Infection related GN, Lupus nephritis
Complement mediated	Atypical HUS, C3 nephropathy
Monoclonal immunoglobulin mediated	PGNMID, Immunotactoid glomerulonephritis

(**GBM**, glomerular basement membrane; **ANCA**, anti-neutrophilic cytoplasmic antibody; **HUS**, hemolytic uremic syndrome; **PGNMID**, proliferative glomerulonephritis with monoclonal immunoglobulin deposits)

Table 7.2: Syndromic Classification of Glomerulonephritis

Clinical Syndrome	Diseases
Nephrotic Syndrome (Proteinuria > 3.5 g/day), Edema, Hypoalbuminemia, Hyperlipidemia	Minimal Change Disease, Focal Segmental Glomerulosclerosis, Membranous Nephropathy, Amyloidosis, Diabetic Nephropathy
Nephritic Syndrome (Renal Failure, Hypertension, Proteinuria, Hematuria with RBC casts)	Infection related glomerulonephritis, Lupus Nephritis, IgA Nephropathy, Shunt Nephritis, Endocarditis, Atypical HUS
Rapidly progressive Glomerulonephritis	Anti GBM disease, ANCA vasculitis (Granulomatous polyangiitis, eosinophilic granulomatosis with polyangiitis, microscopic polyangiitis), Pauci-immune vasculitis, IgA vasculitis (Henoch Schoenlein purpura), Infective endocarditis, Lupus Nephritis

(**GBM**, glomerular basement membrane; **ANCA**, anti-neutrophilic cytoplasmic antibody; **HUS**, hemolytic uremic syndrome)

Clinical Presentation:

Glomerulonephritis usually presents with facial and pedal oedema, hypertension, proteinuria, hematuria (gross or microscopic), and renal dysfunction.

Table 7.3: Clinical Presentations of Glomerulonephritis

Clinical Presentation	Description
Asymptomatic	Incidentally detected proteinuria (150mg to 3g/day), Microscopic hematuria (> 3–5 dysmorphic RBC/high power field)
Macroscopic hematuria	Episodic, may be associated with infections and varying degrees of proteinuria
Nephritic syndrome	Acute onset edema, Proteinuria, Hypertension, Renal dysfunction with hematuria
Nephrotic syndrome	Proteinuria > 3.5grams/day, Edema, Hypoalbuminemia, Hyperlipidaemia
Rapidly progressive glomerulonephritis	Renal failure progressing over days to weeks with proteinuria and hematuria. Extra-renal features of vasculitis may be noticed
Chronic glomerulonephritis	Asymptomatic most often. Hypertension and Renal failure with shrunken smooth kidneys on ultrasonogram

Evaluation:

Evaluation for glomerulonephritis involves a quartet of a good history and clinical examination, basic investigations, special tests, and a kidney biopsy. In addition, genetic analysis in special cases provides valuable information regarding certain diseases and helps to plan further therapy.

Kidney Biopsy:

The role of a kidney biopsy is often crucial in the diagnosis of glomerulonephritis. There is frequent overlap in the presenting features, and a specific diagnosis is important to plan therapy. Hence, any patient with suspected glomerular pathology should be referred to a nephrologist at the earliest to obtain a kidney biopsy and initiate treatment. All kidney biopsies are evaluated by light microscopy and immunofluorescence.

Glomerular pathology includes features of active glomerulonephritis such as endocapillary proliferation, vasculitis, and crescent formation. Some glomerular pathologies may present with less 'active' lesions such as thickening of the basement membrane or mesangial proliferation. Immunofluorescence studies are useful in obtaining the exact diagnosis. In some cases of glomerular disease, light microscopy and immunofluorescence studies may be normal, despite evidence of glomerular involvement on urine analysis (nephrotic proteinuria in minimal change disease). In such cases, electron microscopy is essential in the diagnosis of the underlying condition. Electron microscopy also helps in identifying the site of the immune deposit, which in turn provides the appropriate diagnosis.

Genetic Testing

The role of genetic testing is useful in diagnosis and prognostication. A disease like focal segmental glomerulosclerosis may have a genetic component and testing is essential (in the appropriate clinical context) to avoid unnecessary immunosuppression, since genetic diseases do not respond to immunosuppressive therapy. It may also help in risk stratification to predict the risk of recurrence of the disease in the new kidney after kidney transplantation. Genetic testing is also helpful in cases that present at a stage where a kidney biopsy is not possible.

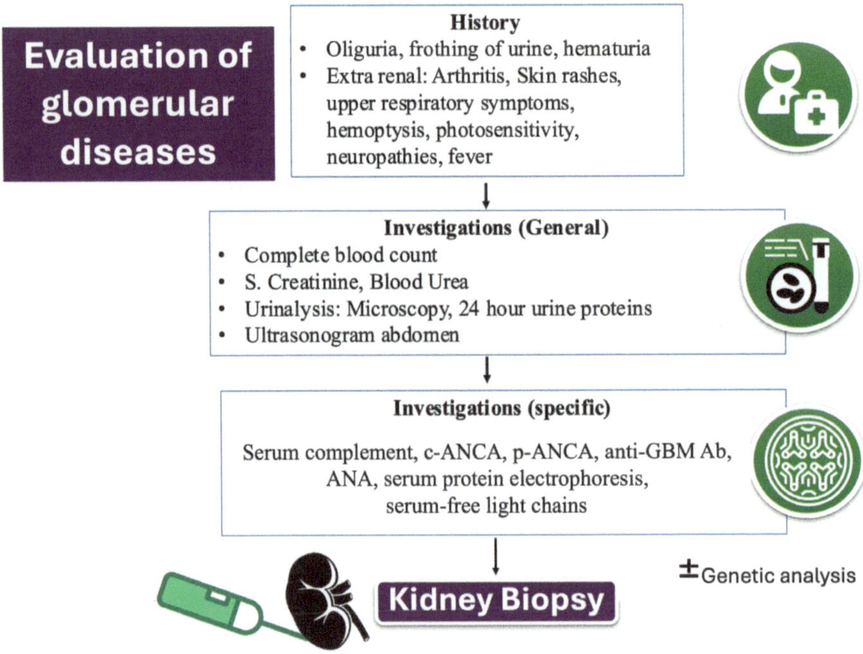

Figure 7.6: Flowchart for the Diagnostic Evaluation of Glomerular Diseases

Treatment:

Treatment of glomerulonephritis may be divided into general measures and specific treatments.

General measures: Optimization of blood pressure control, management of renal failure, renal replacement therapy, if needed, control of edema and hypoalbuminemia with diuretics and albumin infusions, treatment of coexisting infections, and correction of anemia.

Specific measures: These are based on the diagnosis obtained by a kidney biopsy. Various combinations of the following are used.

- Immunosuppressive drugs, including corticosteroids
- Plasma exchange
- Intravenous immunoglobulin

Immunosuppressive Regimens:

Commonly used agents are steroids, cyclophosphamide, mycophenolate mofetil, and rituximab in varying combinations, depending on the disease entity. Immunosuppressive regimens are divided into two phases—an induction phase and a maintenance phase. The induction phase is a period of heightened immunosuppression to achieve control of the disease activity as fast as possible. Once this is achieved—either completely or partially—the next phase of treatment is the maintenance phase, where an attempt to maintain control of the activity of the disease is made through the means of prolonged immunosuppression. Patients are regularly monitored for disease activity and side effects of the drugs, and relapses, if any, are treated. A re-biopsy may be considered in certain cases to assess the extent of improvement or the possibility of a relapse. During this phase of immunosuppression, the patient is prone to infective complications. A high index of suspicion for atypical infections like invasive fungal diseases should be maintained. A balance between adequate immunosuppression and prevention of infections is essential. Prophylaxis for common opportunistic infections like Pneumocystis jirovecii may be given during the induction phase.

Immunosuppressive drugs have side effects such as diabetes, hypertension (steroids), cytopenia, impaired fertility, and hemorrhagic cystitis (mycophenolate mofetil, cyclophosphamide). These should be monitored during therapy.

Renal Replacement Therapy:

In some cases of severe glomerulonephritis, renal function may remain abnormal and progress to end-stage renal disease despite immunosuppressive efforts. Such patients are commenced on renal replacement therapy (hemodialysis or peritoneal dialysis). They can be considered for renal transplant as a definitive form of renal replacement therapy.

Few diseases (focal segmental glomerulosclerosis, membranoproliferative glomerulonephritis, and IgA nephropathy) may recur in the new kidney after transplant, with varying degrees of severity. Appropriate counseling and planning of treatment modalities are needed in these cases.

References:

1. Hricik DE, Chung-Park M, Sedor JR. Glomerulonephritis. N Engl J Med. 1998 Sep 24;339(13):888-99.
2. Sethi S, De Vriese AS, Fervenza FC. Acute glomerulonephritis. Lancet. 2022 Apr 23;399(10335):1646-1663.
3. Jurgen Floege,Richard J Johnson. Introduction to glomerular in Comprehensive Clinical Nephrology, ed.John Feehally, Jurgen Floege, Marcello Tonelli, Richard J Johnson. 7th edition. 2023

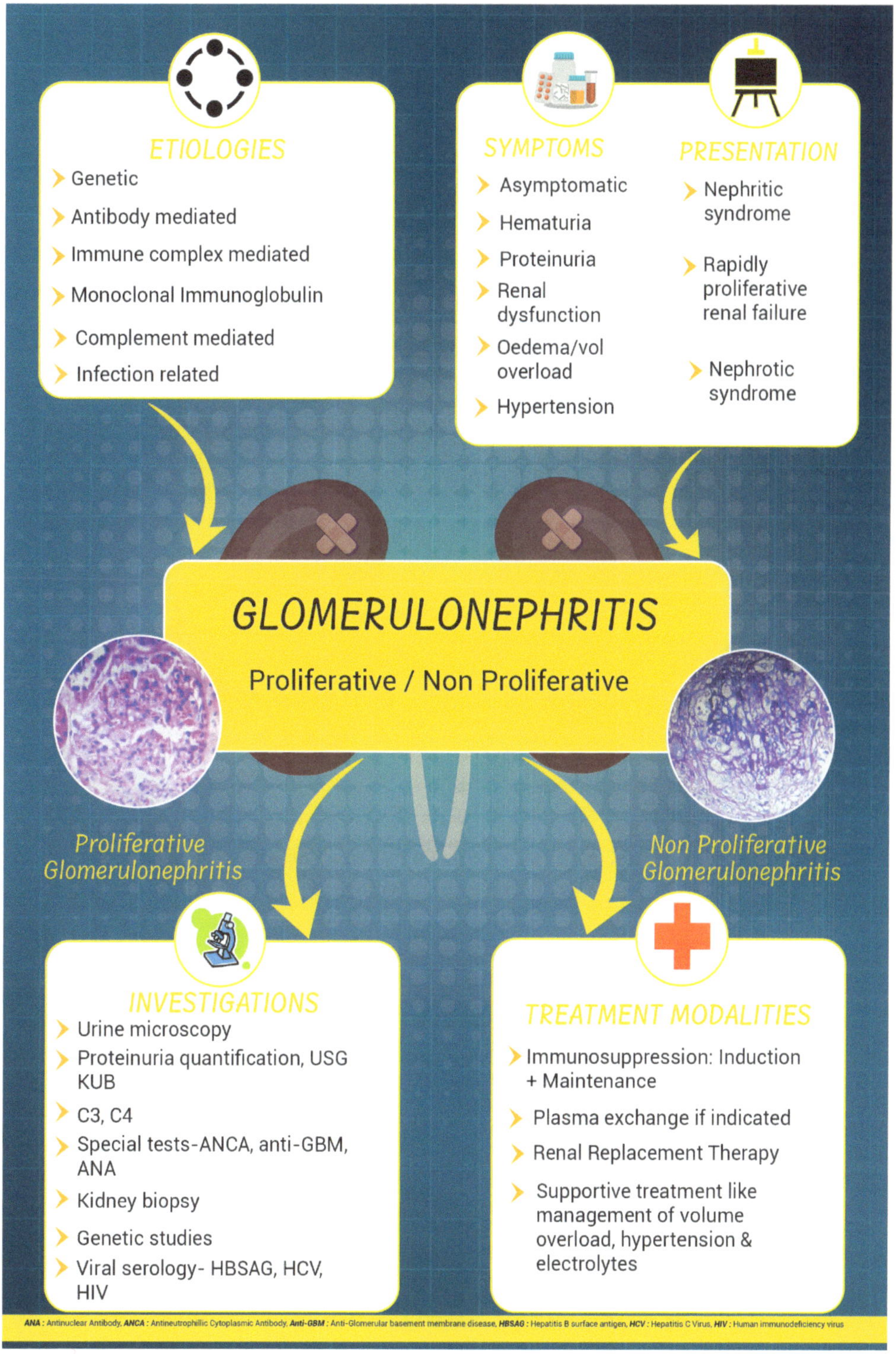
ETIOLOGIES
Genetic
Antibody mediated
Immune complex mediated
Monoclonal Immunoglobulin
Complement mediated
Infection related
SYMPTOMS
Asymptomatic
Hematuria
Proteinuria
Renal dysfunction
Oedema/vol overload
Hypertension
PRESENTATION
Nephritic syndrome
Rapidly proliferative renal failure
Nephrotic syndrome
GLOMERULONEPHRITIS
Proliferative / Non Proliferative
Proliferative Glomerulonephritis
Non Proliferative Glomerulonephritis
INVESTIGATIONS
Urine microscopy
Proteinuria quantification, USG KUB
C3, C4
Special tests-ANCA, anti-GBM, ANA
Kidney biopsy
Genetic studies
Viral serology- HBSAG, HCV, HIV
TREATMENT MODALITIES
Immunosuppression: Induction + Maintenance
Plasma exchange if indicated
Renal Replacement Therapy
Supportive treatment like management of volume overload, hypertension & electrolytes
ANA : Antinuclear Antibody, ANCA : Antineutrophillic Cytoplasmic Antibody, Anti-GBM : Anti-Glomerular basement membrane disease, HBSAG : Hepatitis B surface antigen, HCV : Hepatitis C Virus, HIV : Human immunodeficiency virus

08

LUPUS NEPHRITIS

Dinesh Khullar, Pallavi Prasad

Introduction:

Renal involvement in systemic lupus erythematosus (SLE) is known as Lupus Nephritis (LN) and is common with an estimated prevalence varying between 30–60% depending on the race (more common in the Black race, Hispanics & Asians versus Caucasians). Although SLE is most common in women of reproductive age group, the risk of renal involvement in SLE is higher in children, adolescents, and males.

Clinical Presentation of SLE and LN

The 2019 ACR EULAR classification system enlists clinical and immunological domains on the basis of which a patient with positive ANA (≥ 1:80 by IF) may be classified as a case of SLE (Table 8.1). The renal domain of this criteria includes proteinuria > 0.5 g/24 hours and biopsy proven class II, III, IV, V LN. A class III or IV lesion of LN has been assigned the highest score and alone is diagnostic of SLE in a patient with positive ANA, even if other clinical and immunological criteria are not met.

Table 8.1: EULAR/ACR 2019 Classification Criteria of LN

<table>
<tr><td colspan="4">Entry criterion: ANA 1:80 by IF on Hep- 2 cells or equivalent test. Use the classification criteria for SLE below only if the entry criterion is met</td></tr>
<tr><td>Clinical Domains</td><td>Score</td><td>Immunological Domains</td><td>Score</td></tr>
<tr><td>Constitutional fever</td><td>2</td><td>Antiphospholipid antibodies (APLA)
Anti-cardiolipin or
Anti-beta-glycoprotein or
Lupus anticoagulant</td><td>2</td></tr>
<tr><td>Hematologic
Leukopenia
Thrombocytopenia
Autoimmune hemolysis</td><td>
3
4
4</td><td>Complement proteins
Low C3 or Low C4
Low C3 and Low C4</td><td>
3
4</td></tr>
<tr><td>Neuropsychiatric
Delirium
Psychosis
Seizure</td><td>
2
3
5</td><td>SLE specific antibodies
AntidsDNA or AntiSm antibody</td><td>
6</td></tr>
<tr><td>Mucocutaneous
Non-scarring alopecia
Oral ulcers
Subacute cutaneous LE
Acute cutaneous LE</td><td>
2
2
4
6</td><td></td><td></td></tr>
<tr><td>Serosal
Pleural/pericardial effusion
Pericarditis</td><td>
5
6</td><td></td><td></td></tr>
<tr><td>Musculoskeletal
Joint involvement</td><td>
6</td><td></td><td></td></tr>
<tr><td>Renal
Proteinuria > 0.5 g/d
Class II or V LN
Class III or IV LN</td><td>
4
8
10</td><td></td><td></td></tr>
<tr><td colspan="4">↓
Classify as SLE with a score of 10 or more if entry criterion is met</td></tr>
</table>

Clinical presentation of lupus nephritis includes various presentations like asymptomatic urinary abnormality, nephritic syndrome, nephrotic syndrome, and rapidly progressive renal failure. The most common presentation is nephritic syndrome. Proteinuria is the most important urinary finding in LN and is present in 100% of the patients, followed by microscopic hematuria seen in 80%.

Most patients of LN may suffer from flares of the disease intermittently after their first presentation. These flares may be classified clinically as nephritic flares or proteinuric flares.

Nephritic flare consists of > 30% rise in serum creatine along with active urine sediment. Proteinuric flare is defined as the doubling of urine protein creatinine ratio to > 1 g/g in a patient with previous complete renal response and to 2g/g in a patient with previous partial response to therapy.

Screening of SLE Patients for LN

All patients of SLE should undergo a urine examination and blood tests to rule out renal involvement at the time of diagnosis of SLE and periodic screening subsequently, which should be done at least once in 3 months in patients with a high risk of development of LN (male, pediatric age group, serologically active disease, etc.). Testing should also be done in all patients with suspected lupus flares.

Urine examination should include a routine analysis and microscopy along with a 24-hour urinary quantification for proteinuria. Urinary microscopic examination in SLE often reveals a "telescoped urine", meaning that all kinds of cells and casts may be present in a single urine sample. Blood tests for renal involvement include blood urea and serum creatinine. These tests should be done apart from other immunological markers like AntidsDNA, complement levels deemed necessary for a follow-up of the patient.

Indications for Kidney Biopsy in Lupus Nephritis:

Classification of lupus nephritis is based on histopathological findings. Hence, biopsy is an important cornerstone for diagnosis of lupus nephritis.

Indications of a kidney biopsy in SLE:

- Proteinuria > 500 mg/24 hours
- Active urinary sediment (active urine sediment includes hematuria > 5 RBCs per HPF, leukocyturia > 5 WBCs per HPF in the absence of infection, or RBC and WBC casts)
- Abnormal renal function, which cannot be explained by any other cause.

Ideally, separate kidney biopsy cores should be sent for light microscopy (LM), immunoflourescence (IF), and electron microscopy (EM). Classes of lupus nephritis based on biopsy are described in Table 8.2.

Table 8.2: Classes of Lupus Nephritis on Kidney Biopsy with Common Clinical Presentation

Class on Biopsy	Biopsy Findings	Common Clinical Presentation
Class I (Minimal mesangial LN)	Normal glomeruli by LM, but mesangial immune deposits by immunofluorescence IF and EM	Asymptomatic urinary abnormality Proteinuria + Hematuria+-
Class II (mesangioproliferative LN)	Mesangial matrix expansion or mesangial hypercellularity by LM	Asymptomatic urinary abnormality Proteinuria+ Hematuria +

Class on Biopsy	Biopsy Findings	Common Clinical Presentation
Class III (focal LN)	Endo-capillary or extra-capillary hypercellularity involving < 50% of all glomeruli on light microscopy	Nephritic syndrome Proteinuria ++ Hematuria ++ Raised serum creatinine+-
Class IV (diffuse LN)	Endo- or extra-capillary hypercellularity involving ≥50% of all glomeruli on LM	Nephritic syndrome Proteinuria++ Hematuria++ Raised serum creatinine +
Class V (membranous LN)	Membranous thickening of glomerular capillary walls on LM with subepithelial deposits by EM	Nephrotic syndrome Proteinuria +++ Hematuria- Raised serum creatinine +-
Class VI (advanced sclerosing LN)	≥90% of glomeruli globally sclerosed on LM without residual activity	Chronic kidney disease Proteinuria ++ Hematuria- Raised serum creatinine ++

Class III and IV are the most common classes of LN on biopsy. Class V may be found in addition with Class III/IV, in which case it should be specified as Class III+V or Class IV+V.

All biopsies are also given an activity and a chronicity score, depending on the type of lesions on the biopsy. Signs of activity include fibrinoid necrosis, cellular crescents, endocapillary hypercellularity, neutrophils, hyaline deposits, and interstitial inflammation (scores for fibrinoid necrosis and cellular crescents are double that of other lesions). Signs of chronicity include interstitial fibrosis, tubular atrophy, fibrous crescents, and glomerulosclerosis.

Other pathologies that are less commonly found in LN but are not found in this classification are: Thrombotic microangiopathy, Lupus podocytopathy, and Interstitial or Vascular involvement by LN. Lupus podocytopathy, a rare presentation found in < 1% of all LN biopsies, needs to be differentiated from Class I LN (both may appear normal on LM) by the presence of nephrotic range proteinuria and diffuse foot process effacement on electron microscopy [with or without mesangial deposits but an absence of sub-endothelial and sub-epithelial deposits].

Treatment of LN

The treatment of LN depends on the class as seen on the biopsy.

Class I and Class II LN: Immunosuppressive therapy in patients with Class I or Class II LN should be guided by extra-renal manifestations of SLE. Patients with nephrotic range proteinuria with lupus podocytopathy should be treated with corticosteroids as recommended for minimal change disease/FSGS.

Class III and Class IV LN: In patients with active Class III or IV LN, treatment consists of an induction and a maintenance phase.

Induction/Initial therapy: In the induction phase, treatment should initially be with glucocorticoids plus either intravenous cyclophosphamide or mycophenolate. Methylprednisolone pulse 0.25–0.5g per day may be given for 1–3 days, followed by oral prednisolone at 0.5–1mg/kg/d (tapered gradually over 3–6 months). According to recent guidelines, low-dose corticosteroids should be used and one should consider early tapering of the dose.

Mycophenolate mofetil (MMF): Where mycophenolate is chosen as the first line therapy, the dose can be initiated at 500 mg twice daily of mycophenolate mofetil and then gradually increased to a total dose of 2–3 g/day (depending on tolerability) and should be continued for 6 months with close monitoring of WBC and platelet counts.

IV Cyclophosphamide: It may be given as a low-dose or a high-dose regimen. The low-dose regimen consists of 6 doses of 500 mg cyclophosphamide given every 15 days. In patients with a high risk of renal failure (reduced GFR, histological presence of cellular crescents/fibrinoid necrosis, or severe interstitial inflammation), high-dose cyclophosphamide may be given (0.5–1 g/m^2 monthly for 6 months).

Other first line agents: Triple immunosuppressive therapy consisting of a CNI (tacrolimus/cyclosporine/voclosporine) with reduced-dose mycophenolate and corticosteroid (multitarget therapy), belimumab with MMF or low dose IV cyclophosphamide may be used on a case-by-case basis. Belimumab with either mycophenolate mofetil (MMF) OR low dose IV Cyclophosphamide and MMF with CNI are other first line combinations that can be used as induction. MMF with CNI combination should only be used when eGFR >45ml/min/1.73m^2.

Choice of induction agent: Mycophenolate mofetil should be the preferred agent for patients at a high risk of infertility, patients who have prior cyclophosphamide exposure, and patients of Asian, Hispanic, or African ancestry.

Maintenance therapy: Maintenance therapy is recommended with MMF at a dose of 1 g per day. Azathioprine 1.5–2 mg/kg/day may be used as a second-line alternative to mycophenolate. The total duration of induction plus the maintenance therapy should be a minimum of 3 years in patients with Class III/IV LN, although some centers prefer to continue it for up to 5 years or even longer.

Class V LN: In patients with low-level proteinuria, Class V LN should be treated with renin-angiotensin system (RAS) blockers and immunosuppression should be guided by other systemic manifestations of SLE. In patients with nephrotic syndrome, a combination of a glucocorticoid with another agent (MMF/cyclophosphamide/calcineurin inhibitor/azathioprine) may be used.

Adjunctive non-immunosuppressive treatment for all classes of LN: All patients must be treated with hydroxycholoroquine (HCQ) at 5 mg/kg/day to reduce lupus flares. Patients should have a screening retinal examination before starting HCQ and once a year, subsequently. Protection from UV light with the use of sunscreen agents with an SPF > 50, the use of RAS blockers, and vaccination should be considered in all patients.

Refractory LN: Patients who do not respond to one induction agent can be given a trial of an alternative agent. Patients without response to both induction agents (refractory LN) may be treated with multi-target therapy, addition of rituximab, or extended therapy with cyclophosphamide.

Pregnancy in LN: LN patients should be counseled to avoid pregnancy while the disease is active or when treatment with teratogenic drugs (cyclophosphamide or MMF) is ongoing, and for at least 6 months after LN becomes inactive. Pregnancy in patients with LN may be associated with complications like preeclampsia, pre-term delivery, and IUGR. Agents like steroids, HCQ, azathioprine, and calcineurin inhibitors may be used to treat LN flare during pregnancy. Aspirin should be added in all pregnant patients with LN.

APLA in LN: APLA antibodies may be present in 30–50% cases of LN. Some patients may develop a full-blown APLA syndrome with thrombotic complications. Patients with APLA syndrome should be treated with anticoagulants.

Long-term Complications in LN: LN is a relapsing disease and patients may have nephritic or proteinuric flares, which need to be treated with immunosuppression. Patients who have a poor response to therapy develop chronic kidney disease, and may require renal replacement therapy. Patients are also prone to infections, cardiovascular diseases, and osteoporosis, and should be monitored for the same and appropriately treated.

Transplantation in LN: Kidney transplantation should be considered in LN patients with kidney failure. SLE is quiescent in most patients with End stage renal disease (ESRD) and there is a low risk of recurrence of LN in the graft.

References:

1. Kidney Disease: Improving Global Outcomes (KDIGO) Glomerular Diseases Work Group. KDIGO 2021 Clinical Practice Guideline for the Management of Glomerular Diseases. Kidney Int. 2021 Oct;100(4S): S1-S276. doi: 10.1016/j.kint.2021.05.021. PMID: 34556256.
2. Bertsias GK, Tektonidou M, Amoura Z, et al Joint European League Against Rheumatism and European Renal Association–European Dialysis and Transplant Association (EULAR/ERA-EDTA) recommendations for the management of adult and paediatric lupus nephritisAnnals of the Rheumatic Diseases 2012;**71:**1771-1782.
3. Bajema IM, Wilhelmus S, Alpers CE, Bruijn JA, Colvin RB, Cook HT, D'Agati VD, Ferrario F, Haas M, Jennette JC, Joh K, Nast CC, Noël LH, Rijnink EC, Roberts ISD, Seshan SV, Sethi S, Fogo AB. Revision of the International Society of Nephrology/ Renal Pathology Society classification for lupus nephritis: clarification of definitions, and modified National Institutes of Health activity and chronicity indices. Kidney Int. 2018 Apr;93(4):789-796. doi: 10.1016/j.kint.2017.11.023. Epub 2018 Feb 16. PMID: 29459092.

4. Aringer M, Costenbader K, Daikh D, Brinks R, Mosca M, Ramsey-Goldman R, et al. 2019 European League Against Rheumatism/American College of Rheumatology Classification Criteria for Systemic Lupus Erythematosus. Arthritis Rheumatol. 2019 Sep;71(9):1400-1412. doi: 10.1002/art.40930. Epub 2019 Aug 6. PMID: 31385462; PMCID: PMC6827566.
5. Khullar D, Prasad P(eds). Lupus Nephritis: Pathogenesis to Current Management. New Converse Healthcare Communications;2019.

LUPUS NEPHRITIS

CLINICAL PRESENTATION

SLE with

- Nephritic syndrome or
- Nephrotic syndrome or
- Asymptomatic urinary abnormality or
- Chronic kidney disease or
- Rapid progressive renal failure

INDICATIONS OF BIOPSY

In a patient with SLE having

- Proteinuria >500mg/day
- Active urine sediment
- Renal dysfunction without any other cause

INVESTIGATIONS

- Urine Routine & Microscopy- >Proteinuria, Hematuria, RBC/ WBC casts
- Kidney function tests- >raised creatinine
- SLE specific antibodies- >+ for ANA, AntidsDNA, APLA, others
- Complement profile - Low C3 &/or C4

TREATMENT TO BE GIVEN IN ALL CLASSES OF LN

- Hydroxychloroquine
- UV B light protection with sunscreen > 50 SPF
- Blood pressure control
- RAS blockers
- Dyslipidemia management
- Screen for Herpes zoster,TB, HIV, HBV, HCV
- Pneumocystis jirovecii prophylaxis
- Vaccination
- Fertility preservation (with cyclophosphamide)

TREATMENT AS PER CLASS OF LN

Class I, II

- Normal/Minimal proteinuria
- Microscopic hematuria +/-
- Normal creatinine
- Hypertension uncommon

Treatment:

- Immunosuppression guided by extra renal manifestations of SLE
- NEPHROTIC PROTEINURIA: Rule out lupus podocytopathy

Class III, IV (with/without Class V)

- Hematuria
- Proteinuria
- Reduced eGFR
- Nephrotic syndrome +/-
- Low C3
- High dsDNA

Treatment:

- INDUCTION: Steroids + MMF/ Cyclophosphamide/Calcineurin inhibitor+MMF/B cell targeting biologics.
- MAINTENANCE - Steroids + MMF/Aza

Class V

- Nephrotic syndrome
- Microscopic hematuria
- Hypertension
- Normal/reduced eGFR

Treatment:

- NON NEPHROTIC PROTEINURIA - RAS blockers
- NEPHROTIC SYNDROME- Steroids+ Cyclophosphamide/MMF/Aza/CNI/ B cell targeting biologics

Class VI

- Slowly progressive renal failure with proteinuria
- Bland urinary sediment

Treatment:

- Manage as CKD
- RRT planning

ANA: Anti Nuclear Antibody, ***AntiDNA:*** Anti double stranded DNA body, ***APLA:*** Anti phospholipid antibodies, ***AZA:*** Azathioprine, ***CNI:*** Calcineurin inhibitors, ***CKD:*** Chronic Kidney Disease, ***eGFR :*** Estimated Glomerular Filtration Rate, ***HBV :*** Hepatitis B Virus, ***HCV :*** Hepatitis C Virus, ***HIV :*** Human immunodeficiency virus, ***LN :*** Lupus Nephritis, ***MMF :*** Mycophenolate mofetyl, ***RAS:*** Renin angiotensin aldosterone system, ***RBC:*** Red blood cell, ***RRT:*** Renal replacement therapy, ***SLE:*** Systemic lupus erthromatosis, ***TB:*** Tuberculosis, ***WBC:*** White blood cell, ***UV :*** Ultraviolet

SECTION 3

Acute Kidney Injury

09

ACUTE KIDNEY INJURY: DEFINITION, CAUSES, PATHOPHYSIOLOGY

Smriti Sinha, Vijay Kher

William Osler in his Textbook for Medicine (1909), described Acute Bright's Disease to be "as a consequence of toxic agents, pregnancy, burns, trauma, or operations on the kidneys."

Acute Kidney Injury (AKI) is the term that has now replaced acute renal failure or acute kidney disease. Acute kidney injury is an abrupt worsening of kidney functions that occurs within hours or days. It is characterized by swelling of the body, decreased urine output, vomiting, and dyspnoea.

It is defined as:

- increase in serum creatinine by 0.3mg/dl within 48hrs; or
- increase in serum creatinine to 1.5 times baseline over 7 days; or
- urine volume less than 0.5ml/kg/hr over 6 hours.

Table 9.1: KDIGO Staging of AKI as per the Severity of Kidney Injury

Stage	Serum Creatinine	Urine Output
1	1.5–1.9 × baseline Or > 0.3 mg/dl increase	< 0.5 ml/kg/h for 6–12 h
2	2.0–2.9 × baseline	< 0.5 ml/kg/h for ≥ 12 h
3	3.0 × baseline Or Increase in serum creatinine to > 4.0 mg/dl Or Initiation of renal replacement therapy Or In patients younger than 18 yr, decrease in estimated glomerular filtration rate < 35 ml/min/1.73 m^2	< 0.3 ml/kg/h for ≥ 24 h Or Anuria for ≥ 12 h

Novel Biomarkers of AKI

Serum creatinine is not a sensitive biomarker for AKI. The rise of serum creatinine can be delayed by 8 to 48 hrs, during which the kidney injury occurs unchecked. Hence, novel biomarkers like tissue inhibitor of metalloproteinase 2 (TIMP-2), insulin-like growth factor-binding protein 7 (IGFBP7), hepcidin, kidney injury molecule 1 (KIM-1), neutrophil gelatinase-associated lipocalin (NGAL), and cystatin C are being researched for earlier AKI detection and prognostication.

Incidence and Risk Factors:

The incidence of AKI has been increasing over the last few decades. AKI occurs in an estimated one in five adults, and one in three children are hospitalized with acute illness. AKI in hospitalized patients is associated with higher mortality and longer hospital stay. Patients who recover from AKI are at a high risk of developing chronic kidney disease (CKD) in the future. Risk factors for AKI include diabetes, heart failure, hypertension, volume depletion, sepsis, hyperuricemia, age > 60 yrs, and underlying CKD.

Table 9.2: Risk Factors of AKI

Risk factors for AKI
1. Old age
2. Diabetes
3. Obesity
4. Cardiovascular disease
5. Chronic kidney disease
6. Chronic liver disease
7. Chronic obstructive pulmonary disease
8. Hypoalbuminemia
9. Dehydration
10. Anemia
11. Drugs: Diuretics, Angiotensin Receptor Blockers, ACE inhibitors, Contrast agents

Causes of AKI

The etiology of AKI can be divided into prerenal, intrinsic, and postrenal AKI. (Table 9.3). In India, the most common causes of AKI in tertiary care centers include sepsis and nephrotoxic drugs. However, in poorer rural regions, the causes include tropical infectious diseases like malaria, leptospirosis, dengue fever, infectious diarrhea, snake bites, use of natural medicines, and poor obstetric care. Pregnancy-associated AKI accounts for 3–5% of all AKIs. Most cases occur in the 3rd trimester and postpartum and include preeclampsia/eclampsia, puerperal sepsis, and postpartum hemorrhage (PPH). Atypical HUS/TMA and Acute fatty liver of pregnancy are comparatively rare and underdiagnosed due to the lack of awareness.

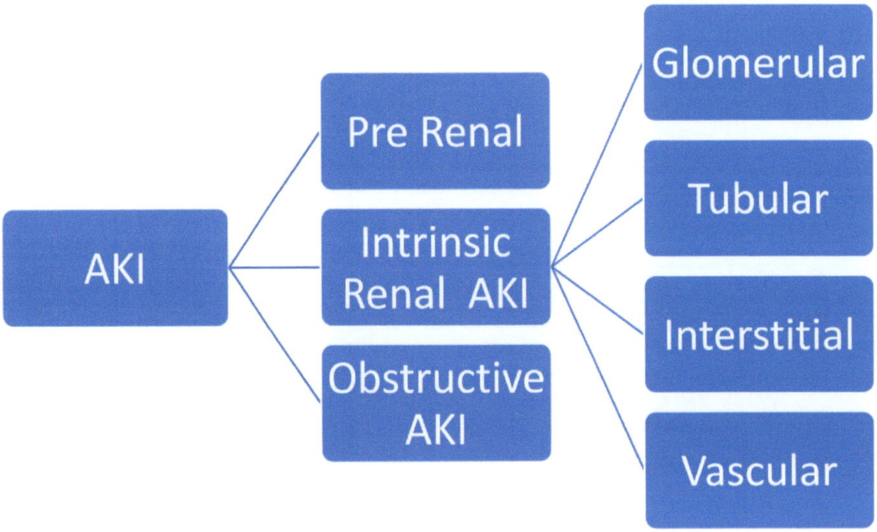

Figure 9.1: Classification of AKI

Table 9.3: Classification and Etiology of AKI

Prerenal	Hypovolemia	Hemorrhage Gastro-Intestinal losses (diarrhea vomiting) Over-diuresis Third space loss (burns, peritonitis, pancreatitis)
	Impaired cardiac function	Heart failure Pulmonary embolism Pericardial tamponade
	Systemic vasodilatation	Sepsis Cirrhosis Anaphylaxis Hepatorenal syndrome
	Intrarenal hemodynamic changes	Drugs: Cyclosporine NSAIDs, RAS Blockers Hypercalcemia Hepatorenal syndrome

Intrinsic	Tubular	Renal ischemia (most prerenal causes can lead to ATN if unchecked) Nephrotoxic drugs Exogenous: Contrast, antibiotics-vancomycin, amphotericin, amikacin, acyclovir, herbal medicines, heavy metals, anticancer drugs – cisplatin, carboplatin Endogenous toxins myoglobin, hemoglobin
	Glomerular	Acute glomerulonephritis (Infection related, IgA nephropathy, membranoproliferative, lupus nephritis, complement mediated) Vasculitis (Paucimmune, anti GBM, immune complex mediated) Thrombotic microangiopathic Anemia
	Interstitium	Infections Sarcoidosis Malignancy Medications: Antibiotics – penicillin, cephalosporins, quinolones, sulphonamides, rifampicin, allopurinol, diuretics, NSAIDs, and many more drugs)
	Vascular	Renal artery thrombosis Renal vein thrombosis Vasculitis Atheroembolism Drugs: Bevacizumab, mitomycin, gemcitabine
Postrenal		Nephrolithiasis Blood clots Papillary necrosis Prostate hypertrophy Improperly placed catheter Bladder, prostate, or cervical cancer Retroperitoneal fibrosis

ATN: Acute tubular necrosis, NSAIDS:Non-steroidal anti-inflammatory drugs, RAS: Renin-angiotensin system

Pathophysiology of AKI

AKI is characterized by a series of pathological changes, which leads to a decrease in the glomerular filtration rate (GFR).

Prerenal AKI:

In prerenal AKI, there is impaired renal perfusion leading to a fall in GFR. The glomerulus has an autoregulatory system, wherein it can maintain the GFR when the Systolic Blood Pressure fluctuates between 80 to 150 mmhg. A mild decrease in renal perfusion is counteracted in individual glomeruli by afferent arteriole vasodilatation and efferent vasoconstriction. The afferent arteriolar vasodilates via medial smooth muscle relaxation (myogenic reflex) to increase the blood flow. Vasodilatory prostaglandins like prostacyclin and prostaglandin E2 also act at the afferent arteriolar level to mediate vasodilation. That is why prostaglandin inhibitors like NSAIDS can blunt this effect and precipitate AKI, especially in volume-depleted states. The efferent arterioles, on the other hand, undergo vasoconstriction to increase the glomerular hydrostatic pressure. This is mainly mediated by Angiotensin II. Drugs like ACE inhibitors and angiotensin receptor blockers (ARBs) can blunt this effect and cause AKI, especially in CKD kidneys, which depend on glomerular autoregulation to maintain their GFR. Uncorrected and prolonged prerenal AKI can further lead to ischemic ATN.

Intrinsic AKI:

Intrinsic AKI pathophysiology more often is complicated and multifactorial. ATN is the most common cause of AKI in hospital settings and occurs most commonly due to renal hypoperfusion, sepsis, and nephrotoxic drugs. The medullary part of the kidney receives most of its blood supply from the vasa recta and is more hypoxic as compared to the cortex. Hence, medulla is the most vulnerable to ischemic injuries. Ischemia leads to the depletion of ATP, causing the more metabolically active segments in relatively ischemic parts of the kidney, like the S3 segment of the proximal tubule and thick medullary ascending limbs, to be most susceptible to ischemic injury.

In the initiation phase, nephrotoxins and/or ischemia cause injury to the endothelium and tubular epithelial cells, leading to cell death by apoptosis or necrosis. In sub-lethally injured cells, there is disruption of the actin cytoskeleton of the cells and loss of polarity of cells, which is characterized by migration of NA/K ATPase channel from the basolateral surface to the cytoplasm or apical surfaces. As a result, there is lesser reabsorption of sodium and chloride at the proximal part and increased distal delivery of sodium and chloride to macula densa cells. This activates the tubulo-glomerular feedback system, leading to decreased renal blood flow and GFR. Injured cells also have poor adhesion to other tubular cells, leading to cell detachment and sloughing into the tubular lumen. The sloughed cells can mix with tamm-horsfall protein and produce granular casts. Loss of tubular cell adhesions leads to increased back-leak of the filtrate into the interstitium, causing a decrease in measure GFR.

In AKI, activation of the inflammatory process contributes to both local damage and fibrosis as well as damage to other organs (organ cross talk). There is activation of both innate and adaptive immunity, especially during reperfusion, leading to further injury.

The recovery phase of ATN can take from 2 weeks to 12 weeks. Recovery from ATN requires the restoration of tubular cell number and coverage of the denuded tubular basement membrane. The existing viable tubular cells undergo differentiation and proliferation into newer mature polar tubular cells. The inflammatory cells (neutrophils and M1 monocytes) are replaced by M2 monocytes that help with epithelial cell repair. Excessive fibrosis during the healing phase, especially in severe AKI, can lead to chronic kidney disease.

Nephrotoxic AKI:

Due to the high blood flow to the kidney and exposure to toxins, which are excreted via the renal route, kidneys become highly susceptible to injury via certain toxins. Nephrotoxins can cause direct tubular injury, interfere with renal hemodynamic, cause allergic reactions leading to acute interstitial nephritis, and cause intratubular obstruction.

Post-obstructive AKI:

In post-obstructive AKI, obstruction of the renal pelvis, ureters, bladder, or urethra can lead to an increase in intratubular pressure, which opposes glomerular filtration pressure leading to a fall of GFR. In normal bilateral kidneys, bilateral ureters must be obstructed for AKI to occur. In solitary functioning, kidney blockage of the same ureter leads to AKI. Obstructive uropathy should be the first to be ruled out as most causes are correctable and reversible.

The complications and management of AKI will be discussed in the next chapter.

References:

1. Koyner JL. Assessment and diagnosis of renal dysfunction in the ICU. Chest. 2012;141(6):1584–1594.
2. Rewa, O., Bagshaw, S. Acute kidney injury—epidemiology, outcomes and economics. Nat Rev Nephrol 10, 193–207 (2014). https://doi.org/10.1038/nrneph.2013.282
3. Chertow GM, Burdick E, Honour M, et al. Acute kidney injury, mortality, length of stay, and costs in hospitalized patients. J Am Soc Nephrol. 2005; 16(11):3365–3370
4. Coca SG, Yusuf B, Shlipak MG, et al. Long-term risk of mortality and other adverse outcomes after acute kidney

injury: a systematic review and meta-analysis. Am J Kidney Dis. 2009;53(6):961–973

5. Vairakkani R, Fernando ME, Sujith S, Harshavardhan TS, Raj TY. Acute Kidney Injury in a Tertiary Care Center of South India. Indian J Nephrol. 2022 May-Jun;32(3):206-215. doi: 10.4103/ijn.IJN_481_20. Epub 2021 Dec 30. PMID: 35814315; PMCID: PMC9267077.
6. Prakash J, Prakash S, Ganiger VC. Changing epidemiology of acute kidney injury in pregnancy: A journey of four decades from a developing country. Saudi J Kidney Dis Transpl. 2019 Sep-Oct;30(5):1118-1130. doi: 10.4103/1319-2442.270268. PMID: 31696851.

ACUTE KIDNEY INJURY

DEFINITION

Increase in serum creatinine by 0.3mg/dl within 48hrs; or increase in serum creatinine to 1.5 times baseline over 7 days or urine volume less than 0.5ml/kg/hr over 6hours

RISK FACTORS

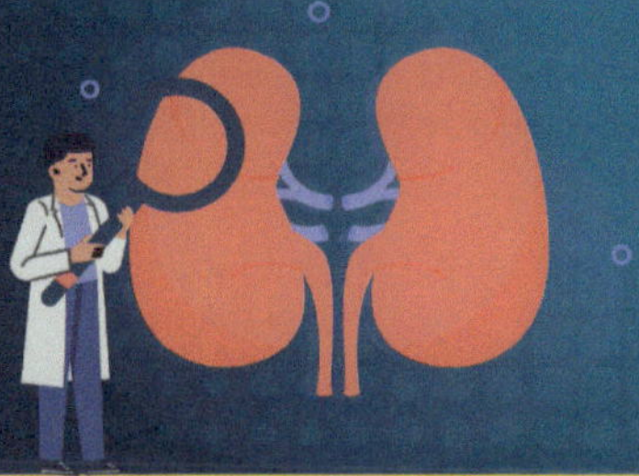

- Old Age
- Underlying CKD
- Diabetes
- Cardiovascular Disease
- COPD
- CLD

CAUSES

PRE RENAL AKI

- Haemorrhage
- Shock
- Diarrhoea
- Heart Failure
- Hepatorenal syndrome
- Excessive diuretics

INTRINSIC AKI

- Glomerular: RPGN, IgAN, MPGN
- Tubular: Ischaemia: shock, sepsis
- Nephrotoxins: Antibiotics, anticancer drugs, Contrast media, myoglobin, hemoglobin
- Interstitial: Infections, malignancy, drugs
- Vascular: vasculitis, drugs

POST RENAL AKI

- Nephrolithiasis
- Papillary necrosis
- BPH
- Uretheral stricture
- Bladder/cervical/ rectal cancer

MISCELLANEOUS CAUSES: Snake bite associated with AKI, Pregnancy associated with AKI, sepsis, kidney involvement in malignancies

AKI **:** Acute Kidney Injury, ***BPH*** **:** Benign prostatic hyperplasia, ***CKD*** **:** Chronic Kidney Disease, ***CLD*** **:** Chronic Liver Disease, ***COPD*** **:** Chronic obstructive pulmonary disease, ***IgAN*** **:** Immunoglobulin A Nephropathy, ***MPGN*** **:** Membranoproliferative glomerulonephritis, ***RPGN*** **:** Rapidly progressive glomerulonephritis

10

AKI: COMPLICATIONS AND MANAGEMENT

Manjuri Sharma, Amit Roy

Introduction:

Acute kidney injury (AKI) is characterized by an acute decrease in renal function that can be multifactorial in its origin and is associated with complex pathophysiological mechanisms. KDIGO defines AKI as any of the following: increase in serum creatinine by 0.3 mg/dL or more within 48 hours, or increase in serum creatinine to 1.5 times baseline or more within the last 7 days, or urine output less than 0.5 mL/kg/h for 6 hours.

AKI complicates 5–15% of hospitalizations and can reach up to 50–60% in critical care patients. Its consequences extend beyond the immediate term, impacting various aspects of patient health such as hospital stay duration, healthcare costs, in-hospital mortality as well as long-term outcomes like increased risks of cardiovascular events, progression to chronic kidney disease (CKD), and overall mortality. The acute loss of kidney function triggers disturbances in fluid, electrolyte, and acid-base balance as well as hematologic, gastroenterologic, and immunologic functions. This chapter focuses on the common complications encountered in AKI and their management strategies.

Section 1: Complications of AKI:

1. **Metabolic and Electrolyte Imbalances**

    i. **Hyperkalemia:** Hyperkalemia arises from impaired potassium excretion or increased cellular breakdown, as observed in conditions like rhabdomyolysis, hemolysis, tumor lysis syndrome, and severe burn injury. While mild hyperkalemia is often asymptomatic, higher levels can lead to electrocardiographic abnormalities such as tall T waves, PR interval prolongation, flattened P waves, widened QRS complexes, and intraventricular conduction defects.

    ii. **Metabolic Acidosis:** AKI is complicated by metabolic acidosis, with a widening of the serum anion gap due to the retention of phosphates, sulfates, and organic anions.

    iii. **Hyponatremia:** Hyponatremia can occur due to impaired free water excretion and is more prevalent in AKI associated with heart failure, liver failure, or diuretic use. Excessive water intake or administration of hypotonic saline or dextrose solutions can trigger severe hyponatremia, leading to cerebral edema, seizures, and other neurologic abnormalities.

    iv. **Mineral and Uric Acid Homeostasis:** Hyperphosphatemia is caused by reduced excretion or continuous release as seen in rhabdomyolysis, severe burns, hemolysis, or tumor lysis syndrome. Hypocalcemia in AKI is due to the skeletal resistance to the actions of parathyroid hormone, reduced levels of 1,25-dihydroxyvitamin D, and Ca^{2+} sequestration in injured tissues. Hypermagnesemia is common in oliguric AKI and reflects the impaired excretion of ingested magnesium-dietary magnesium, magnesium-containing laxatives, or antacids. Asymptomatic hyperuricemia is typical in established AKI. Higher levels suggest increased production of uric acid and may point to a diagnosis of acute urate nephropathy.

2. **Cardiovascular Complications:** Extracellular volume overload is a consequence of impaired salt and water excretion in AKI, leading to manifestations like mild hypertension, increased jugular venous pressure, pulmonary vascular congestion, pleural effusion, ascites, peripheral edema, increased body weight, and potentially life-threatening pulmonary edema.
3. **Gastrointestinal:** Nausea, vomiting, GI bleeding, and anorexia may complicate AKI.
4. **Neurologic:** CNS-related signs of uremic burden are common in AKI, and they include lethargy, somnolence, seizure, and cognitive impairment.
5. **Hematologic:** Anemia in AKI is multifactorial, resulting from inhibited erythropoiesis, hemolysis, bleeding, hemodilution, and reduced red blood cell survival.
6. **Infection:** Infection is the most common and serious complication of AKI, occurring in 50% to 90% of the cases and contributing to up to 75% of deaths. It can arise from defects in host immune responses or repeated breaches of mucocutaneous barriers due to therapeutic interventions like IV cannulas, mechanical ventilation, or bladder catheterization.

Section 2: Complications During Recovery from AKI

During the recovery phase of AKI, robust diuresis can pose complications by causing intravascular volume depletion and potentially delaying the restoration of kidney function. This diuretic response is primarily attributed to osmotic diuresis triggered by the retention of urea, as well as the excretion of accumulated salt and water that occurred during the AKI episode.

Additionally, the delayed recovery of tubular re-absorptive function compared to glomerular filtration contributes to the wastage of salt, further exacerbating the risk of intravascular volume depletion and impeding the timely recovery of kidney function.

Section 3: Long-term Consequences of AKI

3.1. CKD Development and/or Progression: AKI increases the risk of CKD by 8-fold and the risk of end-stage kidney disease by 3-fold. The risk of CKD is also higher in relation to the severity of AKI and even higher in patients who require dialysis. Factors associated with a higher risk of CKD following AKI were previous increased baseline serum creatinine, male gender, older age, diabetes, previous CVD, hypoalbuminaemia, AKI severity, duration, and recovery pattern of AKI, and recurrent AKI episodes.

3.2. Hypertension, Cardiovascular Disease, and Stroke: A retrospective cohort study identified a 22% increase in the risk of presenting with a blood pressure of > 140/90 mmHg in those who had AKI compared with individuals who did not experience AKI after adjustments for demographic factors, precedent health status, and cardiovascular risk factors. AKI increases the risk of subsequent heart failure by 58%, myocardial infarction by 40%, and stroke by 15%.

Section 4: Management of AKI-associated Complications:

- **Fluid Overload:** Fluid overload can be managed by restricting salt and water intake and by using diuretics. Higher doses of loop diuretics or a combination therapy with thiazide and loop diuretics may be necessary. Ultrafiltration or dialysis may be required for volume management when conservative measures fail. Hyponatremia and Hypernatremia: Hyponatremia associated with a fall in effective serum osmolality can be corrected by a restriction of water intake. Conversely, hypernatremia is treated by the administration of water, hypotonic saline solutions, or hypotonic dextrose-containing solutions.

- **Hyperkalemia:** Mild hyperkalemia (< 5.5 mmol/L) can be managed by restricting dietary potassium, discontinuing potassium supplements, and potassium-sparing diuretics. If K+ > 5.5–6.5 mmol/L, administration of exchange resins (sodium polystyrene sulfonate) and loop diuretics can be considered. For severe hyperkalemia with accompanying electrocardiographic manifestations, intravenous administration of calcium gluconate can counteract the cardiac and neuromuscular effects of hyperkalemia. Intravenous insulin (10–20 U of regular insulin) with dextrose (25–50 gm) facilitates potassium entry into cells, reducing extracellular potassium concentration. Beta adrenergic agonists, such as inhaled albuterol (10–20 mg by nebulizer), promote rapid potassium uptake into the intracellular compartment. If conservative measures fail, emergency hemodialysis is the treatment of choice.
- **Metabolic Acidosis:** Metabolic acidosis usually does not require treatment unless serum HCO^3 concentration is < 15 mmol/L or pH < 7.20. Severe acidosis can be corrected with oral or IV bicarbonate. Hemodialysis is indicated for oliguric or anuric patients with volume overload and severe metabolic acidosis (pH < 7.1). Target levels are serum bicarbonate 20–22 mEq/L and pH > 7.2.
- **Disturbances of Calcium, Phosphate, Magnesium, and Uric Acid:** Hypocalcemia typically does not require treatment unless symptomatic. Hyperphosphatemia can be managed by restricting dietary phosphate intake and

using oral phosphate binders (calcium acetate, sevelamer carbonate, lanthanum carbonate). Hypermagnesemia can be prevented by avoiding magnesium-containing medications such as antacids and limiting magnesium in parenteral nutrition. Hyperuricemia is usually mild and does not require specific intervention.

- **Nutritional Management:** AKI patients are at a risk of malnutrition due to inadequate nutrient intake and increased catabolic rate. The goal of nutritional management is to provide enough calories to preserve lean body mass, prevent starvation ketoacidosis, and support healing and tissue repair. KDIGO recommends a total caloric intake of 20 to 30 kcal/kg/day and dietary protein intake of 0.8 to 1.0 g/kg/day in patients without a need for dialysis and 1.0–1.5 g/kg/day in patients on dialysis.
- **Anemia:** Severe anemia is generally managed with blood transfusions. However, transfusion is usually not required for patients with a hemoglobin concentration > 7 g/dL. The role of erythropoiesis-stimulating agents in AKI is uncertain.

Section 5: Renal Replacement Therapy in AKI

The timing to start RRT remains controversial. The AKIKI trial (Artificial Kidney Initiation in Kidney Injury) found that early initiation of RRT, within 6 hours of meeting KDIGO stage 3 AKI criteria, did not reduce mortality or affect hospital stays and renal recovery. KDIGO recommends initiating RRT when life-threatening imbalances in fluid, electrolyte, and acid-base status occur. Indications for initiation of RRT in AKI are summarized in Box 10.1. Modalities of RRT in AKI include intermittent hemodialysis (HD), continuous RRT (CRRT), slow low-efficiency dialysis (SLED), or peritoneal dialysis(PD).

Absolute Indications

- Volume overload unresponsive to diuretic therapy
- Persistent hyperkalemia despite medical therapy
- Severe metabolic acidosis
  Overt uremic symptoms—encephalopathy, pericarditis, uremic bleeding diathesis

Relative Indications

- Progressive azotemia without uremic manifestations
  Persistent oliguria

Box 10.1: Indications for the Initiation of RRT in AKI

Section 6: Follow-up Care After AKI

KDIGO and ADQI recommend that patients should be followed by a nephrologist at least 3 months after an AKI episode to assess kidney recovery and/or progression to CKD. The follow-up assessment should include kidney function and proteinuria, medication reconciliation, patient education on nephrotoxic avoidance, and strategies to prevent CKD progression.

References:

1. Goyal A, Daneshpajouhnejad P, Hashmi MF, et al. Acute Kidney Injury. [Updated 2023 Feb 19]. In: StatPearls [Internet]. Treasure Island (FL): StatPearls Publishing; 2023 Jan.
2. Joana Gameiro, Filipe Marques. et al. Long-term consequences of acute kidney injury: a narrative review. Clinical Kidney Journal, 2021, vol. 14, no. 3, 789–804.
3. Chertow, G.M.; Burdick, E.; Honour, M.; Bonventre, J.V.; Bates, D.W. Acute Kidney Injury, Mortality, Length of Stay, and Costs in Hospitalized Patients. J. Am. Soc. Nephrol. 2005, 16, 3365–3370.
4. Coca SG, Singanamala S, Parikh CR. Chronic kidney disease after acute kidney injury: a systematic review and meta-analysis. Kidney Int 2012; 81: 442–448.
5. Wald R. Chronic dialysis and death among survivors of acute kidney injury requiring dialysis. JAMA 2009; 302: 1179.

6. Hsu, C. Y. et al. Elevated BP after AKI. J. Am. Soc. Nephrol. 27, 914–923 (2016).
7. Odutayo, A. et al. AKI and long-term risk for cardiovascular events and mortality. J. Am. Soc. Nephrol. 28, 377–387 (2017).
8. Gaudry,S.;Hajage,D.;Schortgen,F.; et al. Initiation Strategies for Renal-Replacement Therapy in the Intensive Care Unit. N. Engl. J. Med. 2016, 375, 122–133.
9. Khwaja, A. KDIGO Clinical Practice Guidelines for Acute Kidney Injury. Nephron 2012, 120, c179–c184.
10. Wang, A.Y.; Bellomo, R. Renal replacement therapy in the ICU. Curr. Opin. Crit. Care 2018, 24, 437–442.
11. Bagshaw SM, Wald R. Strategies for the optimal timing to start renal replacement therapy in critically ill patients with acute kidney injury. Kidney Int. 2017;91[5]:1022–1032.

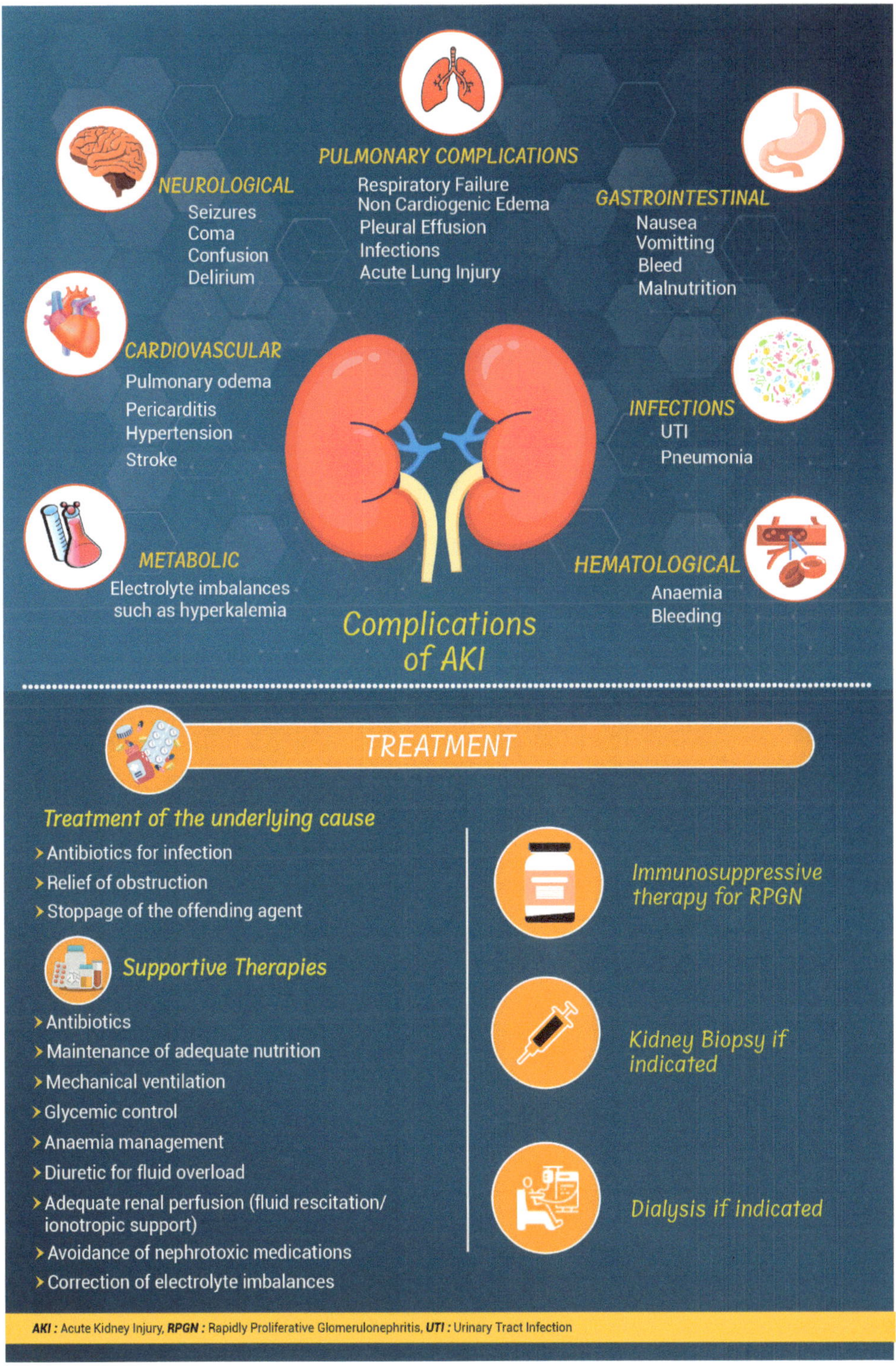

PULMONARY COMPLICATIONS
Respiratory Failure
Non Cardiogenic Edema
Pleural Effusion
Infections
Acute Lung Injury
NEUROLOGICAL
Seizures
Coma
Confusion
Delirium
GASTROINTESTINAL
Nausea
Vomitting
Bleed
Malnutrition
CARDIOVASCULAR
Pulmonary odema
Pericarditis
Hypertension
Stroke
INFECTIONS
UTI
Pneumonia
METABOLIC
Electrolyte imbalances
such as hyperkalemia
HEMATOLOGICAL
Anaemia
Bleeding
Complications of AKI
TREATMENT
Treatment of the underlying cause
Antibiotics for infection
Relief of obstruction
Stoppage of the offending agent
Supportive Therapies
Antibiotics
Maintenance of adequate nutrition
Mechanical ventilation
Glycemic control
Anaemia management
Diuretic for fluid overload
Adequate renal perfusion (fluid rescitation/ ionotropic support)
Avoidance of nephrotoxic medications
Correction of electrolyte imbalances
Immunosuppressive therapy for RPGN
Kidney Biopsy if indicated
Dialysis if indicated
AKI : Acute Kidney Injury, RPGN : Rapidly Proliferative Glomerulonephritis, UTI : Urinary Tract Infection

11

DRUGS AND KIDNEY DISEASE

Anirban Ganguli, Narinder Pal Singh

Introduction:

Drug-induced kidney disease (DIKD) is a significant contributor to acute kidney injury (AKI), comprising 19–26% of cases among hospitalized patients, and can result in severe consequences such as chronic kidney disease (CKD), dialysis dependence, prolonged hospital stays, and escalated healthcare expenses.

Clinical Manifestations of Drug-Induced Kidney Disease:

Timely identification of drug-induced kidney disease (DIKD) necessitates careful attention to the patient's clinical history, particularly their drug history, potential risk factors, urine output, and relevant biochemical tests such as serum creatinine, blood urea nitrogen, urine microscopy, and proteinuria. It is important to note that the serum creatinine levels may not always accurately reflect renal disease, as elevated levels can be caused by drugs that inhibit renal tubular creatinine secretion (e.g., trimethoprim, tyrosine kinase inhibitors, fenofibrates), and is known as "pseudo-acute kidney injury (AKI)". In such cases, more specific glomerular filtration rate (GFR) biomarkers like serum cystatin C can be utilized to determine actual renal function deterioration. To facilitate the recognition of DIKD, four phenotypes have recently been established, based on guidelines from the International Serious Adverse Event Consortium (Table 11.1).

These phenotypes categorize DIKD into AKI, glomerular disorder, tubular disorder, and nephrolithiasis/crystalluria, considering the known mechanisms of nephrotoxicity, disease progression timeline, and clinical setting. The progression of DIKD can vary depending on the mechanism of drug injury, duration of drug exposure, the temporal profile of serum biomarkers (such as serum creatinine), and the timeliness in identifying the culprit agent. DIKD can generally be classified into three timeframes: acute (< 7 days), subacute (injury occurring beyond 7 but < 90 days), and chronic (> 90 days).

Mechanisms of Drug-Induced Kidney Disease:

Mechanisms causing DIKD can be broadly classified into two types: Type A and Type B reactions (Table 11.2).

Type A reactions are dose-dependent and predictable, based on the pharmacological properties of the drug. They can be managed by reducing drug exposure through dose reduction or withdrawal. Examples include aminoglycosides or colistin nephrotoxicity. The specific risk factors for developing a particular drug reaction are unknown, but genetic factors may influence drug metabolism and elimination, predisposing individuals to type A reactions.

Table 11.1: Standardized Clinical Syndromes Associated with Drug Induced Kidney Disease (adapted from Mehta et al. Kid Int 2015)

	Acute Kidney Injury	Glomerular Disorder	Nephrolithiasis	Tubular Dysfunction
Clinical Terminology	Acute Tubular Necrosis (ATN), Acute Interstitial Nephritis (AIN)	Hematuria, Proteinuria	Crystalluria, Ultrasound, Findings of stone with or without obstruction	Renal Tubular Acidosis (RTA), Fanconi syndrome, Syndrome of Inappropriate Antidiuretic Hormone (SIADH), Diabetes Insipidus (DI), Hypophosphatemia
Primary Criteria	Rise in Scr that presents or progresses to stage 2 (KDIGO) which is 2–2.9 × higher than reference Scr OR Decline by at least 50% from peak Scr over 7 days in relationship to changes in drug dosing adjustment or discontinuation within 2 weeks	Biopsy-proven drug-induced glomerular disease (done within 4 weeks of stopping the drug) AND **Proteinuria** as defined by 24 h urine collection > 1 g protein or Urine Dipstix > 2+ protein or urine:protein creatinine ratio(UPCR)> 0.8 g/g **Hematuria** as defined by > 50 RBC per HPF	Must be new onset following drug exposure with no prior history of nephrolithiasis No congenital etiology for nephrolithiasis **If obstructive**, rise in Scr that presents or progresses to stage 2 (KDIGO) or higher **If non-obstructive**, then Urinalysis with crystals and ultrasound with stone	Renal phosphate loss or tubular hypophosphatemia OR/AND Renal glucosuria i.e., urinalysis with 3+ glucose without hyperglycemia (Fanconi's syndrome) OR/AND Hyperchloremic metabolic acidosis (RTA) OR/AND Euvolemic hyponatremia (SIADH) OR/AND Hypernatremia on multiple occasions and/or polyuria > 3 liters/ day(DI)

	Acute Kidney Injury	Glomerular Disorder	Nephrolithiasis	Tubular Dysfunction
Secondary Criteria	Oliguric or urine output < 0.5ml/kg/h for 12 hrs at least (KDIGO-2012) **Urinalysis findings:** – granular and muddy casts consistent with ATN – urinary eosinophils (possible AIN) – proteinuria < 1 g/d – fractional excretion of sodium (FeNa) > 1% AND/OR Clinical symptoms for AIN: fever, rash, and joint pains	RBC casts, dysmorphic RBCs in urine microscopy Absence of secondary disorders that can cause glomerulonephritis such as Diabetes mellitus, Systemic Lupus Nephritis, post-infectious causes, and hepatitis Microangiopathic changes in blood smear, elevated serum LDH, low serum haptoglobin (thrombotic microangiopathy)	**Crystals on urine microscopy** – sheaves of wheat: sulfa drugs – yellow or golden brown annular: methotrexate – needle and fan shaped: indinavir – thin needles: acyclovir – calcium oxalate: iv ascorbate or orlistat – plate or geometric shapes: foscarnet – flat or wedge prisms with rosette formation: sodium phosphate	Tubular hypophosphatemia- fractional excretion of phosphate (FePO4) > 5% Hypomagnesemia- Serum magnesium < 1.2 mg/dl Hypouricemia-Serum uric acid <2mg/dl Tubular proteinuria - 24h urine < 1 g protein or UPCR < 0.8 or dipstix < 2+ protein Diabetes insipidus • Serum osmolality > 300 mOsm/kg • Urine osmolality < 100mOsm/kg • Urine sodium < 10 mEq/l

Type B reactions are immune-mediated, idiosyncratic, and unpredictable. Acute interstitial nephritis from proton pump inhibitors or crescentic glomerulonephritis from hydralazine use are typical examples. Type B reactions involve complex immunological sensitization to drugs acting as haptens or antigens. Additionally, pre-renal AKI can be seen with the use of diuretics due to hypovolemia or from Renin Angiotensin Aldosterone System (RAAS) blockade due to a drop in GFR from efferent arteriolar dilation, especially in the backdrop of reduced renal blood flow from shock or hypovolemia.

Risk Factors for Drug-Induced Kidney Disease:

Various risk factors, modifiable and non-modifiable, influence DIKD beyond individual drug characteristics.

Modifiable risks include:

- Volume depletion
- Hypotension
- Exposure to other nephrotoxic substances
- High drug doses, and incorrect dosing.

Non-modifiable risks include:

- age,
- pre-existing kidney disease,
- liver disease, diabetes,
- heart failure,
- critical illness,
- immune compromise.

Unfortunately, prediction tools for nephrotoxicity risk are not widely available except the Mehran score, which has been recently validated in predicting contrast-associated acute kidney injury after percutaneous interventions. This score considers several clinical factors present at the time of intervention along with the volume of IV contrast in determining the risk of AKI and dialysis post AKI.

Some Selective Drugs Causing Kidney Disease

Non-steroidal Anti-inflammatory Drugs (NSAIDs)

NSAIDs nephrotoxicity occurs through various mechanisms. Type A reaction, which is most common, results from the inhibition of prostaglandin endoperoxide synthase enzyme cyclooxygenase (COX-1-expressed constitutively and COX-2 in inflammatory cells), which lowers renal PGE2 levels. PGE2 is a vasodilator, increasing renal arterial blood flow and maintaining GFR by afferent arteriolar vasodilation, especially in the setting of decreased systemic perfusion from hypovolemia, shock, or congestive heart failure. Reduced PGE2 levels could lead to afferent arteriolar vasoconstriction and a subsequent decline in GFR (pre-renal AKI), while decreased renal blood flow could cause downstream ischemic tubular injury.

Additionally, PGE2 inhibition disrupts tubular sodium reabsorption and water excretion, leading to sodium and water retention. Type B reaction from NSAIDs is rarely seen but typically manifests as acute interstitial nephritis (AIN) with significant proteinuria resulting from T-cell activation and immune-mediated podocyte damage.

Antibiotics

Antibiotics are an important cause of DIKD with multiple mechanisms being involved as listed in Table 11.2. Aminoglycosides such as gentamicin, tobramycin, and amikacin are common culprits, causing dose-dependent reductions in renal function in up to 20% of the cases. These agents primarily induce proximal tubular toxicity. Intravenous vancomycin is also associated with direct proximal tubular toxicity, typically occurring after 4–8 days of therapy. Close monitoring of the renal function is crucial as toxicity can be observed at recommended trough levels (15–20 mg/L). Polymyxins (colistin and polymyxin B), which are used in multidrug-resistant gram-negative infections, exhibit one of the highest rates of dose-dependent nephrotoxicity, leading to acute tubular necrosis and proteinuria. The antifungal amphotericin-B (AmB) acts as a potent tubule toxin, disrupting cell membranes and causing distal tubular acidosis (Type 1). AmB's adverse effects also include decreased GFR, hypokalemia, hypomagnesemia, and nephrogenic diabetes insipidus. Cumulative dose (> 600 mg) is a critical risk factor for AmB nephrotoxicity. Trimethoprim (present in combination with sulfamethoxazole) has already been mentioned to cause pseudo-AKI and, in some cases, hyperkalemia by inhibiting the epithelial Na channel in principal cells. Tenofovir, an antiviral agent, is associated with proximal tubular dysfunction, which may progress to chronic kidney disease if not promptly recognized and managed. Indinavir primarily induces asymptomatic nephrolithiasis, while acyclovir can lead to acute interstitial nephritis due to crystalluria. Risk factors for acyclovir nephrotoxicity include rapid intravenous infusion and higher doses of the drug (> 1500 mg/m^2). Type B reactions in the form of acute interstitial nephritis have been observed with certain beta-lactam antibiotics (particularly nafcillin and methicillin), albeit rarely with cephalosporins, carbapenems, monobactams, sulfa drugs, and fluoroquinolones (especially ciprofloxacin).

Conventional Cancer Chemotherapeutics

Most of these agents cause DIKD through Type A reaction with prototypes being platinum-based compounds such as cisplatin. Besides AKI, cisplatin can also cause hypomagnesemia, nephrogenic diabetes insipidus, proximal tubulopathy, and rarely, thrombotic microangiopathy. Among alkylating agents, ifosfamide is the most nephrotoxic and is associated with proximal tubular dysfunction (Fanconi's Syndrome), which can occasionally be irreversible. Methotrexate, an anti-folate agent, typically develops AKI from crystalline nephropathy. Thrombotic microangiopathy (TMA) is typically seen with gemcitabine and mitomycin C and is a Type A reaction that results from direct endothelial injury.

Targeted Anti-Cancer Agents

Targeted anti-cancer agents are a class of medications that specifically target molecules or pathways involved in the growth and survival of cancer cells. Potential nephrotoxicity from these agents is listed in Table 11.3. Vascular endothelial growth factor (VEGF) pathway blockade leads to the inhibition of endothelial cell proliferation and widespread endothelial dysfunction, leading to HTN, proteinuria, and TMA. Recently, immune-checkpoint inhibitors have revolutionized cancer treatment with their mechanism of action being to enhance an immune response to tumor antigens by binding to inhibitory receptors such as cytotoxic T-lymphocyte-associated protein 4 and programmed death protein 1 or its ligand on T-cells. Since immune activation is non-selective, this can also lead to auto-immune damage to various organs, including the kidney where it may result in AIN, and rarely in glomerular diseases such as podocytopathies.

Calcineurin Inhibitors (CNI)

Medications in this class include tacrolimus and cyclosporine A, and have been extensively used following transplantation and for treating auto-immune diseases. Nephrotoxicity is a major concern with these agents since they can cause afferent arteriolar vasoconstriction, leading to a reversible drop in GFR, and endothelial damage, leading to hypertension and TMA. Chronic toxicity results in tubular ischemia, leading to tubule-interstitial fibrosis and CKD. Key to avoiding CNI nephrotoxicity is reducing drug exposure by dosing based on target trough levels and limiting the duration of therapy.

Proton Pump Inhibitors (PPI)

DIKD associated with PPIs is a rare Type B reaction, resulting in AIN, which may be seen anytime from days to months after initiation of therapy. Patients often have non-specific symptoms making diagnosis challenging and necessitating the need for a renal biopsy. The incidence is higher in those with multiple drug allergies, autoimmune diseases, newly initiated on PPI, or those > 65 years. Additionally, long-term use of PPI has also been associated with 36% and 42% higher incidence of CKD and End-Stage Kidney Disease(ESKD) than non-users. Treatment involves prompt discontinuation of PPIs and the use of short-duration high-dose corticosteroid therapy.

Management of Drug-Induced Kidney Disease:

Management aspects of DIKD are highlighted in Table 11.4 and encompass a combination of prevention and treatment strategies tailored to the specific renal syndrome. This begins with a risk assessment, involving a comprehensive review of the patient's medication history to identify potential nephrotoxic drugs or combinations thereof and promptly stop the agent to avoid irreversible renal damage. Additionally, a timely nephrology consultation is crucial when managing patients at high risk of DIKD, or those with suspected or confirmed renal injury. Patient education is essential to ensure an understanding of the importance of adhering to the prescribed medication regimens, promptly reporting any unusual symptoms or changes in urine output, and seeking medical attention if any concerns arise.

Conclusion:

Drug-induced kidney disease (DIKD) presents a significant clinical challenge, as its consequences can be severe, potentially leading to end-stage kidney disease, if not promptly managed. DIKD can occur through various mechanisms, including direct toxicity, immune-mediated injury, and drug-induced alterations in the renal blood flow. Preventive measures play a crucial role, involving careful drug selection, proper dosage consideration, and addressing additional risk factors. In cases of DIKD, timely discontinuation of the responsible drug and appropriate supportive care are essential to minimize further renal damage and mitigate complications that may arise thereof.

Table 11.2: Common Drugs Associated with Drug Induced Kidney Disease and Their Mechanisms

Drug	Time Course	Genetic Mechanisms	AKI		Glomerular Disease		Tubular Disease		Nephrolithiasis	
			Type A	Type B	Type A	Type B	Type A	Type B	Type A	Type B
Abacavir	Acute/SA	HLA								
Acyclovir	SA	OAT								
Aminoglycosides	Ac/SA	Megalin/cathepsin/ caspase								
Ampicillin	SA	HLA								
Amphotericin	Ac/SA	-								
Anabolic Steroids	SA/chronic	-								
Atazanavir	SA	-								
Bevacizumab	SA	VEGF								
Ceftazidime	SA	HLA								
Cidofovir	Acute	OAT								
Cisplatin	SA/chronic	OAT								
Ceftazidime	SA	HLA								
Colistin	SA	OCT								
Didanosine	SA	OAT/mitochondria								
Flouroquinolones	SA	HLA								
Foscarnet	SA	NaPO4 transport								

Drug	Time Course	Genetic Mechanisms	AKI		Glomerular Disease		Tubular Disease		Nephrolithiasis	
			Type A	Type B	Type A	Type B	Type A	Type B	Type A	Type B
Hydralazine	SA/chronic	HLA								
Ifosphamide	SA/chronic	OAT								
Indinavir	SA	OCT								
Lithium	SA/chronic	VA receptors								
Methotrexate	Acute/Chronic	-								
Nafcillin/Methicillin	SA	HLA								
Pamidronate(iv)	SA	-								
Piperacillin/tazobactam	Acute/SA	HLA								
Propylthiouracil	SA/chronic	HLA								
Rifampicin	SA	HLA								
Ritonavir	SA	MRP-2,4, PGP								
Sodium phosphate(oral)	Acute/Chronic									
Sulfadiazine, sulphamethoxazole	Acute/SA	HLA								
Tacrolimus/calcineurin inhibitors	Acute/SA	CYP 3A								
Tenofovir	SA	OAT								
Vancomycin	Acute/SA	Oxidative stress, HLA								
Zolindronate(iv)	Acute/SA	-								

Abbreviations: CYP: cytochrome P450, HLA: human leukocyte antigen, iv: intravenous, MRP: multidrug resistance-associated protein, NSAIDs: nonsteroidal anti-inflammatory drugs, OAT: organic anion transporter, OCT: organic cation transporter, PGP: p-glycoprotein, SA: subacute.

Table 11.3: Targeted Anti-cancer Agents and Immune-therapy Nephrotoxicity

Medication Class	Mechanism of Action	Renal Syndromes	Management Strategies
VEGF pathway inhibitors	Anti-VEGF receptor antibodies (bevacizumab, aflibercept), Anti-VEGF antibodies (ramucirumab)	TMA, FSGS/MCD	Drug discontinuation RAAS blockade Eculizumab for TMA
VEGF pathway inhibitors	VEGF-TKI inhibitors (axitinib, pazopanib, sorafenib, regorafenib, sunitinib)	TMA (sunitinib) ATN (sunitinib/ sorafenib) Hypophosphatemia, hypocalcemia, hyponatremia, hypokalemia (regorafenib)	Drug discontinuation RAAS blockade Eculizumab for TMA
EGFR pathway Inhibitors	EGFR-TKI inhibitors (erlotinib, gefitinib)	MCD/Membranous nephropathy	Drug discontinuation
EGFR pathway Inhibitors	Anti-EGFR receptor, Antibodies (cetuximab, panitumumab)	Hypomagnesemia/ hypokalemia/ nephrotic syndrome	Drug discontinuation
Bcr-abl TKIs	1st generation: Nilotinib, imatinib	Hypophosphatemia, reversible decrease in GFR, ATN	Close monitoring of renal function and dose reduction when Decreased GFR
Bcr-abl TKIs	2nd generation: dasatinib	Proteinuria	Dose reduction or discontinuation. Change to 1st generation Bcr-abl TKI inhibitors

Medication Class	Mechanism of Action	Renal Syndromes	Management Strategies
IFN	Direct effects on podocyte Indirect effects by cytokine release Damage microvascular endothelial cells by inducing apoptosis in a dose-dependent manner	MCD/FSGS/TMA	Drug discontinuation Steroids (MCD/FSGS)
Interleukin-2	Capillary leak syndrome leading to hypovolemia/ hypoperfusion	Hemodynamically mediated AKI, ATN	Volume resuscitation
CAR-T therapy	CRS, capillary leak syndrome	Hemodynamic mediated AKI, ATN	Volume resuscitation (capillary leak) Steroids, anti-IL6 therapy: tocilizumab (CRS)
Immune checkpoint inhibitors (CTLA-4 inhibitors, PD-1 inhibitors, PD-L1 inhibitors)	Loss of tolerance, formation of new or reactivated T cells against tumor antigens that cross-react with the kidney, generation of autoantibodies against kidney tissues	ATIN (most common) Podocytopathies	Drug withdrawal Steroids

Abbreviations: AKI: acute kidney injury, ATN: acute tubular necrosis, ATIN: acute tubulointerstitial nephritis, Bcr:abl: breakpoint chain region: Abelson, CAR-T: chimeric antigen receptor T-Cell, CRS: cytokine release syndrome, CTLA-4:cytotoxic T-lymphocyte-associated protein 4, EGFR: epidermal growth factor receptor, FSGS: focal segmental glomerulosclerosis, GFR: glomerular filtration rate, IFN: Interferon, MCD: minimal change disease, PD-1, programmed death protein 1; PD-L1, programmed death-ligand 1, RAAS: renin angiotensin aldosterone system, TKI: tyrosine kinase inhibitor, TMA: thrombotic microangiopathy; VEGF: vascular endothelial growth factor.

Table 11.4: Management of Drug Induced Kidney Disease

Non-specific Measures	Specific Measures
Selectively use nephrotoxic medications when benefits > risks	Use low-osmolar (iopamidol) or iso-osmolar (iodixanol) radiocontrast agent for IV contrast studies
<u>Use a minimal dose of agents</u> – dose adjustment based on GFR (chemotherapeutic agents, aminoglycosides, IV vancomycin, polymyxin B, colistin, IV bisphosphonates) – avoid multiple daily dose-aminoglycosides – monitor drug trough levels (aminoglycosides, vancomycin, calcineurin inhibitors) – avoid exceeding cumulative dose implicated in renal toxicity (amphotericin B) – limit total volume of IV radiocontrast (< 4 ml/kg or less than 2 X baseline GFR)	<u>Specific antidote</u> – amifostine for preventing cisplatin nephrotoxicity – leucovorin for preventing systemic toxicity in methotrexate overdose – glucarpidase (enzyme which inactivates methotrexate) in treating methotrexate toxicity
	Use less nephrotoxic formulations-lipid based or liposomal amphotericin B instead of amphotericin B deoxycholate
<u>Prophylactic volume expansion</u> – prevention of CA-AKI: isotonic saline 1–1.5 ml/kg/hr given 1–6 hours prior to IV contrast injection and 6–12 hours after procedure. Caution in CHF, hypertensive or oliguric or edematous patient – prior to cancer chemotherapeutics <u>Fluid resuscitation therapy</u> – pre-renal settings: post chemotherapy emesis, NSAID, diuretic, RAAS blockade associated AKI	<u>Urinary alkalinization</u> prevention of crystalluria and AKI in patients on methotrexate, sulfadiazine, sulfamethoxazole, triamterene
	Increase IV infusion time (IV bisphosphonates)
Statins used prior to angiographic interventions (if patient not already on) to reduce risk of contrast associated AKI	Use non-nephrotoxic agents in the same class if renal dysfunction (ibandronate instead of pamidronate or zoledronate)
	Recommended drug trough levels – For IV vancomycin- < 15 mg/L (if possible) but not to exceed 20 mg/L
Avoid concomitant use of agents that cause decreased renal perfusion-diuretics, ACE inhibitors, ARBs, mineralocorticoid antagonists, SGLT-2 inhibitors	Hemodialysis – methotrexate toxicity associated with AKI

<table>
<tr><th>Non-specific Measures</th><th>Specific Measures</th></tr>
<tr><td>Avoid medications with systemic accumulation and toxicity caused by a drop in GFR-metformin (lactic acidosis), gabapentin (neurotoxicity), colchicine (neuromyotoxicity), pemetrexed (hematological and gastro-intestinal toxicity)</td><td>Plasmapheresis
– drug-induced TMA (gemcitabine, mitomycin C, mTOR inhibitors, calcineurin inhibitor)</td></tr>
<tr><td>Hemodialysis- renal failure with uremic toxicity due to severe DIKD from any agent</td><td rowspan="2">Terminal complement pathway (Complement 5) inhibitor-eculizumab
– drug-induced TMA (gemcitabine, mitomycin C)</td></tr>
<tr><td>Reduce proteinuria and hypertension associated with glomerular disease with ACE inhibitors, ARBs, mineralocorticoid receptor antagonists</td></tr>
</table>

Abbreviation: ACE: angiotensin converting enzyme, CA-AKI: contrast-induced acute kidney injury, DIKD: drug-induced kidney disease, GFR: glomerular filtration rate, RAAS: renin angiotensin aldosterone system, TMA: thrombotic microangiopathy.

References:

1. Ganguli A, Singh NP. Drug-induced Kidney Disease: Revisited. J Assoc Physicians India. 2024 Jan;72(1):74-80.
2. Mehta RL, Awdishu L, Davenport A, Murray PT, Macedo E, Cerda J, Chakaravarthi R, Holden AL, Goldstein SL. Phenotype standardization for drug-induced kidney disease. Kid Int. 2015 Aug 1;88(2):226-34.
3. Perazella MA, Rosner MH. Drug-Induced Acute Kidney Injury. CJASN 2022;17(8):1220-1233.
4. Morales-Alvarez MC. Nephrotoxicity of Antimicrobials and Antibiotics. Adv Chronic Kidney Dis. 2020 Jan;27(1):31-3.
5. García-Carro C, Draibe J, Soler MJ. Onconephrology: update in anticancer drug-related nephrotoxicity. Nephron. 2023;147(2):65-77.
6. Nochaiwong S, Ruengorn C, Awiphan R et al. The association between proton pump inhibitor use and the risk of adverse kidney outcomes: a systematic review and meta-analysis. Nephrol Dial Transplant. 2018 Feb 1;33(2):331–342.
7. Mehran R, Dangas GD, Weisbord SD. Contrast-associated acute kidney injury. N Engl J Med. 2019 May 30;380(22):2146-55.

DRUG INDUCED KIDNEY DISEASE (DIKD)

PREVENTING DRUG INDUCED KIDNEY DISEASE

Review renal adverse effect profile of each drug before prescribing

↓

Is the patient at high risk for nephrotoxic injury?

↓

Prescribe these drugs after risk-benefit assessment

↓

Prescribe these drugs after risk-benefit assessment & using evidence-based preventive measures

↓

Constant vigilance for renal adverse effects and early drug cessation

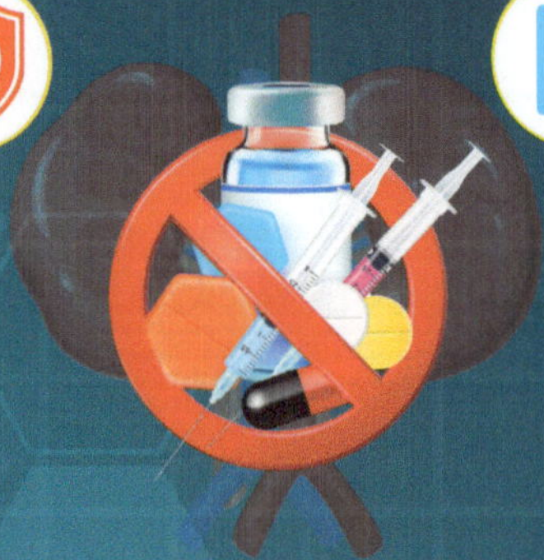

TREATMENT OF POTENTIAL CASE OF DRUG INDUCED KIDNEY DISEASE

Review medication history

↓

Drug induced kidney disease likely

↓

Prompt cessation of potential nephrotoxins

↓

Address coexisting modifiable risks

↓

Supportive therapy including renal replacement herapy

↓

Close follow-up till renal recovery then look for long term sequalae

Drugs can affect different sites of the nephron causing distinct clinical syndromes

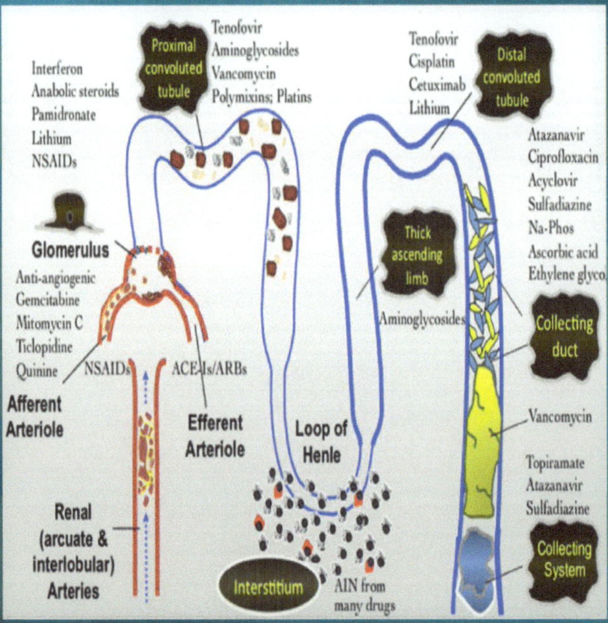

ACEIs : Angiotensin Converting Enzyme Inhibitors, ***AIN :*** Acute Interstitial Nephritis, ***ARBs :*** Angiotensin Receptor Blockers, ***Na-Phos :*** Sodium Phosphate, ***NSAIDS :*** Non Steroidal Anti Inflammatory Drugs

12

RADIOCONTRAST-ASSOCIATED RENAL INJURY

Kulwant Singh, Anupam Prakash

Radiocontrast-associated renal injury is a known cause of acute kidney injury in hospitalized patients who get exposed to contrast agents while undergoing either cardiology or radiology-related procedures. Contrast-associated acute kidney injury (CA-AKI) refers to a broader terminology where AKI occurs after administration of a contrast agent, and may or may not be causally related to the contrast agent. Contrast-induced Nephropathy (CIN) or Contrast-induced Acute Kidney Injury (CA-AKI)—as it is now referred to—is the subgroup of CA-AKI where renal dysfunction can be linked causally to the use of a contrast agent. Thus, CA-AKI includes both CA-AKI as well as other coincidental etiologies like hypovolemia, cardiac dysfunction, and infection, which can also cause renal dysfunction.

Definition and Incidence of CA-AKI

CA-AKI is defined as an absolute increase in serum creatinine of ≥ 0.5 mg/dl or as a relative increase of ≥ 25% from the baseline within 48–72 hours of contrast exposure. CA-AKI is usually transient, with serum creatinine levels peaking at 2–3 days after administration of the contrast agent and returning to baseline within 7–10 days. Newer biomarkers like serum cystatin C and neutrophil gelatinase-associated lipocalin (NGAL) can predict CA-AKI much before the rise of serum creatinine.

Types of Contrast Agents:

The term CA-AKI is generally employed in relation to the use of iodinated contrast media used for a computed tomography (CT) scan. Various contrast agents being used are differentiated based on their osmolality (Table 12.1). Contrast media with high osmolality have higher nephrotoxicity as compared to low and iso-osmolar contrast agents.

Table 12.1: Differentiation of Contrast Agents

Osmolality (mOsm/ kgH2O)	**High-osmolar (1500–2100)**	**Low-osmolar (500–900)**		**Iso-osmolar (290)**
Ionicity	Ionic	Ionic	Non-ionic	Non-ionic
Number of Benzene Rings	Monomer	Dimer	Monomer	Dimer
Viscosity (cP)	8.4	9.5	7.8–11.2	11.1
Iodine Content (mg/ml)	300	320	350–370	320
Example	Diatrizoate (Gastrografin)	Ioxaglate (Hexabrix)	Iohexol (Omnipaque), Iopamidol	Iodixanol (Visipaque)

Pathogenesis of CA-AKI (Figure 12.1)

The pathophysiology of CA-AKI is multifactorial. Intrarenal vasoconstriction, generation of reactive oxygen species, medullary ischemia, and direct tubular damage are the predominant factors that lead to CA-AKI.

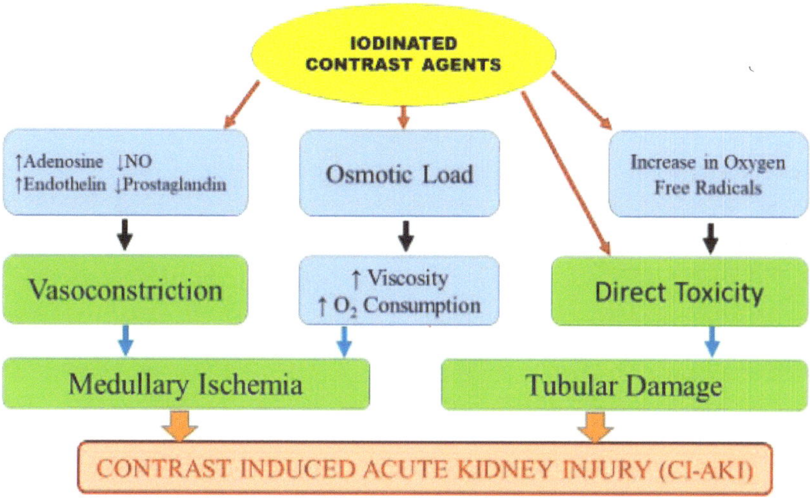

Figure 12.1: Pathogenesis of Contrast-Associated Acute Kidney Injury

Assessment of Risk Factors:

A CA-AKI Consensus Working Panel has shown that the risk of CA-AKI becomes clinically significant when the baseline serum creatinine concentration is ≥ 1.3 mg/dl in men and ≥ 1.0 mg/dl in women, equivalent to an eGFR ≤ 60 ml/min per 1.73 m^2. Apart from pre-existing kidney disease, other major risk factors for developing CA-AKI include diabetes mellitus, congestive heart failure (CHF), advanced age, and intravascular volume depletion. Large volume or high osmolality of the contrast agent is also an important risk factor. Diabetes mellitus acts as a risk multiplier for CA-AKI. Concomitant use of nephrotoxic medications, viz. non-steroidal anti-inflammatory drugs (NSAIDs), aminoglycosides, amphotericin B, high doses of loop diuretics, and antiviral drugs like acyclovir are additional risk factors.

A risk score for the prediction of CA-AKI after a percutaneous coronary intervention has been reported by Mehran et al (Table 12.2).

Table 12.2: Mehran Risk Score for Prediction of CA-AKI

<table>
<tr><th>Risk Factors</th><th>Score</th><th></th><th>Class of Risk (Total Score)</th><th>Risk of CA-AKI</th><th>Risk of RRT Requirement</th></tr>
<tr><td>Hypotension (systolic blood pressure < 80 mm Hg for at least 1 hour requiring inotropic support)</td><td>5</td><td rowspan="10">SUM →</td><td rowspan="3">Low (≤ 5)</td><td rowspan="3">7.5 %</td><td rowspan="3">0.04 %</td></tr>
<tr><td>Use of Intra-aortic balloon pump (IABP)</td><td>5</td></tr>
<tr><td>CHF (NYHA Class III/IV)</td><td>5</td></tr>
<tr><td>Age ≥ 75 years</td><td>4</td><td rowspan="3">Medium (6–10)</td><td rowspan="3">14 %</td><td rowspan="3">0.12 %</td></tr>
<tr><td>Anemia (hematocrit < 39% in men and < 36% in women)</td><td>3</td></tr>
<tr><td>Diabetes mellitus</td><td>3</td></tr>
<tr><td>Contrast media volume</td><td>1 for each 100 ml</td><td rowspan="3">High (11–16)</td><td rowspan="3">26.1%</td><td rowspan="3">1.09%</td></tr>
<tr><td>eGFR ≤ 20 ml/min/1.73m²</td><td>6</td></tr>
<tr><td>eGFR 20–40 ml/min/1.73m²</td><td>4</td></tr>
<tr><td>eGFR 40–60 ml/min/1.73m²</td><td>2</td><td>Very High (≥ 16)</td><td>57.3%</td><td>12.6%</td></tr>
<tr><td colspan="6">IABP – Intra-aortic balloon pump, CHF – Congestive heart failure, NYHA – New York Heart Association, eGFR – estimated glomerular filtration rate, RRT – Renal replacement therapy (e.g. Dialysis).</td></tr>
</table>

Prophylactic Strategies:

First and foremost, we should consider using an alternative and safer modality of imaging that doesn't involve the use of a contrast agent like MRI. In high-risk cases, we should use a minimal quantity of contrast volume and preferably use iso-osmolar contrast agents. Other nephrotoxic drugs like NSAIDs, aminoglycosides, or high-dose loop diuretics should be discontinued prior to administration of radiocontrast.

Fluid Hydration:

Extracellular fluid expansion with intravenous crystalloids like isotonic sodium chloride is the recommended strategy for prevention of renal injury. Recommended regimens for volume replacement for patients undergoing contrast administration include normal saline administered at 1 mL/kg/h for 3–12 hours pre-procedure and continued for 6–12 hours post-procedure. There is no clear evidence to guide the choice of the optimal rate and duration of fluid infusion in CA-AKI prevention. Extracellular volume expansion counteracts both the intrarenal vasoconstriction and the direct tubulotoxic effects of contrast agents that play a role in the pathophysiology of CA-AKI. Volume expansion may also directly reduce cellular damage by dilution of the contrast medium and decrease viscosity, particularly in the medullary tubular segments.

Oral volume expansion may have some benefits, but there is scant evidence to show that it is as effective as intravenous volume expansion. Therefore, hydration with oral fluids alone is not recommended.

"**Renal Guard Therapy**" is an automated and personalized hydration system that has shown superiority in preventing CA-AKI by ensuring a stable urine volume without a reduction in the body's hydration during treatment using contrast media. This system monitors the infusion rate of fluids, urine volume from the catheter, and weight changes. This system allows a high urine flow rate (≥300 mL/h) to be achieved, while simultaneously balancing urine output and venous fluid infusion volume of normal saline to prevent hypovolemia until 4 hours after cardiac catheterization.

The POSEIDON trial showed that left ventricular end-diastolic pressure (LVEDP) guided fluid administration is a safe and effective method of preventing contrast-induced acute kidney injury in patients undergoing cardiac catheterization.

N-acetylcysteine (NAC)

N-acetylcysteine (NAC) is an excellent antioxidant and scavenger of free oxygen radicals. However, it has failed to show conclusive evidence of a protective effect in CA-AKI. Various meta-analyses have shown insignificant results regarding the efficacy of NAC in CA-AKI. NAC is inexpensive and appears to be safe, but it may have some detrimental effects on myocardial and coagulation functions when given intravenously at a higher dosage.

Statins:

The proposed hypothesis for the role of statins in reducing the risk of CA-AKI is because of their anti-inflammatory and antioxidant properties. Various studies, including landmark PROMISS (Prevention of radiocontrast medium induced nephropathy using short-term high-dose simvastatin in patients with renal insufficiency undergoing coronary angiography) study, failed to show any significant benefit with the use of statins. Therefore, the routine use of statins for CA-AKI prevention is not recommended at present.

Role of Other Pharmacological Agents:

Other agents like atrial natriuretic peptide (ANP), ascorbic acid, theophylline, and fenoldopam have failed to show any benefit against CA-AKI, and thus, are not recommended.

There is no conclusive evidence that RAAS inhibitors (ACE inhibitors and angiotensin receptor blockers) increase the risk of CA-AKI. Therefore, discontinuation and reduction in the dosage of these drugs are not required. However, we should temporarily discontinue or reduce the dosage of metformin (biguanides) as it can increase the risk of developing lactic acidosis with a transient impairment in kidney function, which occurs after the use of iodinated contrast agents.

Prophylactic Use of Dialysis Modalities:

Many clinicians perceive that extracorporeal therapies (hemodialysis) can potentially remove contrast agents, and thus, prevent CA-AKI. It could theoretically be anticipated that high-flux membranes used in hemodiafiltration (HDF) modalities should be able to remove contrast molecules more efficiently than low-flux membranes used in routine intermittent hemodialysis (HD). Cruz et al in their meta-analysis of 11 studies (8 of HD and 3 of HDF) concluded that there are no beneficial effects of these modalities as compared to standard fluid hydration.

They, however, showed that hemodialysis actually increased the risk of CA-AKI. This detrimental effect of HD can be explained by the inflammatory mediators and the vasoactive substances that are released when blood cells come in contact with the dialyzer membrane, which often leads to hypotension and renal hypoperfusion. Ultrafiltration can further add to the depletion of intravascular volume, resulting in activation of the sympathetic nervous system and leading to renal medullary ischemia.

There is no conclusive evidence that prophylactic HD or HDF will prevent renal injury, and therefore, these modalities are not recommended. Therefore, HD should only be performed for other routine indications such as hyperkalemia, fluid overload, etc., rather than as a tool for removing contrast agents to prevent CA-AKI.

Table 12.3: Strategies to Prevent Contrast Associated-Acute Kidney Injury

Risk Stratification	Identify high-risk patients – Old age, Diabetes, CHF (Mehran score can be used)
Fluid Hydration	Intravenous fluid hydration – with isotonic sodium chloride Oral fluid hydration alone – Not Recommended Use of "Renal Guard Therapy"
N-acetylcysteine (NAC)	IV NAC– Not Recommended Oral NAC– No conclusive evidence
Contrast Agent	Dose – Minimal Type – Low or Iso – Osmolar contrast agent Intravenous preferred over Intra-arterial
Nephrotoxic Agents	NSAIDs, Aminoglycosides or high-dose loop diuretics, etc., should be stopped
ACE Inhibitors/ ARBs	Reduction of dosage not required
Biguanides (Metformin)	Temporary withdrawal or reduction in dose of biguanides
Prophylactic and post-procedure HD	Not Beneficial
CHF: Congestive Heart Failure, IV: Intravenous, NSAIDs: Non-steroidal anti-inflammatory drugs, ACE: Angiotensin converting enzyme, ARB: Angiotensin receptor blocker, HD: Hemodialysis	

Conclusion:

Pre-existing renal impairment, old age, history of diabetes, heart failure, proteinuria, and hypotension are some important risk factors in the pathogenesis of renal injury. Apart from risk stratification and the use of low and iso-osmolar contrast agents, intravenous fluid hydration with crystalloids is the only recommended strategy for the prevention of CA-AKI. Agents like N-acetylcysteine (NAC), atrial natriuretic peptide, ascorbic acid, theophylline, and fenoldopam have failed to show any proven beneficial role in the prevention of CA-AKI.

References:

1. Davenport MS, Perazella MA, Yee J, Dillman JR, Fine D, McDonald RJ et al. Use of Intravenous Iodinated Contrast Media in Patients with Kidney Disease: Consensus Statements from the American College of Radiology and the National Kidney Foundation. Radiology. 2020;294(3):660-668.
2. AmericanCollegeofRadiology.CommitteeonDrugsandContrast Media. ACR Manual on Contrast Media, Version 2021. 2021. https://www.acr.org/Clinical-Resources/Contrast-Manual (Accessed on February 15, 2021).
3. KDIGO clinical practice guideline for acute kidney injury. Kidney Int Suppl Suppl. 2012;
4. Singh K, Bhargava V, Brar JE, Bhargava M, Kaushal R, Khullar D. Contrast Induced Acute Kidney Injury (CI- AKI) - Myths and Realities. J Assoc Physicians India. 2021;69(11):82-86.
5. Mehran R, Aymong ED, Nikolsky E, Lasic Z, Iakovou I, Fahy M et al. A simple risk score for prediction of contrast-induced nephropathy after percutaneous coronary intervention: development and initial validation. J Am Coll Cardiol. 2004;44(7):1393-1399.
6. Persson PB, Hansell P, Liss P. Pathophysiology of contrast medium-induced nephropathy. Kidney Int. 2005;68(1):14-22.
7. Briguori C, Visconti G, Focaccio A, Airoldi F, Valgimigli M, Sangiorgi GM et al or REMEDIAL II Investigators. Renal

Insufficiency After Contrast Media Administration Trial II (REMEDIAL II): RenalGuard System in high-risk patients for contrast-induced acute kidney injury. Circulation 2011;124(11):1260-1269.

8. Brar SS, Aharonian V, Mansukhani P, Moore N, Shen AY, Jorgensen M et al. Haemodynamic-guided fluid administration for the prevention of contrast-induced acute kidney injury: the POSEIDON randomised controlled trial. Lancet. 2014;383(9931):1814-1823.
9. Xu R, Tao A, Bai Y, Deng Y, Chen G. Effectiveness of N-acetylcysteine for the prevention of contrast-induced nephropathy: A Systematic review and meta-analysis of randomized controlled trials. J Am Heart Assoc 2016;5:e003968.
10. Jo SH, Koo BK, Park JS, Kang HJ, Cho YS, Kim YJ et al. Prevention of radiocontrast medium-induced nephropathy using short-term high-dose simvastatin in patients with renal insufficiency undergoing coronary angiography (PROMISS) trial-a randomized controlled study. Am Heart J. 2008;155(3): 499.e1-8.
11. Goergen SK, Rumbold G, Compton G, Harris C. Systematic review of current guidelines, and their evidence base, on risk of lactic acidosis after administration of contrast medium for patients receiving metformin. Radiology. 2010;254(1):261-269.
12. Cruz DN, Goh CY, Marenzi G, Corradi V, Ronco C, Perazella MA. Renal replacement therapies for prevention of radiocontrast-induced nephropathy: a systematic review. Am J Med. 2012;125(1):66-78.

CONTRAST ASSOCIATED AKI

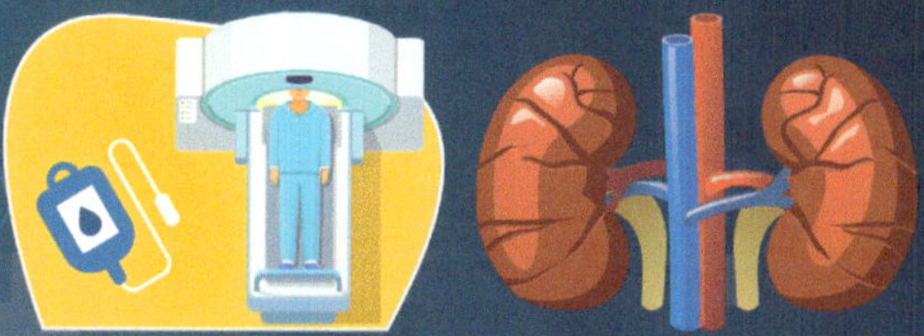

RISK FACTORS

- Pre existing renal dysfunction
- DM, CHF, Old Age, Volume depleted
- High volume or High osmolality of Contrast
- Concomitant use of NSAIDS or Aminoglycosides

PATHOGENESIS

- Renal vasoconstriction ⏭ medullary hypoxia (viscosity and by alterations in NO), endothelin, and/or adenosine.
- Direct cytotoxic effects

CHARACTERISTIC

- 2-3 days after contrast administration and return to baseline within 7-10 days.
- Mostly non-oliguric

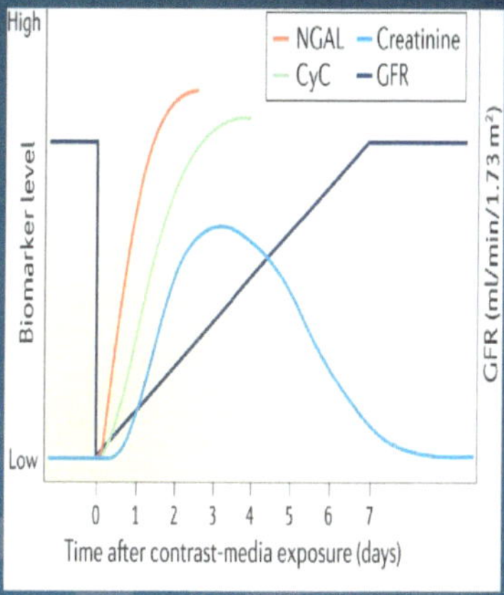

ASSESS CI-AKI RISK →

< 10

- Minimise contrast volume
- Avoid NSAIDS, Diuretics

> 10

- Minimise contrast volume
- Hydration
- Avoid NSAIDS, Diuretics

↓

EMPERICALLY – Isotonic NS @ 1ml/kg/hr 3-12 hours pre-procedure & continue 6-12 hours post-procedure

Meheran Risk Score	
Hypotension	+5
IABP	+5
CHF	+5
Age > 75 years	+4
Anemia	+3
Diabetes	+3
Contrast volume	+1/100ml
	eGFR ml/min
≥60	+0
40-59	+2
20-39	+4
<20	+6

NO role of Prophylactic OR Post Contrast Hemodialysis

AKI : Acute Kidney Injury, ***CHF*** : Congestive Heart Failure, ***CI-AKI*** : Contrast Induced Acute Kidney Injury, ***DM*** : Diabetes mellitus, ***eGFR*** : Estimated glomerular filtration, ***IABP*** : Intra-aortic balloon pump, ***NO*** : Nitric Oxide, ***NSAIDS*** : Non-steroidal anti-inflammatory drugs, ***NS*** : Normal Saline

SECTION 4

Chronic Kidney Disease

13

CKD – DEFINITION, CLASSIFICATION, DIAGNOSIS

Divya Bajpai, Narayan Prasad

Definitions:

Chronic kidney disease (CKD) represents a heterogeneous group of disorders defined by kidney disease improving global outcomes (KDIGO) as abnormalities of kidney structure or function, present for three months, with implications for health. These abnormalities can be broad and include the kidney's excretory, endocrine, and metabolic functions (Box 13.1).

The '3-month' duration criterion is mandatory to distinguish CKD from acute kidney injury (AKI). This duration may be documented based on previous records or inferred based on clinical context. Resolution of the kidney function over weeks to months will confirm the diagnosis of AKI. Thus, longitudinal testing is essential to confirm the diagnosis of CKD, especially in patients with unknown baseline kidney function. Also, during the long course of CKD, patients may have one or more episodes of AKI, which are characteristically reversible, unlike the kidney damage in CKD, which is permanent.

For confirming the diagnosis of CKD, at least one of the following must be present for > 3 months

1. **Marker of kidney damage (one or more)**
   - Albuminuria (Urine albumin excretion rate ≥ 30mg/day, Albumin creatinine ratio ≥ 30 mg/g)
   - Urine sediment abnormalities
   - Electrolyte/acid-base abnormalities due to tubular disorders
   - Abnormalities detected by histology
   - Structural abnormalities detected by imaging
   - History of kidney transplantation
2. **Decreased glomerular filtration rate (GFR) < 60 ml/min/1.73 m^2**

Box 13.1: Diagnostic Criteria for CKD

As these criteria are objective and laboratory-based, the diagnosis of CKD can be made independent of the identification of the causative etiology.

Markers of Kidney Damage:

Out of the markers of kidney damage mentioned in Box 13.1, proteinuria and decreased GFR are the predominant findings that characterize CKD.

A. **Decreased GFR:** The best measurable index for progressive kidney disease is declining GFR, which remains the hallmark of CKD. GFR can be measured by quantifying the clearance of exogenous molecules that are eliminated exclusively by glomerular filtration, e.g., inulin, iohexol, iothalamate, technetium 99m diethylenetriamine pentaacetic acid (99mTc-DTPA), and chromium 51-ethylenediamine tetraacetic acid (51Cr-EDTA). This is known as measured GFR (mGFR).

This method is the gold standard of GFR assessment but is costly and tedious. Thus, its use is restricted to special situations like kidney donor evaluation and cannot be implemented in daily clinical practice where estimated GFR (eGFR) is used. eGFR is based on estimating the clearance of an endogenous filtration marker (e.g., creatinine or cystatin C). A cutoff of eGFR (based on serum creatinine) < 60 ml/min/1.73m^2 is considered to diagnose CKD without other structural and functional damage markers. Patients with CKD with eGFR < 60 ml/min/1.73m^2 have higher incidences of CKD complications like mineral bone diseases, anemia, drug toxicity, cardiovascular diseases, and mortality. This association of complications with the level of eGFR remains valid for all age groups.

GFR Estimation: Commonly used equations for the estimation of GFR are the Modification of Diet in Renal Disease (MDRD) Study equation and the 2009 Chronic Kidney Disease Epidemiology Collaboration (CKD-EPI) equation, as they give an estimation closest to the measured GFR. Both these equations use correction for age, sex, and race as they directly affect serum creatinine. The revised CKD-EPI creatinine equation (2021) is developed from the same data as the 2009 equation but without a coefficient for race and is preferred for use now.

Limitations of Creatinine-based GFR Estimation

There are several circumstances when a change in serum creatinine might not be a true reflection of the change in GFR.

- <u>Variations in creatinine production</u> – Creatinine production varies with dietary intake (vegetarian diet, creatine supplements) or changes in muscle mass (amputation, malnutrition, muscle wasting, muscle building). A meal of cooked meat can acutely increase serum creatinine.

- Variation in creatinine secretion – As the GFR decreases, there is enhanced proximal tubular creatinine secretion, which attenuates the rise in serum creatinine. This keeps the serum creatinine ≤ 1 mg/dl, even when the measured GFR falls to 60 ml/min. Thus, a kidney disease might appear stable if estimated by creatinine-based eGFR. Tubular secretion is significantly high in patients with nephrotic syndrome, leading to over-estimation of GFR. When serum creatinine exceeds 2mg/dl, the secretary process is completely saturated and a relatively rapid rise in serum creatinine is observed.

  Certain drugs increase serum creatinine by inhibiting tubular secretion:

  - Trimethoprim
  - Cimetidine, famotidine
  - Dolutegravir
  - Cobicistat
  - Imatinib and other tyrosine kinase inhibitors

- Extrarenal creatinine excretion – In advanced kidney failure (e.g., eGFR < 15 mL/min per 1.73 m^2), there is intestinal bacterial overgrowth and increased bacterial creatininase activity in the gut. Thus, the serum creatinine concentration is falsely lowered.
- Measurement (assay) issues – If creatinine is estimated by colorimetric method – alkaline picrate method – there can be interference with non-creatinine chromogens (acetoacetate, bilirubin).

Cystatin C – An alternative endogenous filtration marker is cystatin C, which is less affected by muscle mass and is more predictive of subsequent cardiovascular disease and mortality. Cystatin C is filtered at the glomerulus and is not absorbed but is metabolized in the tubules (urinary clearance can't be calculated). Non-GFR determinants of cystatin C (higher fat mass, diabetes, inflammation, hyper-, hypothyroidism, and glucocorticoid use) must be considered while evaluating. For the most accurate estimation of GFR, it is now recommended to use the combined creatinine-cystatin C CKD EPI 2021 equation. As routine use of cystatin C is not practical due to cost and limited availability, it can be used to confirm the GFR when there are anticipated issues with creatinine estimation (e.g., extremes of muscle mass, liver disease, creatine supplements) or when explicit confirmation of GFR is vital (e.g., potential kidney donors). This can be further confirmed with measured GFR, which is the gold standard.

B. **Albuminuria:** Albuminuria, which reflects increased glomerular permeability to macromolecules, is an early marker of kidney damage that can be easily assessed in clinical practice. The most commonly used method is spot (untimed) urine albumin-to-creatinine ratio (ACR) with a 30mg/g cutoff. Patients with a urine ACR > 30 mg/g are at a higher risk for all-cause and cardiovascular mortality, ESKD, AKI, and CKD progression, even when eGFR is normal. It is important to note that apart from primary kidney disease, albuminuria may also reflect the widespread endothelial dysfunction in conditions like hypertension, diabetes, and metabolic syndrome. ACR can also be formulated by converting the protein-by-creatinine ratio (PCR) using various formulas. Timed 24-hour estimation of protein excretion though more accurate may not be feasible in all clinical settings.

C. **Urinary Sediment Abnormalities:** Renal tubular cells, red blood cell (RBC) casts, dysmorphic RBCs, white blood cell (WBC) casts, and coarse granular casts are pathognomonic of kidney damage. Other formed elements and microorganisms can appear in the urine sediment in various kidney and urinary tract disorders, like infections and inflammation.

D. **Imaging Abnormalities:** Imaging with ultrasonography and computed tomography (CT) aids in diagnosing diseases of the renal structure, vessels, and collecting systems. Thus, if significant structural abnormalities (not including simple renal cysts) are persistent for more than three months, CKD is diagnosed.

E. **Tubular Abnormalities (electrolytes, acid-base):** Abnormalities of electrolytes and acid-base disorders may result from abnormal renal tubular reabsorption and secretion. These syndromes are pathognomonic of kidney disease. The conditions are often genetic but can also be acquired due to drugs or toxins. There are usually prominent tubular pathologic lesions.

F. **Pathologic Abnormalities:** A kidney biopsy can reveal abnormalities in the glomeruli, vessels, tubules, and/or interstitium. This must be acknowledged as an important parameter in defining kidney damage, irrespective of eGFR. However, it is important to note that a kidney biopsy is not routinely required to diagnose CKD.

G. **Kidney Transplant Recipients:** Kidney transplant recipients are defined as having CKD, even without other markers of kidney damage and eGFR decline. This is irrespective of the level of GFR or the presence of markers of kidney damage. The rationale is that they usually do have pathologic findings in the biopsy and they have an increased risk of mortality and kidney outcomes compared to the general population, requiring specialized management.

Pediatric Considerations:

The definition mentioned earlier applies to children with some specific considerations. The duration cutoff for ≥ 3 months does not apply to infants < 3 months of age. Normal levels of GFR vary with age, gender, and body size. In health, GFR progressively increases from infancy and approaches the adult mean value by 2 years of age. Thus, in children < 2 years of age, the GFR < 60 ml/min/1.73m^2 criteria does not apply, and an age-appropriate value should be used. A moderate reduction in GFR is defined as age-specific GFR between 1–2 standard deviations below the mean, and severe reduction is > 2SD below the mean. Similarly, age-appropriate cutoffs for albumin excretion rate must be used instead of UACR > 30mg/g.

Staging of CKD

The primary purpose of CKD staging is risk stratification for complications and CKD progression. This can guide appropriate treatment decisions and the intensity of monitoring. After diagnosing CKD based on KDIGO criteria, staging is done based on 3 parameters (Figure 13.1):

a. Cause of CKD (C)
b. GFR categories (G stages)
c. Albuminuria categories (A stage)

This is known as the CGA system of classification.

Prognosis of CKD by GFR and Albuminuria Categories: KDIGO 2012

GFR categories (ml/min/ 1.73m²) Description and range			Persistent albuminuria categories Description and range: A1 Normal to mildly increased <30 mg/g <3 mg/mmol	A2 Moderately increased 30-300 mg/g 3-30 mg/mmol	A3 Severely increased >300 mg/g >30 mg/mmol
G1	Normal or high	≥90	[1 if CKD]	[1]	[2]
G2	Mildly decreased	60-89	[1 if CKD]	[1]	[2]
G3a	Mildly to moderately decreased	45-59	[1]	[2]	[3]
G3b	Moderately to severely decreased	30-44	[2]	[3]	[3]
G4	Severely decreased	15-29	[3]	[3]	[4+]
G5	Kidney failure	<15	[4+]	[4+]	[4+]

Low risk (if no other markers of kidney disease, no CKD)

Moderately increased risk

High risk

Very high risk

No. in parenthesis [] = Frequency of monitoring per year

Figure 13.1: Classification of CKD by GFR and Albuminuria Category and Prognosis [Adapted from KDIGO 2012 Guidelines]

Cause of CKD

KDIGO recommends assigning the cause of CKD based on the presumed pathologic and anatomic findings and the presence of systemic kidney disease, if any (e.g., diabetes, autoimmune diseases like SLE and other vasculitides, polycystic kidney disease, urinary tract obstruction, etc.) This enables specific therapy to manage the cause to prevent further injury (Figure 13.2).

For the overall risk prediction in patients with accomplished CKD, various factors must be considered – GFR stage, albuminuria, CKD etiology, age, control of hypertension, cholesterol levels, smoking status, and presence of other co-morbidities (like heart and liver diseases). Various online risk prediction tools have been developed and validated for the same.

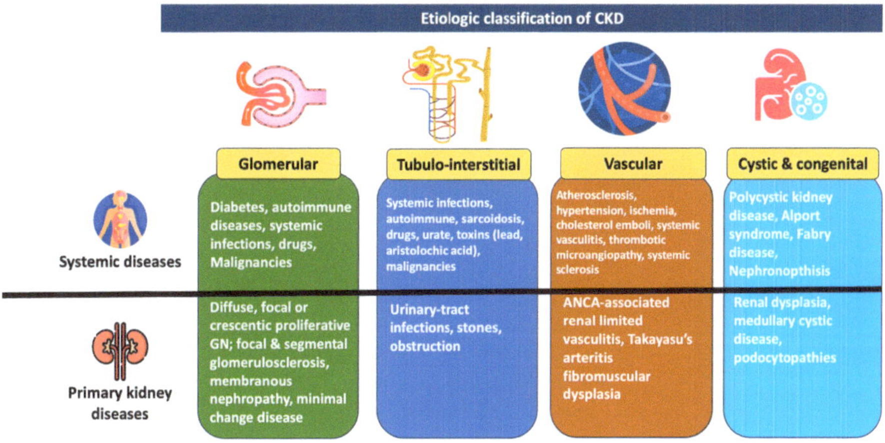

Figure 13.2: Etiologic Classification of CKD

As shown in Figure 13.1, the risk of complications increases progressively with increasing albuminuria and declining eGFR. Low GFR is a stronger predictor of worse CKD outcomes than high albuminuria. Patients on dialysis are subclassified as GFR stage 5D as they require specialized care. As demonstrated in Figure 13.1, the intensity of interventions and frequency of follow-ups increases with increasing CKD stages G and A.

Approach Toward the Diagnosis of CKD

It is essential to understand that most patients with CKD remain asymptomatic until the late stages of the disease. Thus, targeted screening of high-risk groups (e.g., diabetes, hypertension) will be helpful in the early diagnosis of CKD. The following steps are crucial while diagnosing a patient with suspected CKD:

1. **Dialysis triage:** The first step is identifying patients who urgently require dialysis. Patients with presence of refractory pulmonary edema, life-threatening hyperkalemia or metabolic acidosis, uremic encephalopathy, or a pericardial rub should be referred to the emergency department for rapid initiation of dialysis.

2. **Determining the duration of kidney disease:** This can be done by assessing the trend of serum creatinine and/or proteinuria over time. For patients in whom this is unavailable, corroborative evidence like imaging findings of chronic kidney damage and lack of recovery with time points towards the chronicity of damage. Features favoring the acute process are acute onset oligo-anuria, recent symptoms, and rapid doubling of creatinine. It is important to note that the presence of a normal-sized kidney on ultrasound does not exclude chronicity; for example, in diabetic kidney disease, the kidney size is preserved.
3. **Evaluation to identify the etiology:** Targeted history and relevant investigations can point towards the underlying etiology:-

    - Presence of long-standing diabetes or hypertension
    - Presence of peripheral vascular disease or other risk factors for reno-vascular disease like smoking, hyperlipidemia
    - History of systemic disorders like autoimmune diseases, vasculitis, and treatment for the same
    - History of severe AKI or recurrent AKI in the past
    - Family history of inherited renal disorders
    - Presence/history of malignancy
    - Signs and symptoms of urinary tract obstruction and nephrolithiasis
    - Chronic infections like AIDS, Hepatitis B, Hepatitis C, and infective endocarditis
    - History of intake of nephrotoxic medications (e.g., lithium, analgesics, etc.)
    - Exposure to environmental toxins or native to a geography/occupation associated with CKD of unknown etiology (CKDu).

4. **Targeted physical examination**: Physical examination can elicit the etiology of underlying CKD and also point toward the severity of the illness. Signs of volume overload may indicate the presence of concomitant cardiac or liver disease. Also, worsening volume overload is a sign of declining GFR. Signs of long-standing volume depletion (from chronic diarrhea or high-output bowel stoma) may predispose to the progression of CKD. Fundus examination is vital for the presence of diabetic or hypertensive retinopathy. Systemic diseases like lupus will have mucocutaneous and musculoskeletal manifestations.
5. **Targeted investigations**: Urinalysis can give valuable insights about the compartment of the kidney involved. Glomerular lesions will have hematuria, significant proteinuria, and RBC casts. WBC casts, on the other hand, point towards infection. An autoimmune panel (ANA, dsDNA, ANCA, RA factor, anti-CCP, and complement levels) is required to rule out systemic disease. Screening for viral infections is important in all patients. Selected patients must undergo testing for plasma cell dyscrasias. Ultrasonography is necessary to diagnose urinary tract obstruction, cystic kidney disease, and other congenital abnormalities of the kidney and urinary tract (CAKUT). Functional studies like radioisotope imaging help us in quantifying kidney damage. Urological evaluation (cystoscopy, urine flow rate, and urodynamic study) is essential in patients with CKD due to bladder dysfunction. Kidney biopsy may be warranted in selected patients to diagnose CKD and its prognostication.

Indications for Nephrology Evaluation:

Indications for referral to a nephrologist are mentioned in Box 13.2. Patients with eGFR < 30 ml/min/1.73m^2 require preparation for the possible onset of end-stage kidney disease.

This involves discussing the choice of kidney replacement therapy (dialysis and transplantation). All attempts must be made in such patients to preserve the upper limb and central veins for vascular access creation. Evidence suggests that patients referred late to a nephrologist are less likely to initiate dialysis with a functioning fistula. Primary care physicians can work in conjecture with the nephrologist to delay the progression of CKD. This is now easily possible over tele-visits. As these patients with CKD are at a risk for other complications, referral to other appropriate specialists (e.g., cardiologists) should also be considered.

In an adult with CKD, indications for consultation with a nephrologist include:

1. eGFR < 30 mL/min/1.73 m^2
2. Persistent UACR ≥ 300 mg/g or UPCR ≥ 500 mg/g
3. Abnormal urine microscopy (cellular casts, microscopic hematuria, sterile pyuria)
4. Presence of systemic autoimmune disease
5. Large cystic kidneys or family history of polycystic kidney disease
6. Presence of plasma cell dyscrasias
7. Relatively rapid loss of kidney function (eGFR decline > 5 mL/min/1.73 m^2/year or decline > 25%)
8. Inability to identify a presumed cause of CKD, especially in younger patients (may need a kidney biopsy)
9. Difficult to manage complications – hyperkalemia, metabolic acidosis, anemia, mineral bone disease
10. Resistant hypertension
11. Recurrent or extensive nephrolithiasis, recurrent urinary infections
12. Planning to conceive or pregnant
13. Hereditary kidney disease, such as alport syndrome, or autosomal dominant interstitial kidney disease
14. Planning to initiate drugs that may cause AKI or worsen proteinuria (e.g., chemotherapy)
15. Worsening of symptoms
16. Planning for renal transplant

Box 13.2: Patients with CKD That Warrant a Referral to a Nephrologist

References:

1. KDIGO 2012 Clinical Practice Guideline for the Evaluation and Management of Chronic Kidney Disease. Kidney Int Suppl 2013; 3:136.
2. Stevens LA, Coresh J, Feldman HI, et al. Evaluation of the modification of diet in renal disease study equation in a large diverse population. J Am Soc Nephrol 2007; 18:2749.
3. Delgado C, Baweja M, Crews DC, et al. A Unifying Approach for GFR Estimation: Recommendations of the NKF-ASN Task Force on Reassessing the Inclusion of Race in Diagnosing Kidney Disease. J Am Soc Nephrol 2021; 32:2994.
4. Shlipak MG, Matsushita K, √Ñrnl√∂v J, et al. Cystatin C versus creatinine in determining risk based on kidney function. N Engl J Med 2013; 369:932.
5. National Kidney Foundation. K/DOQI clinical practice guidelines for chronic kidney disease: evaluation, classification, and stratification. Am J Kidney Dis 2002; 39:S1.
6. Chronic Kidney Disease Prognosis Consortium, Matsushita K, van der Velde M, et al. Association of estimated glomerular filtration rate and albuminuria with all-cause and cardiovascular mortality in general population cohorts: a collaborative meta-analysis. Lancet 2010; 375:2073.
7. Weaver RG, James MT, Ravani P, et al. Estimating Urine Albumin-to-Creatinine Ratio from Protein-to-Creatinine Ratio: Development of Equations using Same-Day Measurements. J Am Soc Nephrol 2020; 31:591.
8. Mahmoodi BK, Matsushita K, Woodward M, et al. Associations of kidney disease measures with mortality and end-stage renal disease in individuals with and without hypertension: a meta-analysis. Lancet 2012; 380:1649.
9. Astor BC, Eustace JA, Powe NR, et al. Timing of nephrologist referral and arteriovenous access use: the CHOICE Study. Am J Kidney Dis 2001; 38:494.
10. Avorn J, Winkelmayer WC, Bohn RL, et al. Delayed nephrologist referral and inadequate vascular access in patients with advanced chronic kidney failure. J Clin Epidemiol 2002; 55:711.

11. Kinchen KS, Sadler J, Fink N, et al. The timing of specialist evaluation in chronic kidney disease and mortality. Ann Intern Med 2002; 137:479.

12. National Institute for Health and Clinical Excellence (NICE) National Collaborating Centre for Chronic Conditions. Chronic kidney disease. Early identification and management of chronic kidney disease in adults in primary and secondary care, 2008. http://www.nice.org.uk/nicemedia/live/12069/42119/42119.pdf (Accessed on October 07, 2010).

CHRONIC KIDNEY DISEASE: Diagnosis and Classification

DIAGNOSTIC CRITERA

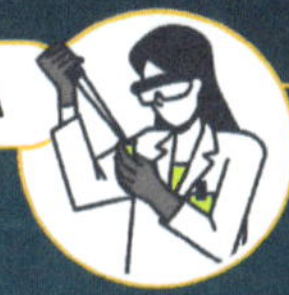

AT LEAST ONE FOR > 3MONTHS

KIDNEY DAMAGE MARKERS

- Albuminuria (UACR>30mg/g)
- Electrolyte, acid-base abnormality
- Urine sediments
- Abnormal imaging
- Abnormal histology
- Kidney transplant recipient

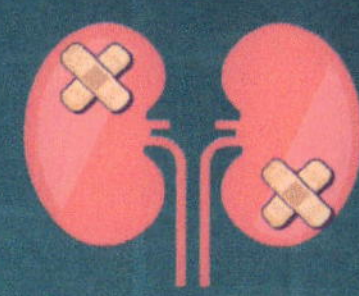

GFR <60ml/min/1.73m2

CKD is classified based on

CAUSES

- Glomerular
- Tubulo-interstitial
- Vascular
- Cystic and Congenital

GFR

MEASURED GFR
Measured using exogenous filtration

ESTIMATED GFR
Calculated using endogenous filtration marker (creatinine cystatin C)

ALBUMINURIA

CKD STAGES AS PER GFR

INCREASING MORTALITY

CV RISKS AS GFR DECLINES

Prognosis of CKD by GFR and albuminuria categories KDIGO 2012				Persistent albuminuria categories Description and range		
				A1	A2	A2
				Normal to mildly increased	Moderately increased	Severely increased
				<30mg/g >3mg/mmol	30-300mg/g 3-30mg/mmol	>300mg/g >30mg/mmol
GFR categories (ml/min per 1.73m²) Description and range	G1	Normal or High	≥90	Low Risk	Moderately increased risk	High Risk
	G2	Mildly decreased	60-89	Low Risk	Moderately increased risk	High Risk
	G3a	Mildly to moderately decreased	45-59	Moderately increased risk	High Risk	Very High Risk
	G3b	Moderately to severely decreased	30-44	High Risk	Very High Risk	Very High Risk
	G4	Severely decreased	15-29	Very High Risk	Very High Risk	Very High Risk
	G5	Kidney Failure	<15	Very High Risk	Very High Risk	Very High Risk

Low Risk (if no other markers of kidney disease, no CKD)	Moderate increased risk	High Risk	Very High Risk

CKD : Chronic Kidney Disease, ***CV :*** Cardiovascular, ***GFR :*** Glomerular filtration rate, ***UACR :*** Urine Albumin-Creatinine Ratio

14

CKD – COMPLICATIONS AND MANAGEMENT

Vali PS, Urmila Anandh

Introduction:

Chronic kidney disease (CKD) is a complex disease whose course is often punctuated by a plethora of complications, which include anemia, bone disease, electrolyte imbalances, fluid overload, and cardiovascular disease. Managing CKD can be challenging and requires a multidisciplinary approach due to its progressive nature and wide range of complex pathophysiological alterations. Though major complications of CKD are less likely to manifest prior to stage 3, it is prudent to formulate a comprehensive approach to monitor for and manage all the potential complications.

The overarching objective of this chapter is to provide a comprehensive exploration of discernment, approaches, and therapeutic strategies employed in navigating these complications.

Anemia:

Anemia in CKD is a consequence of progressive loss of renal reserve and is predominantly due to erythropoietin deficiency.

Chronic inflammation and blunted iron availability are the common contributing factors. Other less common yet plausible causes of anemia in CKD include Hyperparathyroidism, , blood loss, precursor deficiencies, shortened RBC life span, inflammation, bone marrow suppression due to 'uremia' and plasma cell disorders. Diabetic patients are at increased risk of developing and experiencing severe anemia at an earlier stage of CKD. Stage 3 chronic kidney disease patients with diabetes mellitus are three times more likely to suffer from anemia.

The objective of anemia evaluation in CKD is akin to anemia evaluation in the non-CKD population, but with more emphasis on iron deficiency and occult blood loss in view of their more common occurrence. It is prudent to identify and correct other correctable causes of anemia in general, viz., deficiencies of iron, vitamin B12, and folate before treating patients with Erythropoietins. Measurement of serum erythropoietin levels is usually not indicated, as its deficiency is relative and has no impact on therapeutic decisions.

- **Erythropoiesis-stimulating agents (ESAs)** such as erythropoietin and darbepoetin constitute the core therapy for correcting and preventing anemia in CKD. ESAs are usually indicated when Hb falls less than 10 g/dl and are best avoided when Hb > 13 g/dl. Studies have consistently demonstrated an increased risk of stroke and thromboembolic complications with higher Hb levels.
- As per KDIGO guidelines, **intravenous (IV) iron therapy** is needed when transferrin saturation (TSAT) is ≤ 30% and ferritin is ≤ 500 ng/ml (500 µg/l). Oral iron is considered ineffective in dialysis patients but can be tried in non-dialysis patients for a period of 1–3 months prior to starting IV iron. Though debated, it is considered best to avoid IV iron in the presence of active infections.

- **Blood transfusions and erythrocyte transfusions** are usually reserved for severe cases of anemia (Hb <7 g/dl) or when other treatment options have failed.
- **Hypoxia-inducible factor (HIF) and prolyl hydroxylase (PH) enzyme inhibitors** are a novel class of agents for anemia correction in CKD, which have a favorable effect on iron availability in CKD patients. Desidustat is the only HIF-PH inhibitor currently approved in India.

Cardiovascular Complications:

Cardiovascular (CV) complications are the leading cause of mortality among CKD patients, with the severity of the burden inversely proportional to GFR. In comparison with the control population without CKD, stage 5 patients have a higher risk of CV disease, which is due to various traditional and non-traditional risk factors. CV disorders in CKD contain a spectrum of traditional atherosclerotic disorders, viz., coronary artery disease and stroke, and non-atherosclerotic disorders such as left ventricular hypertrophy, valvular heart disease, and arterial calcifications.

Coronary Artery Disease (CAD):

Antiplatelet and lipid-lowering medications are the cornerstones of the management of CAD. Statins become less beneficial as CKD progresses and dialysis patients have no discernible benefit. Despite the fact that revascularization reduces cardiovascular symptoms, it appears to confer a small survival benefit to CKD patients with a high cardiovascular risk at baseline.

Heart Failure (HF):

Almost 50% of the patients with HF have coexisting CKD, denoting a close association between CKD and HF. The common symptomatology of HF and CKD makes the diagnosis of HF difficult.

The treatment of heart failure in CKD includes the use of diuretics, renin-angiotensin-aldosterone system (RAAS) blockers, beta-blockers, and SGLT-2 inhibitors. Angiotensin receptor-neprilysin inhibitors (ARNIs) are used in those with eGFR > 30 ml. Serum creatinine elevations up to 30% after initiating ACEi ARBs or ARNIs are deemed acceptable. Dialysis and ultrafiltration are needed if pharmacological therapy fails.

CKD-Mineral and Bone Disorder (CKD-MBD)

Hyperphosphatemia and a deficiency of 1,25-dihydroxyvitamin D3 lead to a cascade of events that result in the development of secondary hyperparathyroidism, and ultimately, renal bone disease. These biochemical aberrations, in conjunction with well-defined histological changes, are referred to as CKD-mineral and bone disorders. Markers of CKD-MBD need to be monitored once eGFR falls below 45 mL/min/1.73 m^2.

The key to effective management of secondary hyperparathyroidism is phosphate control. In the early stages of CKD, protein restriction and limiting dairy products, especially processed ones with a high phosphate content, would be sufficient. Eventually, a majority will need oral phosphate binders that bind with dietary phosphate in the gut. Phosphate binders can be calcium based (calcium carbonate and acetate) or non-calcium based. Sevelamer carbonate, a nonabsorbable, calcium-free polymer, in doses of 2.4 to 4.8 g/day is an effective phosphate binder without the risk of hypercalcemia. Ferric citrate and superferric oxyhydroxide are iron-containing phosphate binders.

Administration of active vitamin D analogues such as calcitriol, alfacalcidol, doxercalciferol, and paricalcitol are important in the management of CKD-MBD. However, correction of (native) vitamin D deficiency is the initial step in the treatment.

Hypercalcemia, hyperphosphatemia, and adynamic bone disease are the potential side effects of vitamin D analogues. Therefore, active vitamin D therapy needs to be closely monitored.

Calcimimetic agents (cinacalcet), which target calcium-sensing receptors on the parathyroid gland, are indicated in dialysis patients who have hyperparathyroidism, not responding to vitamin D analogues.

Patients who have refractory hyperparathyroidism may require parathyroidectomy.

Metabolic Acidosis:

Metabolic acidosis is a common complication of chronic kidney disease (CKD) and can be caused by several factors such as impaired renal acid excretion, retention of organic acids, and loss of bicarbonate. Correction of metabolic acidosis is shown to reduce the progression of CKD, mitigate hyperkalemia, improve metabolic bone disease, and fight against protein catabolism.

KDIGO recommends oral bicarbonate supplementation for CKD patients with serum bicarbonate levels below 22 mmol/L. Patients initiated on sodium bicarbonate need to be monitored for the worsening of hypervolemia in view of its sodium component. Refractory metabolic acidosis is an indication for initiation of dialysis.

Volume Overload:

The inability to excrete sodium and fluid excess is a challenge with decreasing GFR. Volume overload manifests as hypertension, heart failure (CHF), left ventricular hypertrophy (LVH), and edema.

Salt and fluid restriction reduces the deleterious effects of fluid overload. Loop diuretics are the agents of choice for treating hypervolemia, but refractory and life-threatening fluid overload are indications for initiating dialysis. It is worth noting that the maximum effective doses of loop diuretics increase as GFR drops. The dose of intravenous frusemide in CKD patients is increased from 80 mg to 200 mg as the GFR falls below 30 ml/min/1.73 m^2.

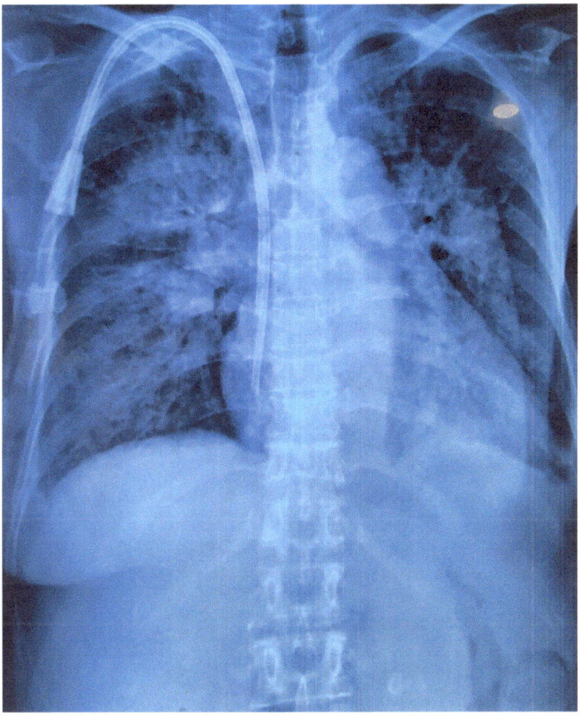

Figure 14.1: Shows Chest X-ray (AP View) Suggestive of Volume Overload in an ESKD Patient on Maintenance Hemodialysis Who Had Missed His Regular Sessions of Hemodialysis

Hyperkalemia:

Hyperkalemia is the most common electrolyte disorder encountered in CKD, whose incidence increases as the GFR drops. Hyperkalemia has been conventionally classified into mild (5.1–6 mmol/l), moderate (6–7 mmol/l), and severe (≥7 mmol/l).

Assessment of hyperkalemia needs a good dietary and medication (ACEi, ARBs, potassium-sparing diuretics, and NSAIDs) history. We should also look for cell and tissue breakdown (hemolysis, rhabdomyolysis, tumor lysis, etc.). Diabetic kidney disease patients are disproportionately prone to hyperkalemia in view of Type-4 renal tubular acidosis.

Arrhythmias secondary to hyperkalemia (tall, tented T waves, prolonged PR intervals, attenuation of P waves, and broadening of the QRS complex), can be potentially life-threatening.

Urgent management is necessary in patients with dysrhythmias, cardiac conduction defects, and muscle weakness/paralysis. Patients with any degree of hyperkalemia with ongoing tissue breakdown such as rhabdomyolysis, hemolysis, gastrointestinal bleeding, acidosis, and oligo-anuria also need urgent therapy.

Initial treatment constitutes the administering of 10 ml of 10% intravenous calcium gluconate over 2 to 3 minutes (membrane stabilization) and 10 units of regular insulin bolus followed by 50 mL of 50% dextrose (25 g of glucose) rapidly (transcellular shift). This lowers serum potassium by 1 mEq/L and the effect lasts for 4–6 hours. It is essential to monitor hypoglycemia for the next 6 hours and administer additional doses of intravenous glucose as needed. Inhalational beta-2 agonists, viz., salbutamol sulphate, provide an additive effect when used along with an IV insulin-dextrose regimen. Salbutamol is given in 10–20 mg doses, nebulized over 10 minutes.

The next modality is to remove potassium. These include loop diuretics, gastrointestinal cation exchangers (patiromer, sodium polystyrene sulfonate [SPS], and sodium zirconium cyclosilicate [SZC]), and dialysis. Loop diuretics, viz., furosemide, can be employed as supplemental anti-hyperkalemic therapy in mild/moderate renal dysfunction. SPS decreases potassium but has gastrointestinal side effects in a few patients. SPS needs to be avoided in patients at high risk of intestinal necrosis (post-operative patients, ileus, bowel obstruction, constipation, and inflammatory bowel disease). The oral dose is typically 15 to 30 g, repeated every 4 to 6 hours, as needed.

Sodium bicarbonate can be considered an adjuvant therapy to treat hyperkalemia and is given as an isotonic solution (150 mEq in 1 L of 5% dextrose in water over 2 to 4 hours). In severe kidney dysfunction, dialysis is often required as a treatment for hyperkalemia.

The treatment principles are summarized in Table 14.1.

Table 14.1: Complications of CKD and Its Management

Complication	Remarks	Treatment
Anemia	Commonly secondary to iron deficiency and reduced erythropoietin production	Iron Erythropoietin, Darbepoetin, CERA and HIF-PHIs Treat other deficiencies
Cardiovascular Complications	Heart failure is common in the later stages of CKD	Salt and fluid restriction, RAAS blockade, ARNI, Flozins, MRAs, Diuretics, Betablockers, Ultrafiltration Coronary evaluation and subsequent intervention in ischemic heart disease
CKD-MBD	Complex interplay between various parameters involved in bone and mineral metabolism	Phosphate binders, Vitamin D supplementation (both active and analogues as clinically indicated), Cinacalcet. Avoid calcium if possible. Evaluate osteoporosis and caution about adynamic bone disease.
Metabolic Acidosis	Important in progressive kidney disease and CKD-MBD.	Sodium bicarbonate. Watch for fluid overload

Complication	Remarks	Treatment
Volume Overload	Clinically significant in later stages of CKD, patients with heart failure.	Salt and fluid restriction. Diuretics and ultrafiltration.
Hyperkalemia	Common because of dietary indiscretions (potassium-rich food, even salt substitutes) and drugs.	Calcium gluconate Insulin dextrose Salbutamol nebulization Sodium polystyrene sulphonate Newer drugs Patiromer Sodium zirconium cyclosilicate Dialysis

Conclusion:

It is imperative on the part of treating clinicians to keep abreast of the dynamic concepts of optimal management of complications of CKD.

References:

1. Kiefer MM, Ryan MJ. Primary Care of the Patient with Chronic Kidney Disease. Med Clin North Am. 2015;99(5):935-952. doi:10.1016/J.MCNA.2015.05.003.
2. Babitt JL, Lin HY. Mechanisms of anemia in CKD. J Am Soc Nephrol. 2012;23(10):1631-1634. doi:10.1681/ASN.2011111078.
3. Fishbane S, Spinowitz B. Update on Anemia in ESRD and Earlier Stages of CKD: Core Curriculum 2018. 2017. doi:10.1053/j.ajkd.2017.09.026.
4. Health N, Survey NE. Chapter 1 : CKD in the General Population. 2015;1:13-24.
5. Dhillon S. Desidustat: First Approval. Drugs. 2022;82(11):1207-1212. doi:10.1007/S40265-022-01744-W.

6. Bello AK, Alrukhaimi M, Ashuntantang GE, et al. Complications of chronic kidney disease: current state, knowledge gaps, and strategy for action. Kidney Int Suppl. 2017;7(2):122-129. doi:10.1016/j.kisu.2017.07.007.
7. Warrens H, Banerjee D, Herzog CA. Cardiovascular Complications of Chronic Kidney Disease: An Introduction. Eur Cardiol. 2022;17. doi:10.15420/ECR.2021.54.
8. Ryan DK, Banerjee D, Jouhra F. Management of Heart Failure in Patients with Chronic Kidney Disease. Eur Cardiol. 2022;17. doi:10.15420/ECR.2021.33.
9. Cannata-Andía JB, Martín-Carro B, Martín-Vírgala J, et al. Chronic Kidney Disease-Mineral and Bone Disorders: Pathogenesis and Management. Calcif Tissue Int. 2021;108(4):410-422. doi:10.1007/S00223-020-00777-1.
10. Hu L, Napoletano A, Provenzano M, et al. Mineral Bone Disorders in Kidney Disease Patients: The Ever-Current Topic. Int J Mol Sci. 2022;23(20):12223. doi:10.3390/IJMS232012223.
11. Johnson, R. J., Floege, J., & Tonelli, M. (2023, March 15). Comprehensive Clinical Nephrology. Elsevier.
12. Melamed ML, Raphael KL. Metabolic Acidosis in CKD: A Review of Recent Findings. Kidney Med. 2021;3(2):267. doi:10.1016/J.XKME.2020.12.006.
13. Andrassy KM. Comments on "KDIGO 2012 Clinical Practice Guideline for the Evaluation and Management of Chronic Kidney Disease." Kidney Int. 2013;84(3):622-623. doi:10.1038/KI.2013.243.
14. Ellison DH. Treatment of Disorders of Sodium Balance in Chronic Kidney Disease. Adv Chronic Kidney Dis. 2017;24(5):332-341. doi:10.1053/J.ACKD.2017.07.003.
15. Yamada S, Inaba M. Potassium Metabolism and Management in Patients with CKD. Nutrients. 2021;13(6). doi:10.3390/NU13061751.

CHRONIC KIDNEY DISEASE

Complications & Management

ANEMIA

- Erythropoietin deficiency: Primary cause
- Rule out iron deficiency & occult blood loss
- ESAs Core therapy
- Avoid high Hb targets

CARDIOVASCULAR DISEASE

- Leading cause of mortality
- Atherosclerotic & non-atherosclerotic
- Coronary Artery Disease management: antiplatelets, lipid-lowering
- Heart failure management: diuretics, RAAS blockers, SGLT-2 inhibitors, ARNI

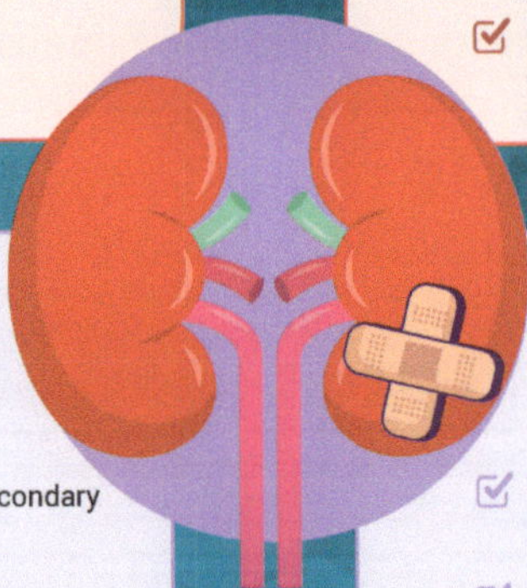

CKD-Mineral & Bone Disorder (CKD-MBD)

- Hyperphosphatemia → Secondary Hyperparathyroidism
- Phosphate control, binders
- Vitamin D analogues, calcimimetic agents
- Consider parathyroidectomy if indicated

Metabolic Acidosis

- Metabolic acidosis → Worsens CKD progression
- Sr Bicarbonate < 22 : Start Alkali therapy
- Monitor for hypervolemia when on alkali

Volume Overloaded

- Sodium and volume excess worsen as eGFR↓↓
- Dietary sodium restriction & optimize fluid intake
- Loop diuretics: cornerstone of treatment
- Dialysis may be required in refractory cases

Hyperkalemia

- Identify contributing causes (RAASi/NSAIDs/Type IV RTA)
- Urgent treatment Muscle weakness/ dysrhythmia/conduction defects
- IV Calcium gluconate, Insulin-dextrose regimen, Beta agonist
- Avoid sodium polystyrene sulfonate in gut disorders
- Rapid removal scenarios: Dialysis

ARNI: Angiotensin receptor/neprilysin inhibitor, ***CKD:*** Chronic Kidney Disease, ***eGFR:*** Estimated glomerular filtration rate, ***ESAs:*** Erythropoiesis stimulating agents, ***Hb:*** Hemoglobin
IV: Intravenous, ***NSAIDs:*** Non steroidal anti inflammatory drugs, ***RAASi:*** Renin angiotensin aldosterone system inhibitors, ***RAS:*** Renin Angiotensin Aldosterone System,
RTA: Renal Tubular acidosis, ***SGLT :*** Sodium glucose cotransporter, ***SR:*** Serum

15

DELAYING PROGRESSION OF CKD

Tanuj Moses Lamech, Natarajan Gopalakrishnan

Introduction:

Chronic kidney disease (CKD) is often characterized by a slow yet relentlessly progressive decline in GFR, eventually resulting in end-stage kidney disease. Several interventions have been studied to slow, or even halt, this decline. These include:

1. Glycemic control in Diabetics
2. Hypertension management
3. Renin-angiotensin-aldosterone system (RAAS) blockade
4. Sodium-glucose cotransporter-2 (SGLT2) inhibitors
5. Correction of chronic metabolic acidosis
6. Avoidance of nephrotoxins
7. Avoidance of infections, including periodontitis
8. Weight loss in Obese or Overweight

Glycemic Control:

There is strong evidence that intensive glycemic control reduces microvascular diseases in both type 1 and type 2 diabetes. Renoprotection has been consistently documented in patients

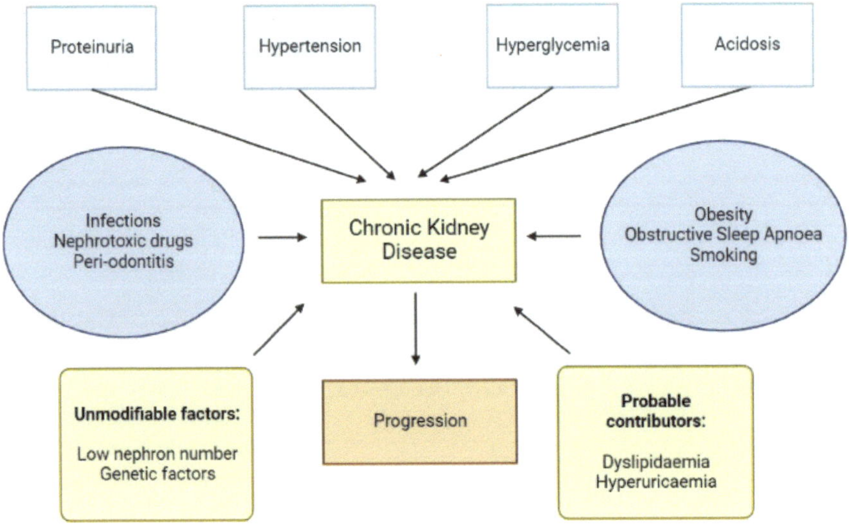

Figure 15.1: Factors Affecting the Progression of CKD

with intensive glucose control, both in the classic trials conducted in the 1990s (UKPDS, DCCT) and in the more contemporary data (ACCORD, ADVANCE, VADT). However, because of the frequent comorbidities in patients with longstanding diabetes and CKD, an individualized HbA1c target ranging from < 6.5% to < 8.0% has been suggested [Figure 15.2].

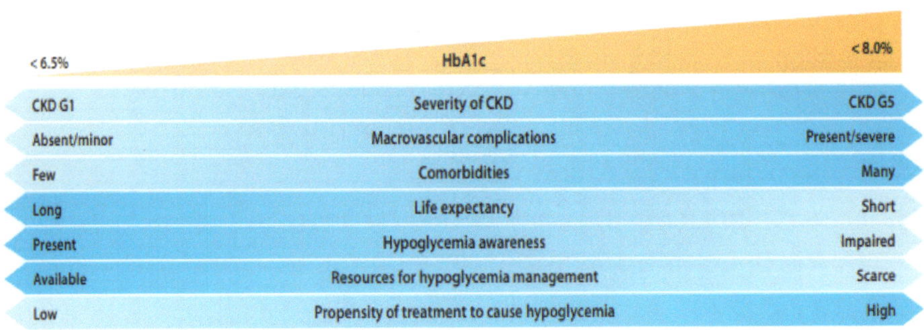

Figure 15.2: Factors Guiding Decisions on Individual Glycated Hemoglobin (HbA1c) Targets

(Source: KDIGO 2022 Clinical Practice Guideline for Diabetes Management in Chronic Kidney Disease)

The most recent KDIGO guidelines (updated in 2022) suggest that metformin and SGLT2 inhibitors be used as the first-line therapy for glucose-lowering.

For patients with proven or presumed diabetic kidney disease, in addition to intensive glucose lowering, additional measures that have been shown to slow the decline in GFR are the use of maximum-tolerated doses of RAAS inhibition, and the nonsteroidal mineralocorticoid receptor antagonist (MRA), finerenone (10–20 mg/day). Notably, however, in terms of renoprotection, the superiority of the non-steroidal MRA – finerenone – over the more readily available steroidal MRA – spironolactone – has not been demonstrated. Careful monitoring for hyperkalemia is mandatory while using MRAs, particularly when combined with RAAS blockers.

Hypertension:

The KDIGO 2021 guideline suggests that a systolic blood pressure of < 120 mmHg, measured using standardized office BP measurement, should be targeted while treating hypertension. However, care should be taken with regard to the technique of BP measurement as this target of < 120 mmHg is potentially hazardous if the BP measurements are obtained in a non-standardized manner.

Furthermore, the first-choice antihypertensive agent for patients with stable CKD should be an angiotensin-converting enzyme inhibitor (ACEi) or an angiotensin II receptor blocker (ARB). It remains unclear whether intensive lowering of blood pressure has an effect on the decline of GFR, but the cardiovascular benefits of this approach remain undisputed, and therefore, blood pressure control should be prioritized for all patients with chronic kidney disease.

Renin-Angiotensin-Aldosterone System (RAAS) Blockade:

Above and beyond their blood pressure-lowering effects, multiple RCTs have unequivocally demonstrated that RAAS blockade slows the progression of CKD in individuals with albuminuria. Care should be taken while initiating and up-titrating these agents, as they may trigger an acute rise in serum creatinine or hyperkalemia. A rise in creatinine of > 30% from the baseline should prompt an evaluation for underlying renal artery stenosis, and the drug should be withdrawn. Serum creatinine and potassium should be monitored 2 weeks after every dose increase. RAAS blockers should be gradually up-titrated to the doses used in trials (Table 15.1), or at least until maximally tolerated. These drugs should be withheld in an acutely ill patient, as hemodynamics in such patients are expected to be unstable and predisposing to AKI. Hyperkalemia from RAAS blockers can be managed by dietary potassium restriction, cessation of other drugs that could potentially contribute to hyperkalemia, use of diuretics, sodium bicarbonate supplementation, or the use of potassium binders. Dual blockade of the RAAS system, with the combined use of an ACEi and an ARB, is to be avoided.

Table 15.1: Different Formulations of Angiotensin-converting Enzyme Inhibitors (ACEi) and Angiotensin II Receptor Blockers (ARBs)

Drug		Starting dose	Maximum daily dose
Angiotensin converting enzyme inhibitors (ACEi)	Enalapril	5 mg once daily	40 mg
	Ramipril	2.5 mg once daily	20 mg
	Lisinopril	5 mg once daily	40 mg
Angiotensin II receptor blockers (ARB)	Telmisartan	40 mg once daily	80 mg
	Valsartan	80 mg once daily	320 mg
	Losartan	50 mg once daily	100 mg

Sodium-Glucose Cotransporter-2 (SGLT2) Inhibitors:

The last decade has witnessed trial after trial of SGLT2 inhibitors, reporting an overwhelmingly positive result, with many terminated prematurely for efficacy – a decidedly rare spectacle in the field of Nephrology. The glucose-lowering ability of the 'flozins' in the setting of diabetes is mediocre at best; their true value is in the prevention of renal and cardiovascular outcomes, prompting Eugene Braunwald to describe them as "the statins of the 21st century."

SGLT2 inhibitors have been shown to delay the progression of proteinuric and non-proteinuric kidney diseases, irrespective of the presence or absence of diabetes. The lower limit of GFR, at which these drugs can be initiated, has been repeatedly challenged and revised, and currently stands at 20 mL/min/1.73 m^2. However, they are continued subsequently even as the GFR continues to decline, and are stopped only when the patient initiates dialysis or receives a kidney transplant. The doses are described in Table 15.2.

An initial rise in serum creatinine is expected on initiating the drug; quite similar to the bump in creatinine seen while initiating RAAS blockade. The important adverse events that have been described are genital mycotic infections, euglycaemic ketosis (which contraindicates the drug in type 1 diabetes mellitus), limb amputations, and urinary tract infections.

It is important to try to achieve reasonable control of blood sugar before initiating an SGLT2 inhibitor, as hyperglycemia predisposes to profound osmotic diuresis when these medications are initiated. This is particularly true if the patient is also on a diuretic, the dose of which might need to be reduced.

Table 15.2: Sodium-glucose Cotransporter-2 Inhibitors (SGLT2i) with Established Kidney and Cardiovascular Benefits

Drug	Dose
Dapagliflozin	10 mg daily
Empagliflozin	10 mg daily (can increase to 25 mg daily, if needed for glucose control)
Canagliflozin	100 mg daily

(Source: KDIGO 2022 Clinical Practice Guideline for Diabetes Management in Chronic Kidney Disease.)

Correction of Metabolic Acidosis:

Multiple lines of evidence support the notion that kidney adaptations that facilitate acid excretion to maintain normal acid-base balance can themselves cause kidney injury. However, clinical data on the renoprotective effects of supplemental sodium bicarbonate has been conflicting. Nevertheless, clinical practice guidelines continue to suggest that metabolic acidosis in CKD should be treated with alkali therapy if serum bicarbonate is < 22 mEq/L. Oral sodium bicarbonate therapy is generally initiated at 1 g/day, but doses of up to 4.5 g/day have been used. Gastrointestinal side effects, however, are common and may be dose-limiting.

Avoidance of Nephrotoxins:

Routine administration of NSAIDs in chronic kidney disease is not recommended, especially among individuals who are taking ACEi/ARB therapy. Proton pump inhibitors are widely used and have been associated with incident CKD in some studies. Similarly, herbal remedies have been associated with numerous renal syndromes and should be discouraged.

Avoidance of Infections, Including Periodontitis:

Systemic or localized infections hasten the decline in GFR in patients with CKD. This is particularly true of diabetics, in whom an infected diabetic foot or an acute episode of pyelonephritis often results in an abrupt decline in GFR, with incomplete recovery or non-recovery, despite eradication of the infection.

A growing body of data supports a strong correlation between periodontitis and kidney disease. However, beneficial effects of treating periodontitis on the decline in GFR have not been demonstrated.

Weight Loss:

Observational data suggest an association between a high BMI and chronic kidney disease. Given the indisputable health benefits of increased physical activity and weight loss, all patients with chronic kidney disease who are overweight should be encouraged to lose weight.

Uric Acid Lowering Therapy:

Serum uric acid levels are frequently elevated in the setting of CKD, and this was, therefore, previously considered a therapeutic target. However, recent data suggests that there is no benefit of urate-lowering therapy in slowing the decline in GFR in patients with CKD, and there was even a signal to harm (though this did not reach statistical significance). Thus, in the contemporary setting, uric acid lowering should only be considered if there is coexistent clinical evidence of gout.

Lifestyle Modifications:

While not shown to directly affect CKD progression, it is nevertheless imperative that all patients be advised regarding smoking cessation, limiting alcohol intake, and restricting salt intake to < 5 g/day.

Since most patients with CKD are on therapeutic RAAS blockade, with or without an MRA, there is an intrinsic tendency to hyperkalemia (particularly in diabetes), and therefore, patients are advised a dietary restriction of potassium. High-potassium foods include tomatoes, beans, potatoes, oranges, mangoes, bananas, spinach, dates, raisins, and salt substitutes. Patients should be advised to focus on moderation and portion size, rather than a complete elimination of high potassium foods from the diet.

Protein restriction in patients with CKD was previously thought to slow GFR decline. However, in the current era of RAAS blockade and SGLT2 inhibition, the added benefit of protein restriction is likely to be negligible. Furthermore, in an Indian context, majority of the adults living in urban areas consume on average 0.6 g/kg/day of protein, with adults in rural areas consuming even less – this is, even at baseline, lower than the suggested 'low protein diet' threshold of 0.8 g/kg/day. Protein restriction in such patients predisposes to malnutrition, and therefore, should not be recommended.

Supplements, Pre-Biotics and Pro-Biotics:

Despite the widespread clinical use of keto-analogues, N-acetylcysteine, taurine, and various pre- and pro-biotics, the evidence for the efficacy of these agents is tenuous at best. In light of the high costs of such medication, along with the polypharmacy that most patients with CKD have to contend with, the use of these medications cannot be recommended.

Conclusion:

There is an extremely high prevalence of CKD in India, not just due to the increasing rates of diabetes, hypertension, and obesity, but also because of the widespread consumption of alternative medicines, and the recently identified "CKD hotspots" that are the epicenters of "CKDu"or CKD of unknown origin. Though most patients with CKD experience an inexorable gradual decline in GFR, the nephrologist of today has several tools to slow this progression, potentially delaying the onset of ESRD by several years. It is incumbent on clinicians to be aware of what works and what doesn't when prescribing medication to patients with chronic kidney disease.

References:

1. Chen, T. K., Sperati, C. J., Thavarajah, S. & Grams, M. E. Reducing Kidney Function Decline in Patients With CKD: Core Curriculum 2021. Am. J. Kidney Dis. 77, 969–983 (2021).
2. Zoungas, S. et al. Effects of intensive glucose control on microvascular outcomes in patients with type 2 diabetes: a meta-analysis of individual participant data from randomised controlled trials. Lancet Diabetes Endocrinol. 5, 431–437 (2017).
3. Rossing, P. et al. Executive summary of the KDIGO 2022 Clinical Practice Guideline for Diabetes Management in Chronic Kidney Disease: an update based on rapidly emerging new evidence. Kidney Int. 102, 990–999 (2022).
4. Neuen, B. L. et al. SGLT2 inhibitors for the prevention of kidney failure in patients with type 2 diabetes: a systematic review and meta-analysis. Lancet Diabetes Endocrinol. 7, 845–854 (2019).
5. Meraz-Muñoz, A. Y., Weinstein, J. & Wald, R. eGFR Decline after SGLT2 Inhibitor Initiation: The Tortoise and the Hare Reimagined. Kidney360 2, 1042–1047 (2021).
6. Raphael, K. L. Metabolic Acidosis in CKD: Core Curriculum 2019. Am. J. Kidney Dis. 74, 263–275 (2019).
7. Mohebbi, N. et al. Sodium bicarbonate for kidney transplant recipients with metabolic acidosis in Switzerland: a multicentre, randomised, single-blind, placebo-controlled, phase 3 trial. The Lancet 401, 557–567 (2023).
8. Chen, T. K., Knicely, D. H. & Grams, M. E. Chronic Kidney Disease Diagnosis and Management: A Review. JAMA 322, 1294–1304 (2019).

9. Gonzalez-Martin, G. et al. The dirty little secret of urate-lowering therapy: useless to stop chronic kidney disease progression and may increase mortality. Clin. Kidney J. 13, 936–947 (2020).
10. Ray S, Singh AK, Mukherjee JJ, et al. Protein restriction in adults with chronic kidney disease, with or without diabetes: Integrated Diabetes and Endocrine Academy (IDEA) consensus statement for Indian patients. Diabetes Metab Syndr. 2023 May;17(5):102785.
11. Obeid, W., Hiremath, S., & Topf, J. M. (2022). Protein Restriction for CKD: Time to Move On. Kidney360, 3(9), 1611–1615.

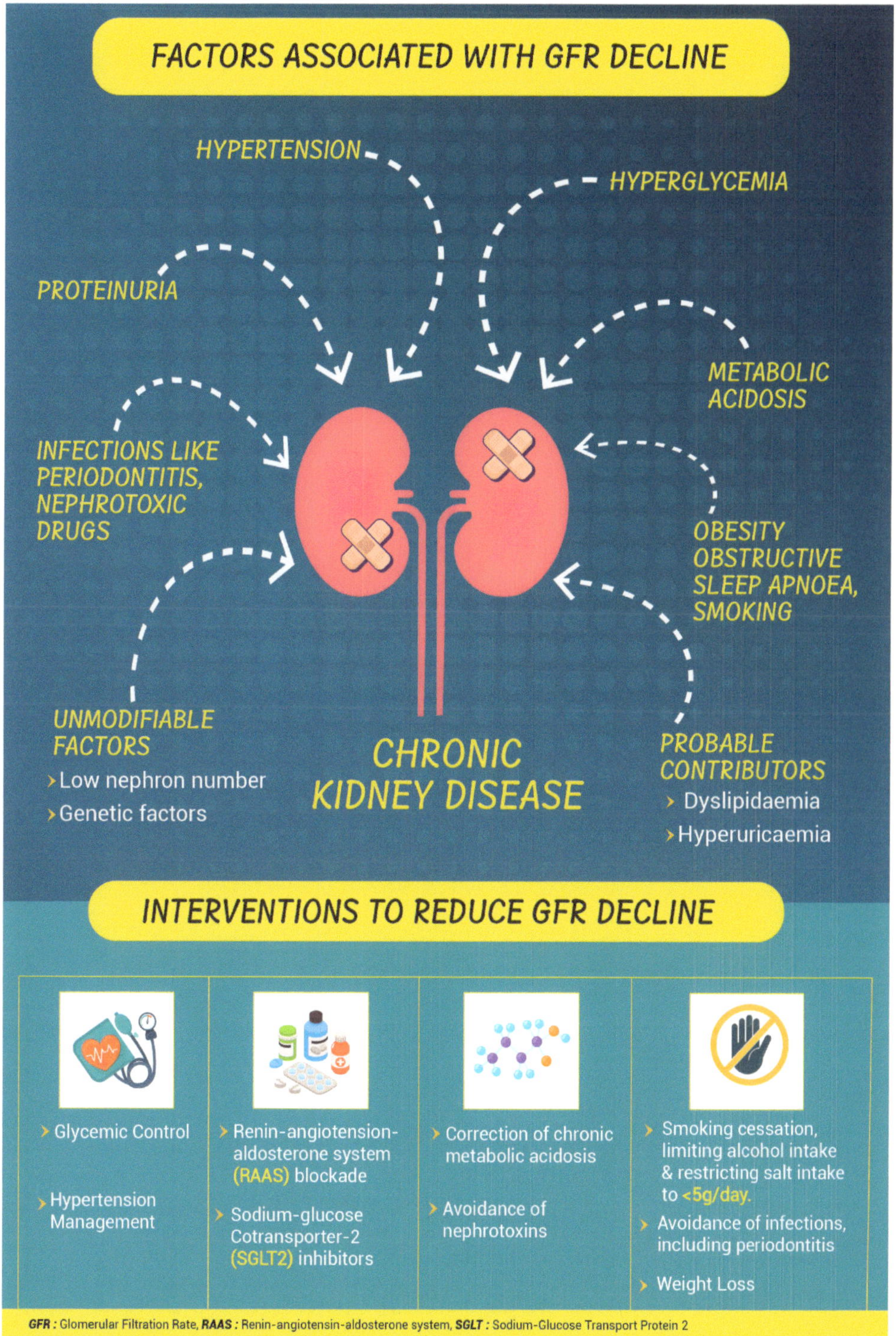

GFR : Glomerular Filtration Rate, ***RAAS :*** Renin-angiotensin-aldosterone system, ***SGLT :*** Sodium-Glucose Transport Protein 2

SECTION 5

Kidney Disorders in Systemic Diseases

16

KIDNEY DISORDER IN SYSTEMIC DISEASES

Shyam Chand Chaudhary, Arvind Kumar Verma, Avinash Kumar, Shambhavi Sinha, Kamal Kumar Sawlani

Overview: Kidney function is influenced by a wide range of systemic conditions, including acute illnesses and the use of certain medications. It is impossible to encompass all potential causes of renal disease within a single compilation. However, this chapter aims to provide an overview of the prevalent systemic illnesses that can affect the kidneys. The kidney-related systemic diseases can be categorized according to their underlying causes. (Table 16.1).

Hypertensive Nephropathy:

Hypertensive nephropathy, also known as hypertensive nephrosclerosis, is a kidney disease linked to long-standing high blood pressure and is frequently reported to be the second most common cause of end-stage renal disease (ESKD). Persistent

Table 16.1: Systemic Diseases Associated with Kidney Disorders

Metabolic disorder	• Diabetic nephropathy • Hypertensive nephropathy
Immunologically mediated diseases	• SLE • Vasculitis • Rheumatoid arthritis • Goodpasture syndrome • Henoch-schönlein purpura • Scleroderma • Sarcoidosis • Sjogren syndrome • Antiphospholipid syndrome
Infections	• Post infectious GN • Malaria • Leptospirosis • Boreliosis • Scrub Typhus • Rocky mountain spotted fever
Cardiac and liver diseases	• Hepatorenal syndrome • Cardiorenal syndrome • Subacute bacterial endocarditis
Paraproteinaemia and neoplasia	• Multiple myeloma • Amyloidosis • Cryoglobulinemia
Drug and toxins	• Poisoinings such as copper sulphate, • Alternative or over-the-counter drugs

high blood pressure damages tubular cells, triggering epithelial-mesenchymal transition (EMT) and tubulointerstitial fibrosis. Hypertension-related vascular injury involves pre-glomerular arterioles, resulting in ischemic injury to the glomeruli and post-glomerular structures. Direct damage to the glomerular capillaries due to glomerular hyperperfusion, ultimately leading to loss of autoregulation of renal blood flow, resulting in a lower blood pressure threshold for renal damage and a steeper slope between blood pressure and renal damage. Glomerular pathology progresses to glomerulosclerosis, and eventually, the renal tubules may also become ischemic and gradually atrophic. The renal lesion associated with malignant hypertension consists of fibrinoid necrosis of the afferent arterioles.

Patients typically have long-standing hypertension, often accompanied by retinopathy and left ventricular hypertrophy, which precede the onset of proteinuria or impaired kidney function. The likelihood of progressing to kidney failure is directly related to the level of blood pressure control, and episodes of accelerated hypertension (which may go unnoticed) can accelerate the rate of disease progression. Macroalbuminuria (a random urine albumin/creatinine ratio > 300 mg/g) and microalbuminuria (a random urine albumin/creatinine ratio 30–300 mg/g) are the early markers of renal injury. They are also risk factors for renal disease progression and cardiovascular diseases. ACE inhibitors and angiotensin II receptor blockers (ARBs) are the drugs of choice for kidney protection in patients with proteinuric chronic kidney disease.

Systemic Vasculitis:

Typically presents as rapidly progressive glomerulonephritis (RPGN), which includes acute kidney injury (AKI), hematuria, and proteinuria. It involves inflammation and necrosis of blood vessels, which can occur in various disorders. Systemic vasculitis can either be a primary autoimmune disorder or a secondary manifestation of another underlying condition such as infection, malignancy, and chronic inflammatory disorder, or be drug-related.

Vasculitic syndromes commonly affect the kidneys, leading to tissue infarction, loss of kidney function, and rapid progression to end-stage renal disease within a matter of weeks or months. Small-vessel vasculitides, particularly ANCA-associated vasculitis, are the most frequent cause of renal vasculitis. ANCA-associated vasculitis encompasses three syndromes: granulomatosis with polyangiitis (formerly Wegener's granulomatosis), microscopic polyangiitis, and eosinophilic granulomatosis with angiitis (formerly Churg-Strauss syndrome).

In medium- and larger-vessel vasculitides, renal involvement is less common. Polyarteritis nodosa (ANCA-negative) and Kawasaki's disease, which are medium-vessel disorders, rarely affect the kidneys. Likewise, in large-vessel disorders, such as giant cell arteritis and Takayasu's arteritis, renal disease is rare.

Glucocorticoids play a crucial role in the initial treatment of renal vasculitis; however, their effectiveness is restricted, and long-term maintenance therapy should incorporate alternate-day dosing whenever feasible.

Antiphospholipid Syndrome:

APS nephropathy primarily occurs as a result of thromboses in renal arteries, veins, intraparenchymatous arteries, and glomerular capillaries. About 50% of the patients with APS nephropathy exhibit renal involvement with proteinuria.

Histologically, APS nephropathy is characterized by thrombotic microangiopathy (TMA), along with commonly observed chronic vaso-occlusive lesions such as fibrous intimal hyperplasia, focal cortical atrophy, and fibrous occlusions of arteries. The most prevalent antibodies in patients with APS nephropathy are anticardiolipin and lupus anticoagulants.

In patients with systemic lupus erythematosus (SLE), who have antiphospholipid antibodies (APL), it is crucial to differentiate kidney failure caused by SLE nephritis (an immune-complex disease) from kidney failure caused by APS-related TMA. In such cases, a renal biopsy is necessary. SLE nephritis requires immunosuppressive therapy, while APS nephropathy is typically managed with anticoagulants.

Table 16.2: Different Types of Vasculitis with Renal Involvement

ANCA positive small vessel vasculitis	Granulomatosis with polyangiitis	• Necrotizing and granulomatous vasculitis • Primary renal manifestation of GPA is rapidly progressive glomerulonephritis (RPGN). • RPGN can lead to CKD or end-stage renal disease (ESRD). • Initially, renal involvement is seen in only 10–20% at presentation. • However, approximately 80% of patients eventually develop renal involvement within two years of disease onset. • Renal signs include microscopic hematuria, often with erythrocyte casts. • Non-nephrotic proteinuria is usually present
	Microscopic polyangiitis	• Necrotizing vasculitis. • Clinical manifestations of MPA result from the activation of primed neutrophils and MPO-ANCA with receptors on the endothelial surface. • 80% to 100% of individuals experiencing some form of glomerulonephritis at the onset or during the progression of the disease. • Presentation varies, ranging from asymptomatic hematuria and sub-nephrotic proteinuria to a rise in serum creatinine or overt renal failure. • Remission in MPA is achieved using a combination of glucocorticoids and cyclophosphamide. • Plasmapheresis is effective in severe renal disease and pulmonary hemorrhage
	Eosinophilic granulomatosis with angiitis	• Vasculitis is characterized by small- to medium-sized systemic necrotizing vasculitis. • Eosinophil-rich tissue infiltrates and the presence of granulomatous lesions. • Primarily affects the respiratory system, intrinsic renal injury is not uncommon. • Up to 25% of patients with EGPA have been recorded to experience renal involvement

Table 16.2: Different Types of Vasculitis with Renal Involvement Continued...

ANCA negative small vessel vasculitis	Goodpasture syndrome	• Clinical manifestations associated with the condition include pulmonary hemorrhage, iron deficiency anemia, and progressive renal failure. • Anti-GBM antibodies are present in 90% of cases, and histological examination reveals linear capillary loop staining with IgG and C3, as well as extensive crescent formation.
	IgA vasculitis or Henoch-Schönlein purpura	• Characterized by IgA-dominant immune deposits • Affects small vessels, commonly involving the skin, gastrointestinal tract, joints, and kidneys. • Affects children more frequently than adults. • In adults, more likely to lead to chronic renal disease. • Formation of galactose-deficient IgA1 (Gd-IgA1) and related immune complexes plays a crucial role
Medium size vasculitis	Polyarteritis nodosa	• Inflammation of primarily medium-sized arteries. • Microaneurysms, often involving the renal arteries

Sjogren Syndrome:

Primary Sjögren's Syndrome (PSS) is an autoimmune disorder characterized by lymphocytic infiltration of exocrine glands, leading to sicca symptoms. Renal involvement occurs in 5% of PSS patients and includes interstitial nephritis, clinically manifested by hyposthenuria and renal tubular dysfunction, with or without acidosis. Untreated acidosis may lead to nephrocalcinosis.

Immune complex-mediated disease is expressed with vasculitis affecting primarily small-sized vessels, mainly manifested with purpura and rarely with urticarial rash, skin ulcerations, mononeuritis multiplex, and membranoproliferative glomerulonephritis associated with mixed type II or III cryoglobulinemia.

Treatment depends on the specific condition, ranging from supportive care to immunosuppressive therapy. Around 10–20% of PSS patients with kidney disease develop end-stage kidney disease (ESKD).

Sarcoidosis:

A systemic granulomatous disease, primarily affecting the respiratory system and lymphatic vessels. Direct kidney involvement occurs in < 5% of sarcoidosis patients. It is associated with granulomas in the kidney itself and can lead to nephritis. However, hypercalcemia is the most likely cause of sarcoidosis-associated renal disease and contributes to renal injury, leading to acute tubular necrosis, nephrolithiasis, and nephrocalcinosis. In 1–2% of sarcoidosis patients, acute renal failure may develop as a result of hypercalcemia.

Suspicion of renal involvement arises when patients have elevated serum creatinine, bland urine sediment, or sterile pyuria, along with a known diagnosis or characteristic presentation of extrarenal sarcoidosis. Membranous nephropathy is a common glomerular disease associated with sarcoidosis, often accompanied by the presence of phospholipase A2 receptor (PLA2R) antibodies. Granulomatous tubulointerstitial nephritis is the most frequent renal lesion and can progress to end-stage renal disease in some patients.

Successful treatment of hypercalcemia with glucocorticoids and other therapies often improves, but usually does not totally resolve renal dysfunction.

Systemic Sclerosis:

Renal involvement is common in systemic sclerosis (SSc), an autoimmune vasculopathy associated with dysregulated innate and adaptive immunity. Scleroderma renal crisis (SRC) is a severe complication of SSc with a high mortality rate. Anti-RNA polymerase III antibodies are strongly associated with SRC. While renal biopsy may not be necessary in typical cases, it may be needed in atypical presentations. The use of angiotensin-converting enzyme inhibitors (ACEIs) has significantly improved the prognosis, reducing the 1-year mortality from 85% to 24%. Vasodilating prostaglandins can help control blood pressure and improve renal blood flow. Renal recovery may take up to 24 months, so decisions about renal transplantation should be delayed until that time.

Rheumatoid Arthritis:

Renal involvement in rheumatoid arthritis (RA) is uncommon. It can occur through various mechanisms, including secondary renal amyloidosis, membranous nephropathy, nephrotoxic effects of anti-rheumatic drugs, and extra-articular manifestations known as rheumatoid nephropathy.

Hepatorenal Syndrome (HRS)

Cirrhosis and portal hypertension can set off the neurohormonal cascade, which results in HRS. Vasodilators and cytokines such as nitric oxide and prostaglandins are produced and released, resulting in splanchnic and systemic vasodilation. The systemic drop in circulation pressure activates three distinct compensatory mechanisms in the carotid and aortic arch baroreceptors. These include the renin-angiotensin-aldosterone system, vasopressin release, and sympathetic nervous system (SNS) activation. Cirrhosis progression causes a decrease in cardiac output as well as a decrease in systemic vascular resistance, inducing additional renal vasoconstriction. This causes further renal hypoperfusion, which is exacerbated by renal vasoconstriction, eventually leading to renal failure. In HRS, though the kidney function is compromised yet there is no sign of intrinsic kidney diseases such as proteinuria, hematuria, or abnormal kidney ultrasonography. Hepatorenal syndrome, which comes from functional alterations in the renal circulation and may be treatable with a liver transplant or vasoconstrictor medications, is different from other AKIs. Depending on how severe and rapidly the kidney damage is progressing, there are two distinct types of hepatorenal syndrome. The first – HRS-AKI, is an acute kidney dysfunction, whereas the second – HRS-CKD (chronic kidney disease), is a more chronic kidney dysfunction. Patients with HRS have a very poor prognosis, particularly those with a rapidly progressive course. Due to the poor prognosis, it is challenging to implement liver transplantation in all patients. However, liver transplantation is the best treatment option for suitable candidates. Standard initial treatment consists of vasoconstrictor medications and intravenous albumin administered intravenously. Terlipressin (TP) is recommended, but it has adverse effects.

Cardiorenal Syndrome (CRS)

Cardiorenal syndrome encompasses a spectrum of disorders, involving both the heart and kidneys, in which acute or chronic dysfunction in one organ may induce acute or chronic dysfunction in the other organ. (Table 16.3).

Table 16.3: Classification of CRS Based on the Consensus Conference of the Acute Dialysis Quality Initiative

Phenotype	Nomenclature	Description	Clinical Examples
Type 1	Acute CRS	HF resulting in AKI	ACS resulting in cardiogenic shock and AKI, AHF resulting in AKI
Type 2	Chronic CRS	Chronic HF resulting in CKD	Chronic HF
Type 3	Acute renocardiac syndrome	AKI resulting in AHF	HF in the setting of AKI from volume overload, inflammatory surge, and metabolic disturbances in uremia
Type 4	Chronic renocardiac syndrome	CKD resulting in chronic HF	LVH and HF from CKD-associated cardiomyopathy
Type 5	Secondary CRS	Systemic process resulting in HF and kidney failure	Amyloidosis, sepsis, cirrhosis

(ACS: acute coronary syndrome; AHF: acute heart failure; AKI: acute kidney injury; CKD: chronic kidney disease; CRS: cardiorenal syndrome; HF: heart failure; and LVH: left ventricular hypertrophy.)

HIV infection can lead to a glomerulopathy called collapsing focal segmental glomerulosclerosis (FSGS) or HIV-associated nephropathy (HIVAN). HIVAN can occur during acute or chronic infection, with higher viral RNA levels and lower CD4 T lymphocyte counts seen in chronic cases. Symptoms of HIVAN include proteinuria and renal impairment, sometimes accompanied by edema. Imaging studies may show increased kidney size despite reduced glomerular filtration rate (GFR) and increased echogenicity in some cases. A renal biopsy is necessary for a definitive diagnosis. All HIV-positive individuals should receive combination antiretroviral therapy (ART) to prevent HIV-related CKD. The introduction of ART has significantly reduced the incidence of HIV-associated end-stage renal disease (ESRD) and may prevent HIVAN. ART can lead to a rapid resolution or decrease in proteinuria within 6 months of initiation.

Sepsis is a major cause of acute kidney injury (AKI) in intensive care unit patients, accounting for up to 50% of the cases. The presence of septic AKI is associated with high mortality rates, particularly in those requiring renal replacement therapy. The development of sepsis-associated AKI is driven by the release of molecules from pathogens or injured cells. These molecules, such as lipopolysaccharide, flagellin, lipoteichoic acid, and DNA, activate the innate immune system by binding to toll-like receptors (TLRs) and other immune cell receptors.

Infections can cause a range of kidney problems, from asymptomatic urinary abnormalities to acute kidney injury (AKI) and, rarely, chronic kidney disease (CKD). Malaria, leptospirosis, dengue, scrub typhus, acute gastroenteritis (especially in children), toxic envenomations like snake bites or wasp stings, and certain poisonings are common tropical infections that affect the kidneys. It is now recognized that some patients with infection-related AKI may experience residual damage, leading to the development of CKD.

Paraproteinemias:

Renal disease in paraproteinemias is caused by nephrotoxic monoclonal immunoglobulins. The specific pattern of renal injury depends on factors such as the type, size, pattern, and location of the immunoglobulin deposits in the kidney tissue. In addition to immunoglobulin-related damage, non-immunoglobulin factors such as volume depletion, hypercalcemia, tubulointerstitial nephritis, plasma cell infiltration, hyperviscosity syndrome, and hyperuricemia can also contribute to renal injury. A renal biopsy and comprehensive hematologic evaluation are necessary to establish the link between the paraprotein and renal disease. Recent advancements in treatment, including more effective chemotherapies and stem cell transplantation, have improved the prognosis for renal and overall outcomes in these disorders.

Conclusion:

Renal manifestations of systemic diseases encompass a broad spectrum of conditions, each with distinct pathophysiological mechanisms and clinical implications. Though diabetes mellitus, hypertension, SLE, and vasculitis are commoner systemic diseases associated with renal manifestations, however, infections, cardiac diseases, liver diseases, and paraproteinemias also contribute to the complex landscape of renal manifestations. Moreover, the advancements in understanding these diseases have led to more targeted treatments. Immunomodulatory therapies, angiotensin receptor blockers, and innovative medications like SGLT2 inhibitors have revolutionized the management of various conditions. Overall, recognizing the intricate interplay between systemic diseases and kidney function is essential for improving patient outcomes. Continued research, advancements in diagnostics, and innovative therapies hold the promise of better managing and mitigating the impact of renal manifestations associated with systemic conditions.

References:

1. Freedman BI, Iskandar SS, Appel RG. The link between hypertension and nephrosclerosis. Am J Kidney Dis. 1995;25:207.
2. Barratt J, Topham P, Carr S, Arici M, Liew A. The kidney in systemic disease. In: Barratt J, Topham P, Carr S, Arici M, Liew A, editors. Oxford Desk Reference: Nephrology. 2nd ed. Oxford: Oxford University Press; 2000. p. 188-200.
3. Ntatsaki E, Watts RA, Scott DG. Epidemiology of ANCA-associated vasculitis. Rheum Dis Clin North Am. 2010;36(3):447-61. Epub 2010 Jun 15. doi: 10.1016/j.rdc.2010.04.002.
4. Idolor ON, Guraya A, Muojieje CC, Kannayiram SS, Nair KM, Odion J, Sanwo E, Aihie OP. Renal Involvement in Granulomatosis With Polyangiitis Increases Economic Health Care Burden: Insights From the National Inpatient Sample Database. Cureus. 2021;13(1):e12515. doi: 10.7759/cureus.12515.
5. Doreille A, Buob D, Bay P, Julien M, Riviere F, Rafat C. Renal Involvement in Eosinophilic Granulomatosis With Polyangiitis. Kidney Int Rep. 2021;6(10):2718-2721. doi: 10.1016/j.ekir.2021.07.002.
6. Delbet JD, Parmentier C, Herbez Rea C, Mouche A, Ulinski T. Management of IgA Vasculitis with Nephritis. Paediatr Drugs. 2021;23(5):425-435. doi: 10.1007/s40272-021-00464-0. Epub 2021 Aug 16.
7. Wang H, Sun L, Tan W. Clinical features of children with pulmonary microscopic polyangiitis: report of 9 cases. PLoS One. 2015;10(4):e0124352.
8. Tektonidou MG. Antiphospholipid Syndrome Nephropathy: From Pathogenesis to Treatment. Front Immunol. 2018;9:1181. doi: 10.3389/fimmu.2018.01181.
9. Aiyegbusi O, McGregor L, McGeoch L, Kipgen D, Geddes CC, Stevens KI. Renal Disease in Primary Sjögren's Syndrome. Rheumatol Ther. 2021r;8(1):63-80. doi: 10.1007/s40744-020-00264-x. Epub 2020 Dec 24.
10. Correia FASC, Marchini GS, Torricelli FC, Danilovic A, Vicentini FC, Srougi M, Nahas WC, Mazzucchi E. Renal manifestations of

sarcoidosis: from accurate diagnosis to specific treatment. Int Braz J Urol. 2020;46(1):15-25. doi: 10.1590/S1677-5538.IBJU.2019.0042.

11. Shanmugam VK, Steen VD. Renal disease in scleroderma: an update on evaluation, risk stratification, pathogenesis and management. Curr Opin Rheumatol. 2012;24(6):669-76. doi: 10.1097/BOR.0b013e3283588dcf.
12. Icardi A, Araghi P, Ciabattoni M, Romano U, Lazzarini P, Bianchi G. Coinvolgimento renale in corso di artrite reumatoide [Kidney involvement in rheumatoid arthritis]. Reumatismo. 2003;55(2):76-85. Italian. doi: 10.4081/reumatismo.2003.76.
13. Ng CK, Chan MH, Tai MH, Lam CW. Hepatorenal syndrome. Clin Biochem Rev. 2007;28(1):11-7. PMID: 17603637.
14. Wyatt CM, Klotman PE, D'Agati VD. HIV-associated nephropathy: clinical presentation, pathology, and epidemiology in the era of antiretroviral therapy. Semin Nephrol. 2008;28(6):513-22. doi: 10.1016/j.semnephrol.2008.08.005.
15. Damman K, Tang WW, Testani JM, McMurray JJ. Terminology and definition of changes renal function in heart failure. European heart journal. 2014;35(48):3413-6.
16. Peerapornratana S, Manrique-Caballero CL, Gómez H, Kellum JA. Acute kidney injury from sepsis: current concepts, epidemiology, pathophysiology, prevention and treatment. Kidney Int. 2019 Nov;96(5):1083-1099. Epub 2019 Jun 7. doi: 10.1016/j.kint.2019.05.026.
17. Heher EC, Goes NB, Spitzer TR, Raje NS, Humphreys BD, Anderson KC, Richardson PG. Kidney disease associated with plasma cell dyscrasias. Blood. 2010 Sep 2;116(9):1397-404. Epub 2010 May 12. doi: 10.1182/blood-2010-03-258608.

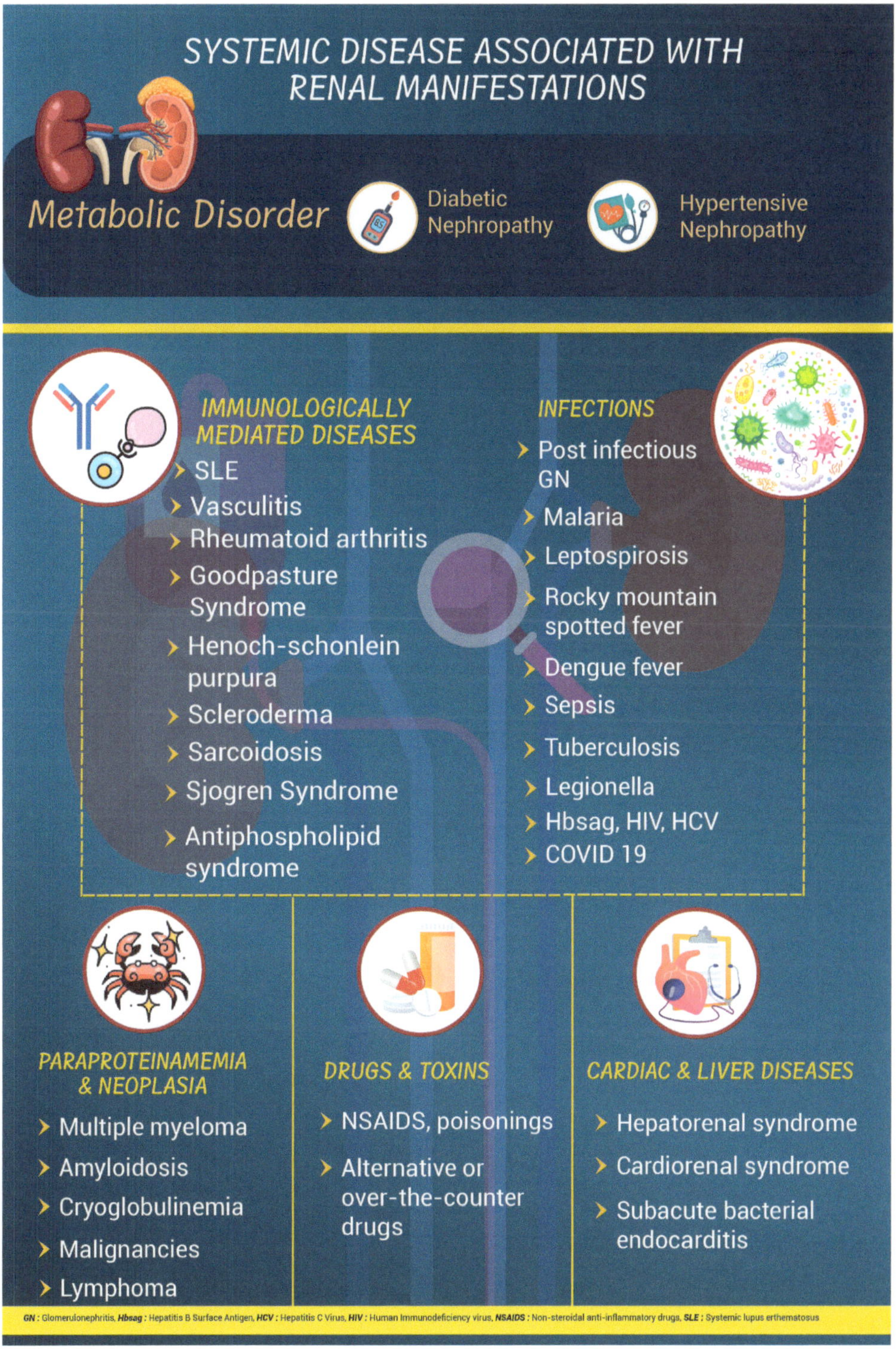
SYSTEMIC DISEASE ASSOCIATED WITH RENAL MANIFESTATIONS
Metabolic Disorder
Diabetic Nephropathy
Hypertensive Nephropathy
IMMUNOLOGICALLY MEDIATED DISEASES
SLE
Vasculitis
Rheumatoid arthritis
Goodpasture Syndrome
Henoch-schonlein purpura
Scleroderma
Sarcoidosis
Sjogren Syndrome
Antiphospholipid syndrome
INFECTIONS
Post infectious GN
Malaria
Leptospirosis
Rocky mountain spotted fever
Dengue fever
Sepsis
Tuberculosis
Legionella
Hbsag, HIV, HCV
COVID 19
PARAPROTEINAMEMIA & NEOPLASIA
Multiple myeloma
Amyloidosis
Cryoglobulinemia
Malignancies
Lymphoma
DRUGS & TOXINS
NSAIDS, poisonings
Alternative or over-the-counter drugs
CARDIAC & LIVER DISEASES
Hepatorenal syndrome
Cardiorenal syndrome
Subacute bacterial endocarditis
GN : Glomerulonephritis, Hbsag : Hepatitis B Surface Antigen, HCV : Hepatitis C Virus, HIV : Human Immunodeficiency virus, NSAIDS : Non-steroidal anti-inflammatory drugs, SLE : Systemic lupus erthematosus

17

DIABETIC KIDNEY DISEASE: NATURAL HISTORY, PATHOGENESIS, AND COMPLICATIONS

Arpita Roy Choudhary, Padmini Sirkanungo

Introduction:

Diabetic kidney disease (DKD) is the leading cause of chronic kidney disease (CKD) in the world and the Indian scenario is no different. As reported by several investigators, it amounts to 30–40% of the CKD population. By 2030, India will have the highest diabetic population in the world. An Indian Council of Medical Research—ICMR-INDIAB—study report identifies a sharp rise in the prevalence of diabetes in both urban and rural populations alike. 30–40% of diabetic patients may develop end-stage kidney disease (ESKD), and the disease progression may be effectively delayed if intervened early. The presence of DKD is also strongly associated with cardiovascular (CV) morbidity and mortality and has a major influence on survival.

This chapter will cover the following issues to increase awareness and ensure early intervention in the course of the disease.

1. Natural history of Type 1 and Type 2 Diabetes Mellitus (DM)
2. Pathogenesis of Diabetic Nephropathy (DN): addressing the three pathways, namely, Hemodynamic, Metabolic, and Inflammatory
3. Possible macrovascular and microvascular complications

Renal involvement in diabetes can be in the form of Diabetic kidney disease, Non-diabetic kidney disease (NDKD), or NDKD superimposed on DKD. "DN" is a diagnosis that refers to specific pathologic structural and functional changes seen in the kidneys of patients with DM (both T1/T2DM). Histological changes are described as predominant glomerular changes in the kidney, while the clinical counterpart is characterized by persistent albuminuria and progressively declining renal function. On the other hand, DKD is a clinical syndrome characterized by overt proteinuria (>200μg/min or 300mg/day) and declining renal function, often preceded by progressively increasing urinary albumin excretion (30–300 mg/day), usually described as incipient diabetic nephropathy.

DKD is a clinical diagnosis based upon the decreased estimated glomerular filtration rate (eGFR) in diabetic patients and proteinuria, either or both, and does not indicate a specific pathological type. It can be from diverse causes, including hypertensive nephrosclerosis and unresolved acute kidney injury. The likelihood that DN is the cause of DKD varies widely, depending upon the clinical circumstances. Increased duration of diabetes, particularly in Type 1 DM, associated with macro or microangiopathic complications, increases the likelihood that DN is the cause of DKD in that patient. Another subset of diabetic patients from 14–25%, may have nonproteinuric DKD due to the high universal use of RAS-blockers to control hypertension in diabetics, or unresolved acute kidney injury, or coexistent obstructive component.

Natural History:

The natural history of diabetic nephropathy in patients of T1DM is best described in the pre-insulin era by Kussman et al (1970) by examining death records of untreated patients with juvenile-onset DM who died from renal failure. The traditional five-stage progression of diabetic nephropathy, given by Mogensen through studies in patients with type 1 diabetes, follows this pattern:

1. **Stage I: Hyperfiltration** – This stage is marked by an increased glomerular filtration rate (GFR) and kidney enlargement, sometimes with a temporary rise in albumin excretion (AER).
2. **Stage II: Silent Nephropathy** – Here, GFR and AER return to normal, though there may be occasional episodes of microalbuminuria (a slight increase in albumin in the urine). Most people with diabetes stay in this stage for life, but about one-third progress further.
3. **Stage III: Incipient Nephropathy** – Microalbuminuria becomes persistent, signaling the start of kidney damage
4. **Stage IV: Overt Nephropathy** – Microalbuminuria worsens into macroalbuminuria (higher levels of albumin in the urine), blood pressure increases, and GFR starts to decline.
5. **Stage V: End-Stage Renal Disease (ESRD)** – GFR continues to drop, leading to kidney failure that requires dialysis or a kidney transplant unless the patient dies, often due to cardiovascular disease (CVD).

Throughout these stages, the progression of albuminuria often coincides with worsening diabetic retinopathy, another major complication of diabetes.

In type 1 diabetes, most patients with microalbuminuria develop macroalbuminuria over 6-14 years. In type 2 diabetes, the progression is less predictable because of the high death rate from cardiovascular disease, which can disrupt the typical course of DN.

Observations revealed that proteinuria appeared 11 to 23 years after the T1DM diagnosis, while serum creatinine begins to increase 13 to 25 years later, and ESKD develops after 18 to 30 years. Over time, more sensitive assays to detect urinary albumin excretion were developed, which helped in detecting microalbuminuria, 30–300 mg/g creatinine. The development of overt proteinuria (macroalbuminuria > 300 mg/g creatinine) in most patients, occurs 5 to 10 years after the diagnosis of DM. Presently, micro-albuminuria and macro-albuminuria are referred to as A2 and A3 respectively, by the KDIGO (Kidney Disease: Improving Global Outcomes) chronic kidney disease (CKD) guideline.

The natural history of diabetic nephropathy in the longitudinally studied population of T2 DM was documented to have essentially similar pathology as in Type 1 DM. However, as the disease onset cannot be ascertained outside a study cohort situation, the patients of T2 DM can have established pathological changes of diabetic nephropathy even at diagnosis. Another important difference is in the cardiovascular (CV) mortality and morbidity spectrum; this macrovascular complication hardly appears before established renal failure in Type 1 DM patients, while it is common to have CV complications in T2DM patients even before the renal disease has appeared. The single best predictor of kidney function deterioration and diabetic nephropathy progression is proteinuria, which when combined with kidney function decline (eGFR), can be comfortably used for risk prediction and intensive target-based management is warranted.

Based on studies of untreated patients with T1DM and Pima Indians with T2DM, the rate of GFR loss can be of the order of 7 to 12 mL/min/1.73 m^2 per year. Treatment with renin-angiotensin system (RAS) inhibitors has reduced this rate of decline to 3 to 6 mL/min/1.73 m^2 per year.

In patients with CKD stage 3 (eGFR ≤ 60 mL/min/1.73 m^2), the risk of death is more than 10 times higher than the risk of progression to ESKD. Once on dialysis, the 5-year survival is less than 40% in these patients, predominantly owing to CVD-associated morbidity and mortality. Also, it has been observed that CKD patients have a 13-fold more chance of dying from other causes rather than progression of ESRD accounting for death, the risk of death from CV disease is 6-fold more.

Pathogenesis:

A complex interaction of multiple mechanisms contributes to the development and progression of DN, which include interaction between hyperglycemia-induced metabolic and hemodynamic changes, oxidative stress, and release of several inflammatory cytokines, together with genetic predisposition, ultimately setting the stage for a kidney injury. In patients with type 1 or type 2 diabetes, the likelihood of developing diabetic nephropathy is markedly increased in those who have a sibling or parent with diabetic nephropathy. The likelihood of the offspring developing overt proteinuria was 14% if neither parent had proteinuria, 23% if one parent had proteinuria, and 46% if both parents had proteinuria. See Table 17.1.

Table 17.1: Pathogenesis of Diabetic Nephropathy

Sl.No	Factor	Pathogenesis
1.	Metabolic factors	Hyperglycemia is crucial, but not the single causative factor. Hyperglycemia can increase VEGF, which can alter the podocyte permeability and may cause proteinuria. Three mechanisms have been postulated: 1) Non-enzymatic glycosylation-based advanced glycation end products (AGEs) formation; 2) Activation of protein kinase C (PKC): Hyperglycemia activates PKC through DAG and oxidative stress; 3) Acceleration of Aldose reductase pathway activation.
	Hemodynamic factor	The renal hemodynamic changes of hyperperfusion and hyperfiltration result from decreased vascular resistance in both afferent and efferent arterioles, more in afferent.
3.	Inflammation	Cytokines like monocyte chemoattractant protein-1 (MCP-1) and TNF-α also have been implicated in the hemodynamic disbalance between vasodilatory and vasoconstrictive mediators, affecting intraglomerular blood flow and glomerular filtration rate.

Pathological Changes:

Pathological classification of Diabetic Nephropathy:

- **Class I:** Glomerular Basement Membrane Thickening
- **Class II:** Mesangial Expansion, subdivided into Mild (IIa) or Severe (IIb)
- **Class III:** Nodular Sclerosis (Kimmelstiel–Wilson lesions)
- **Class IV:** Advanced Diabetic Glomerulosclerosis with Tubular Lesions

As diabetic nephropathy progresses from Class II onwards, concomitant thickening of the tubular basement membrane in nonatrophic tubules becomes noticeable, becoming increasingly prominent in Classes III and IV. This thickening is most effectively visualized using PAS or silver stains.

Interstitial fibrosis and tubular atrophy (IFTA) follow the glomerular changes, eventually leading to ESKD.

Vascular Lesions: Hyalinosis of the efferent arteriole is relatively specific for diabetic nephropathy.

Diabetic nephropathy includes the thickening of the tubular basement membrane (TBM), tubular atrophy, interstitial fibrosis, arteriosclerosis, and the severity of tubulointerstitial changes, which correlate well with the progression of the disease and albuminuria. There can be mesangial matrix expansion that can be diffuse, nodular, or both. Vascular hyalinosis, glomerular capillaries (hyaline caps), and Bowman capsule (capsular drop) can also be seen. Immunofluorescent microscopy typically shows diffuse linear staining for immunoglobulin IgG along glomerular capillaries and TBM.

Complications:

Diabetics account for 45% of the new ESRD patients annually; up to a third of patients with type 2 diabetes develop ESRD and require renal replacement therapy for survival. In type 1 diabetics, 90% have diabetic retinopathy while for type 2 diabetics it varies between 40–60%. While ESKD is commonly associated with DKD, it is important to note that most patients succumb to cardiovascular illnesses and infections before requiring kidney replacement therapy. Common complications associated with DKD are shown in the figure 17.

References:

1. Kumar V, Yadav AK, Sethi J, Ghosh A, Sahay M, Prasad N, Varughese S, Parameswaran S, Gopalakrishnan N, Kaur P, Modi GK, Kamboj K, Kundu M, Sood V, Inamdar N, Jaryal A, Vikrant S, Nayak S, Singh S, Gang S, Baid-Agrawal S, Jha V. The Indian Chronic Kidney Disease (ICKD) study: baseline characteristics. Clin Kidney J. 2021 Aug 13;15(1):60-69. doi: 10.1093/ckj/sfab149. PMID: 35035937; PMCID: PMC8757418.
2. Erdogmus S, Kiremitci S, Celebi ZK, Akturk S, Duman N, Ates K, Erturk S, Nergizoglu G, Kutlay S, Sengul S, Ensari A, Keven K. Non-Diabetic Kidney Disease in Type 2 Diabetic Patients: Prevalence, Clinical Predictors and Outcomes. Kidney Blood Press Res. 2017;42(5):886-893. doi: 10.1159/000484538. Epub 2017 Nov 1. PMID: 29130997.
3. Kausik Umanath and Julia B. Lewis. Update on Diabetic Nephropathy: Core Curriculum 2018. Am J Kidney Dis. 71(6): 884-895. doi: 10.1053/ j.ajkd.2017.10.026.
4. Remuzzi G, et al. Nephropathy in Patients with Type 2 Diabetes NEJM 2002; 346: 1145-51.
5. Kussman MJ, Goldstein HH, Gleason RE. The Clinical Course of Diabetic Nephropathy. JAMA. 1976;236(16):1861–1863. doi:10.1001/jama.1976.03270170027020.

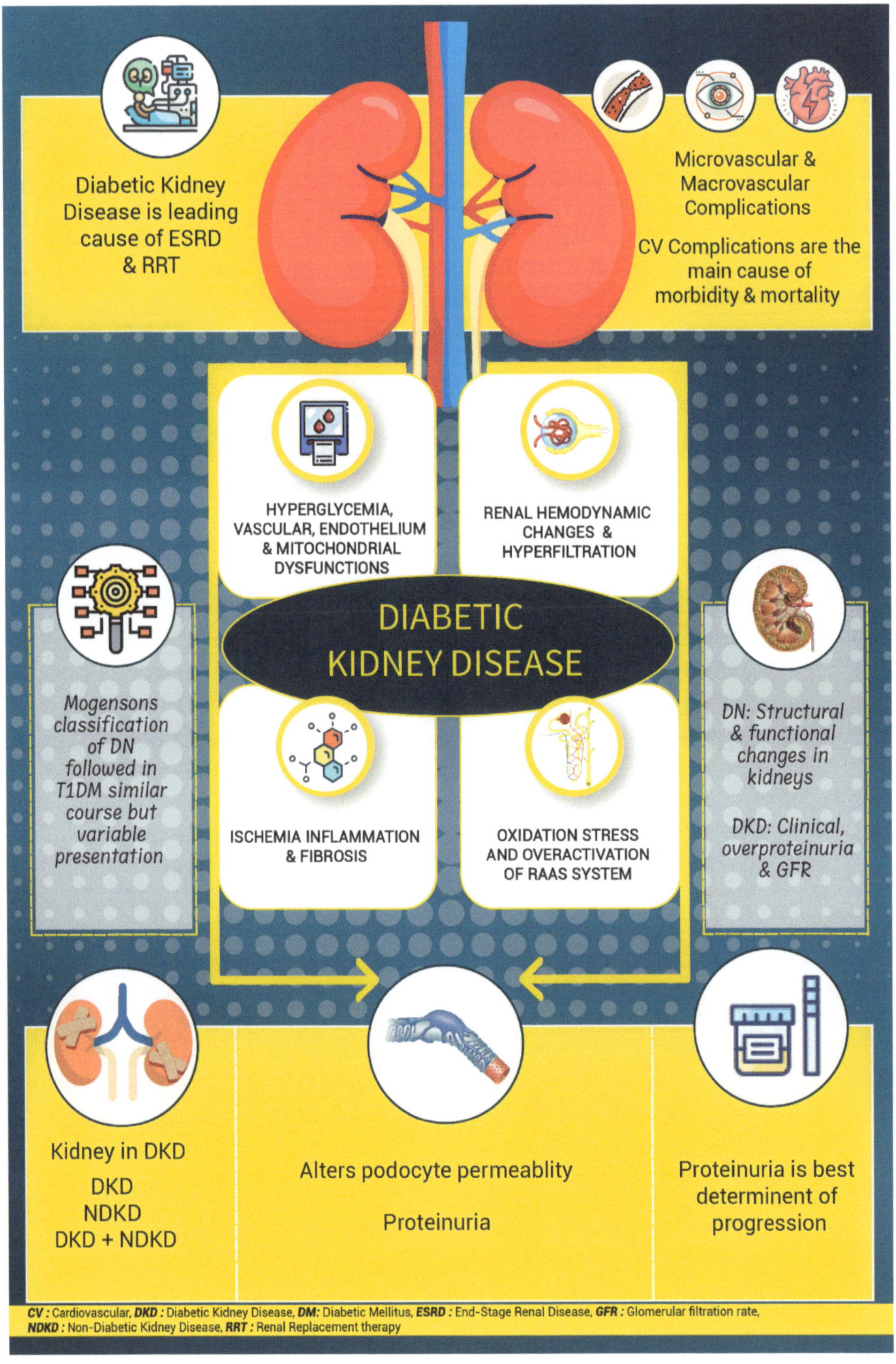
Diabetic Kidney Disease is leading cause of ESRD & RRT
Microvascular & Macrovascular Complications
CV Complications are the main cause of morbidity & mortality
HYPERGLYCEMIA, VASCULAR, ENDOTHELIUM & MITOCHONDRIAL DYSFUNCTIONS
RENAL HEMODYNAMIC CHANGES & HYPERFILTRATION
DIABETIC KIDNEY DISEASE
Mogensons classification of DN followed in T1DM similar course but variable presentation
ISCHEMIA INFLAMMATION & FIBROSIS
OXIDATION STRESS AND OVERACTIVATION OF RAAS SYSTEM
DN: Structural & functional changes in kidneys
DKD: Clinical, overproteinuria & GFR
Kidney in DKD
DKD
NDKD
DKD + NDKD
Alters podocyte permeablity
Proteinuria
Proteinuria is best determinent of progression
CV : Cardiovascular, DKD : Diabetic Kidney Disease, DM: Diabetic Mellitus, ESRD : End-Stage Renal Disease, GFR : Glomerular filtration rate,
NDKD : Non-Diabetic Kidney Disease, RRT : Renal Replacement therapy

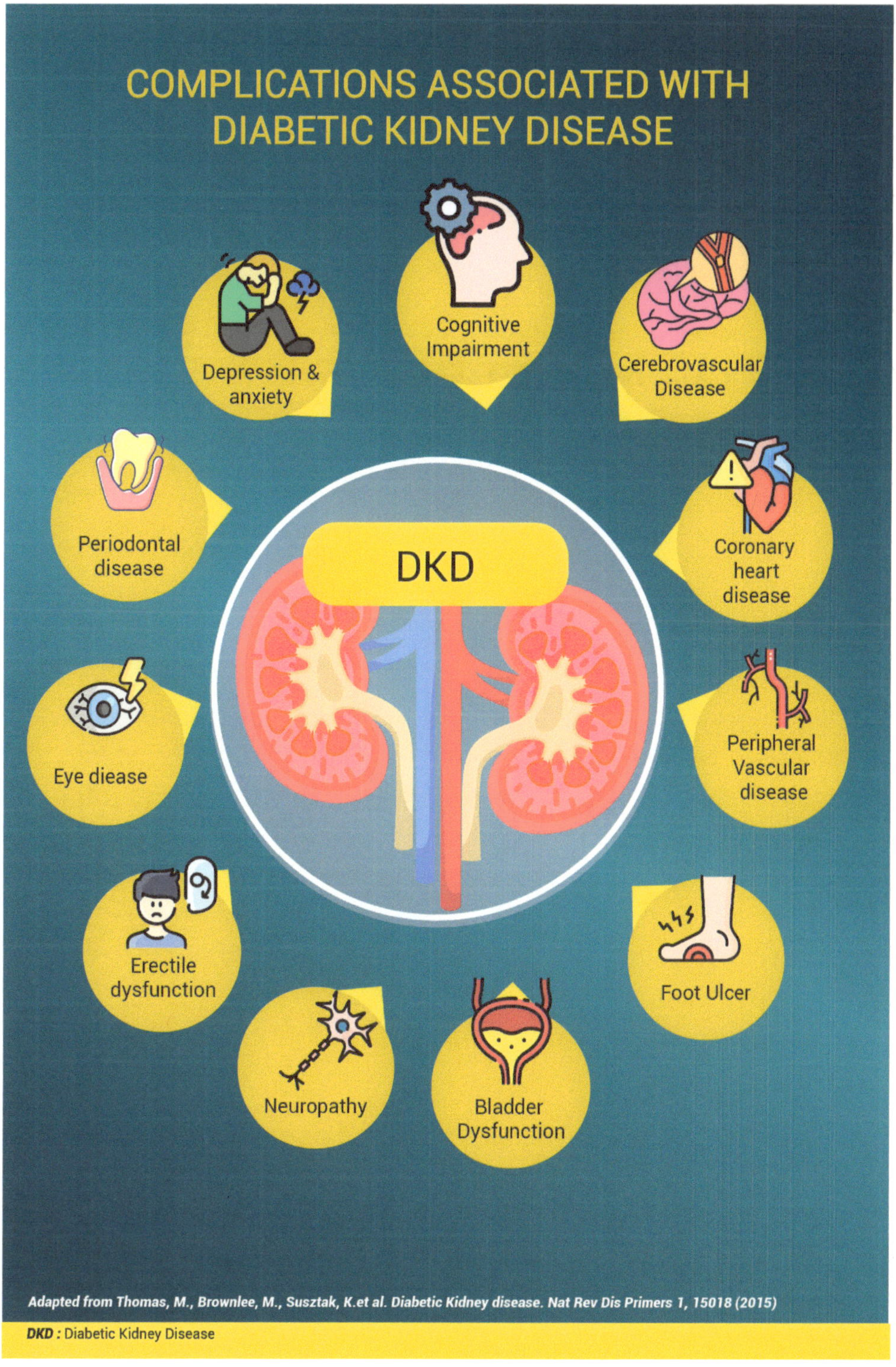

Figure 17: Shows complications associated with diabetic kidney disease.

18

DIABETIC KIDNEY DISEASE – MANAGEMENT

Gurleen Kaur, Narinder Pal Singh, Anish Kumar Gupta

Introduction:

Diabetic kidney disease (DKD) is a significant complication of diabetes mellitus and a leading cause of end-stage kidney disease (ESKD). Effective management of DKD is essential in preventing disease progression and improving patient outcomes. This chapter aims to provide a comprehensive guide for the management of DKD, focusing on the approach and incorporating the latest guidelines and drugs available.

Approach to Diabetic Kidney Disease Management:

Glycemic Control:

Glycemic control, or the management of blood glucose levels, is a critical aspect of the overall treatment strategy for individuals with DKD. American Diabetes Association (ADA) recommends an HbA1c (glycated hemoglobin) goal ranging from < 6.5% to < 8.0% in patients with diabetes and chronic kidney disease (CKD) not treated with dialysis. Glycemic control should be part of a multifactorial intervention strategy that addresses blood pressure control and cardiovascular risk and promotes the use of ACE inhibitors, angiotensin-receptor blockers, statins, and acetylsalicylic acid.

Importance of Achieving and Maintaining Optimal Glycemic Control in DKD

Studies such as the Diabetes Control and Complications Trial (DCCT) and the Action to Control Cardiovascular Risk in Diabetes (ACCORD) trial have demonstrated the long-term benefits of tight glycemic control in reducing the occurrence and risk of DKD progression. Glycemic targets should be individualized based on factors such as age, comorbidities, life expectancy, and presence of complications.

Lifestyle Modifications, Dietary Interventions, and Pharmacological Therapies for Blood Glucose Management

Non-pharmacological intervention involves:

1. Protein intake of 0.8 g protein/kg(weight)/d;
2. Sodium intake to be < 2 g of sodium per day (or < 90 mmol of sodium per day, or < 5 g of sodium chloride per day) in patients with diabetes and CKD;
3. Moderate-intensity physical activity for a cumulative duration of at least 150 minutes per week; and
4. Obesity is a major driver of DKD progression and can contribute to glomerular hyperfiltration via glomerular enlargement. Bariatric surgery might reduce the incidence and long-term progression of CKD.

In recent years, the management of DKD has witnessed significant advancements with the introduction of novel therapeutic agents such as sodium-glucose transport protein 2 (SGLT2) inhibitors and mineralocorticoid receptor antagonist (MRA).

Treatment with both metformin and a SGLT2i would be beneficial in DKD patients with eGFR > 30 ml/min per 1.73 m^2. Long-acting GLP-1 RA is the second drug of choice if the glycemic target is not achieved with metformin/SGLT-2i. MRA also has a potential role in DKD management.

SGLT2 Inhibitors:

SGLT2 inhibitors have demonstrated additional benefits beyond glucose lowering, including renoprotective effects in DKD. The mechanisms through which SGLT2 inhibitors exert their renal benefits are not entirely understood but likely involve their effects on glucose reabsorption, sodium handling, intraglomerular pressure, and oxidative stress.

Reduction in Albuminuria: Albuminuria reduction is independent of glycemic control and blood pressure lowering. The EMPA-REG OUTCOME, CANVAS, and CREDENCE trials demonstrated significant reductions in albuminuria with empagliflozin, canagliflozin, and dapagliflozin, respectively. The reduction in albuminuria is associated with a decreased risk of DKD progression, cardiovascular events, and improved renal outcomes.

Slowing the Progression of DKD: CREDENCE trial evaluated the effects of canagliflozin in patients with DKD, showing a significant reduction in the composite renal outcome of ESKD, doubling of serum creatinine, and renal or cardiovascular death.

Blood Pressure and Cardiovascular Benefits: SGLT2 inhibitors have been shown to lower blood pressure and reduce arterial stiffness, and provide cardiovascular benefits in patients with DKD. These effects are attributed to their diuretic and natriuretic actions, leading to a reduction in extracellular fluid volume and improved endothelial function.

Renin-Angiotensin-Aldosterone System (RAAS) Inhibition:

The renoprotective effects of RAAS inhibitors (ACEIs, ARBs, and MRA) in DKD: Research has shown that RAAS inhibitors prevent proteinuria, kidney fibrosis, and a slow decline of renal function, thus, playing a protective role both in the early and late stages of DKD.

Indications, dosing, and potential side effects of RAAS inhibitors: ACEi or ARB may be prescribed in patients with diabetes mellitus with significant albuminuria, with or without hypertension. Monitor for changes in blood pressure, serum creatinine, and serum potassium within 2–4 weeks of initiation or increase in the dose of an ACEi or ARB. Continue ACEi or ARB therapy unless serum creatinine rises by more than 30% within 4 weeks following initiation of treatment or an increase in dose.

Hyperkalaemia is another biochemical abnormality that needs to be closely monitored in patients on RAAS blockade. Other than in the setting of very high serum potassium levels, when medication needs to be stopped momentarily, every effort should be made to lower the levels using dietary means or through potassium-eliminating diuretics such as thiazides or loop diuretics. Additionally, renal consultation may be sought to allow the safe prescription of this medication in this setting, as well as in complex settings such as symptomatic hypotension, following AKI, or in advanced stages of DKD (eGFR < 15 ml/min per 1.73 m^2) where the risks and benefits of therapy need to be individualized. The combination of an ACEi with an ARB, or the combination of an ACEi or ARB with a direct renin inhibitor, is potentially harmful due to the increased risk of AKI and hyperkalemia.

Considerations for RAAS inhibition in specific patient populations:

- **Pregnancy:** RAAS inhibitors are generally contraindicated during pregnancy as they can harm the developing fetus.
- **Renal artery stenosis:** Patients with bilateral renal artery stenosis (narrowing of the arteries supplying to the kidneys) or stenosis in a solitary kidney may be at risk for AKI, if treated with RAAS inhibitors.
- **Hyperkalemia:** RAAS inhibitors can cause an increase in serum potassium levels (hyperkalemia), especially in patients with pre-existing kidney disease or impaired kidney function.
- **Older adults:** Elderly patients may be more susceptible to the side effects of RAAS inhibitors such as hypotension, renal impairment, or electrolyte imbalances. Close monitoring and cautious dosage adjustment are recommended.

Proteinuria Management:

Significance of proteinuria as a marker of kidney damage and a risk factor for DKD progression:

Proteinuria is a marker of kidney damage and an important risk factor for the progression of DKD as well as cardiovascular morbidity and mortality. The presence of proteinuria suggests dysfunction in the glomerular filtration barrier. A persistent (2 of 3 consecutive urine samples) elevation in urinary albumin to creatinine ratio (UACR, ≥ 30 mg/g [≥ 3 mg/mmol]) and/or a persistent reduction in eGFR (< 60 mL/min/1.73 m^2) in a person with diabetes is a hallmark of DKD. A ratio of protein to creatinine > 100 mg/mmol or a ratio of albumin to creatinine > 60 mg/mmol should be considered as thresholds to indicate a high risk of progression to end-stage renal disease.

There are three categories of albuminuria:

- Stage A1, normal to mildly increased albuminuria: < 30 mg/g (< 3 mg/mmol) UACR in the urine sample.
- Stage A2, moderately increased albuminuria, microalbuminuria: 30–300 mg/g (3–30 mg/mmol) UACR; occurring ≥ 2 times, 3–6 months apart.
- Stage A3, severely increased albuminuria, macroalbuminuria: > 300 mg/g (> 30 mg/mmol) UACR; occurring ≥ 2 times, 3–6 months apart.

Role of RAAS inhibitors and other interventions in reducing proteinuria:

Both ACEI and ARBs are effective and the drugs of choice in reducing protein excretion. Aldosterone-receptor antagonists may also be used alternatively or in combination with either an ACE inhibitor or an ARB to decrease proteinuria.

Sodium restriction, dietary protein management, and adjunctive therapies to manage proteinuria effectively:

Nonpharmacologic therapies are less effective. A protein-controlled diet (maintaining a protein intake of 0.8 g protein/kg(weight)/d), sodium intake of < 2 g of sodium per day (< 5 g of sodium chloride per day) as well as weight reduction may be beneficial in decreasing proteinuria.

Blood Pressure Control:

The control of blood pressure plays a crucial role in slowing the progression of DKD. Several clinical studies and guidelines recommend specific blood pressure targets for individuals with diabetes and DKD. The target blood pressure goal is typically less than 130/80 mmHg, or even lower in certain cases, depending on the individual's overall health and specific risk factors.

Achieving and maintaining optimal blood pressure levels often requires a combination of lifestyle modifications and medication. Lifestyle changes may include adopting a DASH diet plan, engaging in regular physical activity, managing stress, and avoiding tobacco and excessive alcohol consumption.

Medications such as angiotensin-converting enzyme (ACE) inhibitors or angiotensin receptor blockers (ARBs) are commonly prescribed to individuals with DKD to control BP and provide additional kidney protection. MRA may contribute to renal protection by decreasing intraglomerular pressure and mitigating renal injury.

Mineralocorticoid Receptor Antagonist (MRA)

Eplerenone and Finerenone are MRAs and emerging evidence suggests their potential role in DKD management, particularly in patients with albuminuria.

Reduction in Albuminuria: The BEAM and EMPHASIS-HF trials evaluated the effects of eplerenone in patients with heart failure and reduced ejection fraction, a population often affected by DKD. FIDELIO-DKD and FIGARO-DKD demonstrated reduction in proteinuria in patients of Type 2DM with CKD with the use of Finerenone. These trials showed a significant reduction in albuminuria, suggesting the renoprotective and cardioprotective potential of these drugs.

Lipid Management:

- The association between dyslipidemia and increased cardiovascular risk in DKD: Numerous epidemiological studies have consistently shown that dyslipidemia is a significant risk factor for cardiovascular disease (CVD) in DKD.

- Lifestyle modifications and pharmacological interventions (e.g., statins) for lipid management:
- Lifestyle modifications and pharmacological interventions targeting dyslipidemia have shown cardiovascular benefits in DKD. Clinical trials, such as the Collaborative Atorvastatin Diabetes Study (CARDS) and the Study of Heart and Renal Protection (SHARP), have demonstrated the efficacy of statin therapy in reducing cardiovascular events and mortality in DKD patients with dyslipidemia. ADA recommends lipid-lowering therapy with statins in individuals with diabetes, who are over 40 years of age or have additional cardiovascular risk factors, including DKD.
- Individualized treatment goals based on cardiovascular risk factors:

Initiate statin therapy for patients with stage 4 CKD and titrating the dose to achieve an LDL cholesterol level < 2.0 mmol/L and a ratio of total cholesterol to HDL cholesterol < 4.0 mmol/L.

Serial creatinine kinase and alanine aminotransferase should be measured every 3 months for patients with stage 4 chronic kidney disease, who are taking a moderate to high dose of statin (≥ 40 mg/d of simvastatin or atorvastatin, or an equivalent dose of another statin).

Management of Coexisting Conditions:

- Consideration of comorbidities commonly seen in patients with DKD (e.g., hypertension, cardiovascular disease).
- Collaborative care with other healthcare professionals to optimize overall management.
- Integration of multidisciplinary approaches for improved patient outcomes.

Monitoring and Follow-up:

Importance of regular monitoring of renal function, blood pressure, glycemic control, and proteinuria in DKD:

By regularly monitoring these parameters, healthcare providers can detect changes in kidney function, blood pressure, glycemic control, and proteinuria in DKD patients. Early identification of deviations from target values allows for timely interventions and adjustments to treatment plans, aiming to slow the progression of DKD, prevent complications such as hypoglycemia, and improve long-term outcomes. Additionally, patient education regarding self-monitoring and understanding the significance of these parameters empowers individuals to actively participate in their own care and make necessary lifestyle modifications under medical guidance.

Recommended Frequency of Follow-up Visits and Necessary Laboratory Tests:

Glycemic monitoring twice per year (up to 4 times per year if not achieving target or for change in therapy) using hemoglobin A1c (HbA1c) in patients with diabetes and CKD G1–G3b is highly reliable. However, in CKD G4–G5, including treatment by dialysis or kidney transplant, HbA1C offers low reliability, while the use of glucose management indicator (GMI) such as continuous glucose monitoring (CGM) and self-monitoring of blood glucose (SMBG) are highly reliable.

Monitoring proteinuria through urine albumin-to-creatinine ratio (ACR) or protein-to-creatinine ratio (PCR) measurements provides valuable information about kidney damage and the efficacy of treatment.

Monitoring renal function, typically assessed by measuring serum creatinine and eGFR, helps evaluate the progression of DKD.

Strategies for Early Identification and Intervention in Disease Progression:

Implement regular screening protocols for individuals with diabetes, especially those at higher risk for DKD, such as those with long-standing diabetes, poor glycemic control, hypertension, or a family history of kidney disease.

Timely interventions, including glycemic control, BP management, reduction of proteinuria, lipid management, exercise, smoking cessation, and dietary modifications are vital in preserving kidney function, reducing the risk of complications, and improving long-term outcomes for individuals with DKD.

Implement a multidisciplinary approach to DKD management, involving healthcare providers such as endocrinologists, nephrologists, dietitians, and diabetes educators. This ensures comprehensive assessment, individualized treatment plans, and regular follow-up visits to monitor kidney function, blood pressure, glycemic control, and proteinuria.

Educate patients about the importance of regular screenings, self-monitoring of blood glucose, BP control, lifestyle modifications, and adherence to medications. Emphasize the significance of early identification and intervention in preventing DKD progression. Encourage patients to report any symptoms, such as increased thirst, frequent urination, fatigue, or swelling.

Table 18.1: Algorithm for the Management of Diabetic Kidney Disease

Step 1: Diagnosis of Diabetic Kidney Disease
• Confirm the diagnosis of diabetes mellitus based on clinical criteria and laboratory tests (e.g., fasting glucose, oral glucose tolerance test, HbA1c). • Assess for the presence of kidney disease by measuring UACR and eGFR using serum creatinine-based equations. • Confirm the persistence of albuminuria and reduced eGFR on at least 2 occasions, at least 3 months apart.

Step 2: Assess Cardiovascular Risk Factors and Comorbidities • Evaluate and manage CV risk factors: hypertension, dyslipidemia, obesity, smoking, and sedentary lifestyle. • Identify and address comorbid conditions: CVD, retinopathy, neuropathy, and peripheral vascular disease.
Step 3: Optimize Glycemic Control • Set individualized glycemic targets based on patient characteristics (age, comorbidities, hypoglycemia risk). • Encourage lifestyle modifications: dietary changes, regular physical activity, and weight management. • Initiate or adjust antidiabetic medications, considering the efficacy, safety, and patient preferences.
Step 4: Manage Hypertension • Aim for BP control below 130/80 mmHg in patients with DKD. • Implement lifestyle modifications: sodium restriction, weight reduction, regular exercise, and moderation of alcohol consumption. • Initiate antihypertensive medications, preferably ACEIs or ARBs, as the first-line agents for BP management. • Titrate the dose or add additional antihypertensive agents to achieve the target BP.
Step 5: Proteinuria Management • Initiate or optimize the use of ACEIs/ARBs to reduce proteinuria, even in the absence of hypertension. • Consider the use of other antiproteinuric agents such as direct renin inhibitors (e.g., aliskiren) or MRA (e.g., spironolactone, eplerenone), guided by individual patient characteristics and response to treatment. • Monitor UACR regularly to assess the response to therapy and adjust medications accordingly.
Step 6: Lipid Management • Screen and manage dyslipidemia according to established guidelines. • Encourage lifestyle modifications: heart-healthy diet, regular exercise, weight management, and smoking cessation. • Initiate statin therapy based on an individual patient's CV risk profile and lipid levels.

Step 7: Coordinated Care and Monitoring • Collaborate with other healthcare professionals, including endocrinologists, cardiologists, nephrologists, and dietitians, to provide comprehensive care for DKD patients. • Schedule regular follow-ups to monitor glycemic control, BP, kidney function, proteinuria, and lipid profile. • Educate patients about the importance of medication adherence, lifestyle modifications, and self-monitoring of blood glucose.
Step 8: Referral for Advanced Management • Consider referral to a nephrologist for further evaluation and management in cases of rapidly declining kidney function, uncontrolled hypertension, significant proteinuria, or suspected nondiabetic kidney disease.
[**Note:** This algorithm serves as a general guide and should be adapted to individual patient characteristics and local clinical practice guidelines. Regular updates should be made based on emerging evidence and advancements in the management of DKD.]

References:

1. KDIGO 2020 Clinical Practice Guideline for Diabetes Management in Chronic Kidney Disease. Kidney International Supplements. 2020;10(1):e13-e102. Available from: https://kdigo.org/guidelines/diabetes-management-in-ckd/.
2. Perkovic V, Jardine MJ, Neal B, et al. Canagliflozin and renal outcomes in type 2 diabetes and nephropathy. N Engl J Med. 2019;380(24):2295-2306.
3. Heerspink HJL, Stefánsson BV, Correa-Rotter R, et al. Dapagliflozin in patients with chronic kidney disease. N Engl J Med. 2020;383(15):1436-1446.
4. Cherney DZI, Zinman B, Inzucchi SE, et al. Effects of empagliflozin on the urinary albumin-to-creatinine ratio in patients with type 2 diabetes and established cardiovascular disease: An exploratory analysis from the EMPA-REG OUTCOME randomised, placebo-controlled trial. Lancet Diabetes Endocrinol. 2017;5(8):610-621.

5. Bakris GL, Agarwal R, Anker SD, et al. Effect of finerenone on chronic kidney disease outcomes in type 2 diabetes. N Engl J Med. 2020;383(23):2219-2229.
6. De Boer IH, Cherney DZ, Lund SS, et al. Canagliflozin and renal outcomes in type 2 diabetes: Results from the CANVAS Program randomised clinical trials. Lancet Diabetes Endocrinol. 2018;6(9):691-704.
7. Alicic RZ, Johnson EJ, Tuttle KR. SGLT2 inhibitors: nephroprotective and cardioprotective agents in type 2 diabetes mellitus. Curr Opin Nephrol Hypertens. 2021;30(4):470-478.

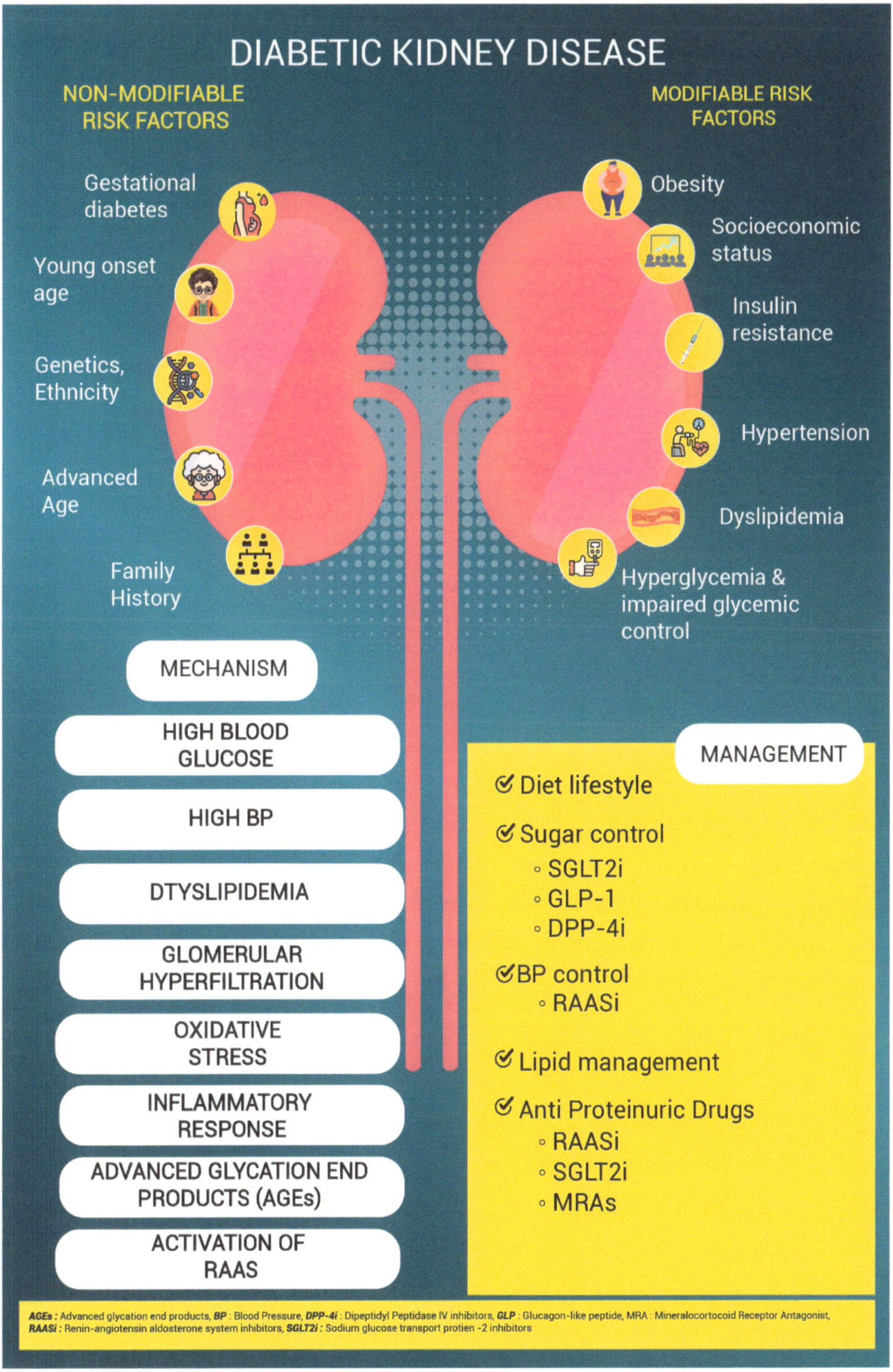
DIABETIC KIDNEY DISEASE
NON-MODIFIABLE RISK FACTORS
Gestational diabetes
Young onset age
Genetics, Ethnicity
Advanced Age
Family History
MODIFIABLE RISK FACTORS
Obesity
Socioeconomic status
Insulin resistance
Hypertension
Dyslipidemia
Hyperglycemia & impaired glycemic control
MECHANISM
HIGH BLOOD GLUCOSE
HIGH BP
DTYSLIPIDEMIA
GLOMERULAR HYPERFILTRATION
OXIDATIVE STRESS
INFLAMMATORY RESPONSE
ADVANCED GLYCATION END PRODUCTS (AGEs)
ACTIVATION OF RAAS
MANAGEMENT
Diet lifestyle
Sugar control
SGLT2i
GLP-1
DPP-4i
BP control
RAASi
Lipid management
Anti Proteinuric Drugs
RAASi
SGLT2i
MRAs
AGEs : Advanced glycation end products, BP : Blood Pressure, DPP-4i : Dipeptidyl Peptidase IV inhibitors, GLP : Glucagon-like peptide, MRA : Mineralocortocoid Receptor Antagonist,
RAASi : Renin-angiotensin aldosterone system inhibitors, SGLT2i : Sodium glucose transport protien -2 inhibitors

19

PULMONARY RENAL SYNDROME

Sujit Suren, Sreejith Parameswaran

Introduction:

The term "pulmonary renal syndrome" describes a clinical syndrome that is characterized by the presence of both diffuse alveolar hemorrhage and glomerulonephritis. It encompasses a group of diseases with distinctive clinical and radiological manifestations, as well as different pathophysiological processes. Pulmonary renal syndrome is a potentially life-threatening condition, defined as the combination of diffuse alveolar hemorrhage (DAH) and rapidly progressive glomerulonephritis (RPGN). It was first described by Goodpasture in 1919.

Pulmonary renal syndrome can be caused by many systemic autoimmune conditions with anti-neutrophil cytoplasm antibodies (ANCA)-associated vasculitis accounting for most cases.

Epidemiology and Pathophysiology:

The pulmonary renal syndrome is associated with several diseases, which can broadly be divided into ANCA-associated vasculitis (AAV) and immune complex-mediated vasculitis. AAV is the most common underlying cause, accounting for 70% of the cases. Anti-GBM disease, an immune complex vasculitis, accounts for up to 20% of the cases, with the remaining 10% of the cases attributable to less common conditions.

Classification of pulmonary renal syndromes into groups based on the underlying pathological process.

I. ANCA-associated vasculitis-Granulomatosis with polyangiitis (GPA), Microscopic polyangiitis (MPA), Eosinophilic granulomatosis with polyangiitis (EGPA).

II. Anti-glomerular basement membrane (GBM) disease.

III. Anti-neutrophil cytoplasm antibodies ANCA-negative vasculitis-IgA disease, Cryoglobulinaemia.

IV. Autoimmune connective tissue disease – Systemic lupus erythematosus (SLE), Polymyositis, Mixed connective tissue disease (MCTD), Systemic sclerosis.

V. Drug-induced vasculitis Cocaine, D-penicillamine.

ANCA: anti-neutrophil cytoplasm antibodies; GBM: glomerular basement membrane.

The specific pathological process depends on the underlying disease. In the majority of pulmonary renal syndromes, small vessel vasculitis affecting the alveoli and glomeruli is responsible. The inflammation arises through neutrophilic infiltration of the vascular endothelium, which affects the arterioles, venules, and capillaries, resulting in vessel wall destruction and necrosis. Necrosis can be fibrinoid or granulomatous in nature.

In the lung, in addition to the small vessel vasculitis and resultant necrosis, a distinct process has been identified within the alveolar wall/interstitium called necrotizing pulmonary capillaritis. It can be distinguished by the marked influx of interstitial neutrophils, which are undergoing leukocytoclastic or fragmentation. Pyknotic cells and nuclear dust accumulate within the lung parenchyma as these neutrophils are constantly undergoing apoptosis. The interstitium fills with these neutrophils, edema, and fibrin thrombi, and eventually undergoes fibrinoid necrosis. The integrity of interstitial capillaries is damaged during this process, allowing the red blood cells to cross the now incompetent alveolar-capillary basement membranes, entering the interstitial space and flooding the alveoli. In the kidney, fibrinoid deposition causes crescentic inflammation in the glomerulus, where inflammatory cells infiltrate Bowman space with epithelial cell hyperplasia and fibrosis.

Clinical Features:

Clinical features vary depending on the underlying etiology. However, DAH and glomerulonephritis are the unifying features. Hemoptysis is the most common manifestation of DAH, but it is absent in up to 30% of the cases. Other common symptoms include cough, dyspnea, and low-grade pyrexia. Acute respiratory failure requiring intubation occurs in 50% of the cases. DAH is more common in GPA (42% of cases), compared with MPA (29%) and EGPA (3%).

Glomerulonephritis should be suspected when hematuria, proteinuria, and active urinary sediment are seen. It can worsen very fast to a rapidly progressive renal failure, requiring renal replacement therapy.

Clinical features of pulmonary renal syndrome are nonspecific and, thus, a high index of suspicion is required. The pulmonary renal syndrome should be considered in those with bilateral pulmonary infiltrates, falling hemoglobin levels, and renal failure. Symptoms of underlying diseases like unexplained sinusitis, mononeuritis multiplex, polyarthralgia, asthma, pericarditis, cerebral ischemia, purpura, and congestive heart failure can also accompany.

Diagnostic Evaluation:

Establishing the diagnosis promptly is crucial as respiratory failure and end-stage renal failure can occur rapidly.

Radiology:

Chest radiograph typically demonstrates bilateral airspace opacities, with or without air bronchograms. These are typically in a perihilar distribution, predominantly affecting the middle and lower zones; however, the chest radiograph can be normal in up to 25% of the cases. The typical features of chest computed tomography (CT) are mixed areas of consolidation and ground glass. When interlobular septal thickening is present, it is usually coarse. Cavitating nodules/masses can be seen in GPA, while airway wall thickening and small non-cavitating nodules are common in EGPA. Multiphase CT angiography can help localize an active bleeding source in large-volume hemoptysis and define the bronchial artery anatomy.

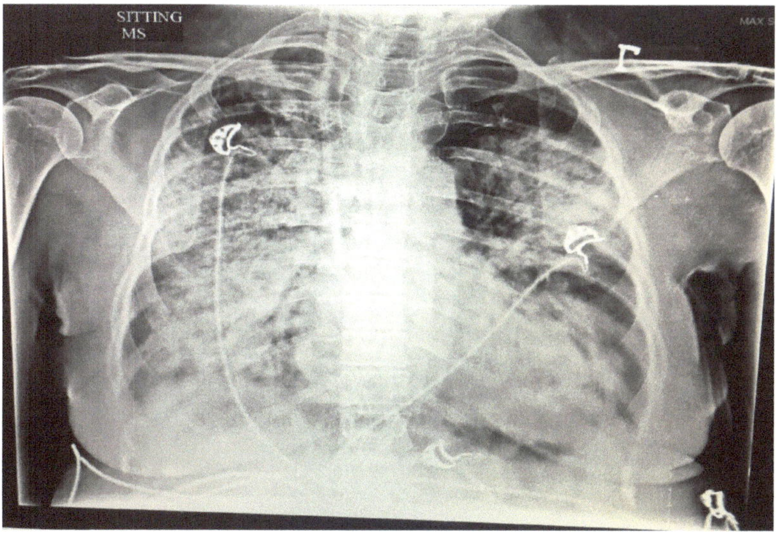

Figure 19.1: Chest X-ray of a Patient with Pulmonary Hemorrhage

Bronchoscopy:

Bronchoscopy can be useful in diagnosing DAH. Bronchoalveolar lavage (BAL) fluid shows increasing blood-stained aspirates in sequential samples (Figure 19.2) with hemosiderin-laden macrophages on cytology. Transbronchial biopsy may be considered for histology but often an alternate site, such as renal biopsy, may confer a lower risk. Bronchoscopy can also be valuable in excluding infection.

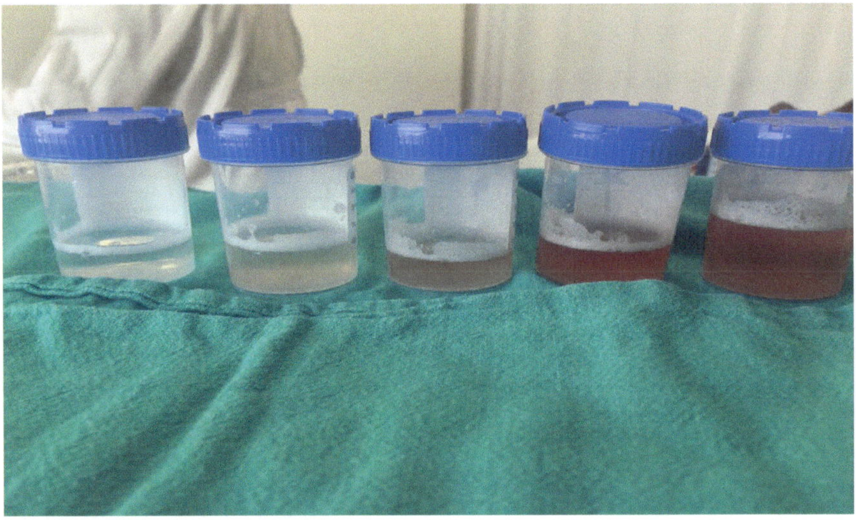

Figure 19.2: Sequential BAL in a Case of Pulmonary Hemorrhage

Laboratory Testing:

A reduction in serum hemoglobin and hematocrit should raise suspicion for DAH, especially when acute in nature. Typically, normochromic normocytic anemia is seen, which is out of proportion to renal failure. Elevated urea and creatinine can signify acute renal injury suggestive of glomerulonephritis. Abnormal platelet count and coagulation studies may indicate bleeding diathesis as a cause of DAH. Peripheral eosinophilia is suggestive of EGPA. Coombs-negative hemolytic anemia with schistocytes or fragmented red cells with thrombocytopenia is suggestive of TTP. Respiratory viral and atypical bacteria PCR along with blood cultures should be evaluated to assess the infectious process.

Urine analysis is essential; proteinuria is always present but rarely in the nephrotic range. Urinalysis can demonstrate dysmorphic red cells, red cell casts, and fragments. Proteinuria is more common than hematuria; however, when both are present, it is highly indicative of glomerulonephritis.

Serology tests are useful in determining the cause.

ANCA-associated vasculitis:

1. Granulomatosis with polyangiitis (GPA) – ANCA positive at 90%; PR3 positive at 75%.
2. Microscopic polyangiitis (MPA) – ANCA positive in 60%; MPO positive in 65%.
3. Eosinophilic granulomatosis with polyangiitis (EGPA) – ANCA positive 30–70%; PR3 positive in 5%, MPO positive in 45%.

Anti-GBM disease Anti-GBM antibodies are 95–100% sensitive and 90–100% specific.

ANCA-negative vasculitis:

1. IgA disease – Nil specific
2. Cryoglobulinaemia – Hepatitis serology; serum cryoglobulins

Autoimmune connective tissue disease:

1. Systemic lupus erythematosus (SLE) – Anti-dsDNA, anti-Smith, anti-C1q antibodies.
2. Antiphospholipid syndrome (APS) – Anti-cardiolipin, lupus anticoagulant antibodies.
3. Rheumatoid arthritis (RA) – Rheumatoid factor, anti-cyclic citrullinated peptides.

4. Mixed connective tissue disease (MCTD) – Anti-RNP.
5. Polymyositis and dermatomyositis – Anti-Jo1, anti-Ro antibodies.
6. Systemic sclerosis – Anti-centromere, anti-Scl70.

ANCA: anti-neutrophil cytoplasm antibodies; GBM: glomerular basement membrane; PR3: proteinase-3; MPO: myeloperoxidase; dsDNA: double-stranded DNA.

Renal Pathology:

There are several variations in renal pathological findings depending on the etiology. Renal biopsies typically demonstrate a focal segmental necrotic glomerulonephritis in anti-GBM and AAV disease, where crescent formation with normal glomerular segments intermixed is seen in > 90% of the cases. Necrosis and crescent formation are typically absent; if crescent formation is present, it typically affects less than 50% of the glomerulus. Furthermore, renal histology can be divided into three immunohistochemical patterns: type 1 antibody-mediated as seen in the anti-GBM disease, type 2 immune complex-mediated as seen in SLE, and type 3 pauci-immune as seen in AAV.

In addition, specific findings can indicate the underlying etiology. Anti-GBM disease can be confirmed by linear deposition of IgG on renal biopsy. Granulomas with necrosis on lung biopsy indicate GPA. Necrotizing vasculitis, eosinophilic tissue infiltration, and extravascular granulomas on lung biopsy indicate EGPA. Lupus nephritis has six phenotypes, generally demonstrating immunofluorescence, strongly positive for immunoglobulins, and complement in a granular pattern. In AAV, immunofluorescence typically reveals minimal antibody deposits, hence, the term pauci-immune.

General Management:

Treatment should be initiated promptly as mortality and morbidity in pulmonary renal syndrome are high. Treatment depends on the underlying cause; however, it is often a combination of glucocorticoid and immunosuppressant. Plasmapheresis can be considered in certain groups. Treatment typically consists of an induction phase followed by a maintenance phase, as shown in Figure 19.3. Optimal treatment is based on the underlying disease process; hence, it is best considered on an individual basis. The initial treatment typically involves a combination of glucocorticoids, immunosuppressive agents (cyclophosphamide, mycophenolate mofetil, azathioprine, Rituximab, methotrexate), and plasmapheresis. Supportive measures such as transfusion, mechanical ventilation, and renal replacement therapy are implemented when needed. The broad-spectrum antimicrobial cover is often given until further workup is performed to exclude infection.

The mechanism of action of plasmapheresis is largely unknown; it likely reduces ANCA titers and removes a large fraction of pro-inflammatory cytokines, complement, and coagulation factors from the systemic circulation. The American College of Rheumatology recommends against the use of plasmapheresis in DAH; however, they suggest consideration in those who are critically ill, have failed to respond to the recommended remission induction therapies, or for those at a higher risk of progression to end-stage renal disease.

Conclusion:

Clinical vigilance is key as the symptom complex is often non-specific. The diversity of these conditions involves a wide range of severity of presentation from the general outpatient clinic to the ICU setting. Often, multidisciplinary input is required.

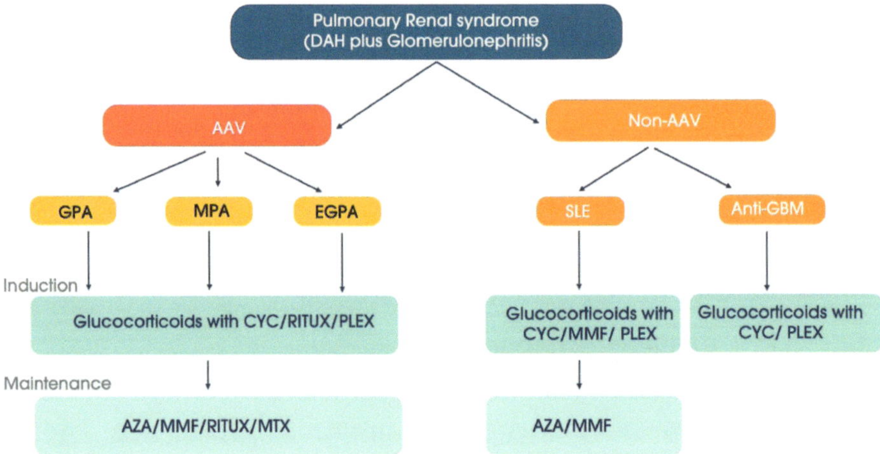

Figure 19.3: Management of Pulmonary Renal Syndrome

DAH: diffuse alveolar hemorrhage; AAV: ANCA-associated vasculitis; ANCA: anti-neutrophil cytoplasm antibodies; GPA: granulomatosis with polyangiitis; MPA: microscopic polyangiitis; EGPA: eosinophilic granulomatosis with polyangiitis; GBM: glomerular basement membrane; SLE: systemic lupus erythematosus; CYC: cyclophosphamide; PLEX: plasmapheresis; MMF: mycophenolate mofetil; AZA: azathioprine; MTX: methotrexate.

Appropriate management of these conditions includes early and accurate diagnosis, exclusion of infection, close monitoring, and specialized immunosuppressive treatment, coupled with plasma exchange in selected cases.

References:

1. Goodpasture EW. The significance of certain pulmonary lesions in relation to the etiology of influenza. Am J Med Sci 1919; 158: 863.
2. West SC, Arulkumaran N, Ind PW, et al. Pulmonary-renal syndrome: a life threatening but treatable condition. Postgrad Med J 2013; 89: 274,Äì283.
3. N. Boyle et al. Breathe 2022; 18: 220208, DOI: 10.1183/20734735.0208-2022.

4. McCabe C, Jones Q, Nikolopoulou A, et al. Pulmonary-renal syndromes: an update for respiratory physicians. Respir Med 2011; 105: 1413‚Äì1421.
5. Papiris SA, Manali ED, Kalomenidis I, et al. Bench-to-bedside review: pulmonary‚Äìrenal syndromes ‚Äì an update for the intensivist. Crit Care 2007; 11: 213.
6. Franks TJ, Koss MN. Pulmonary capillaritis. Curr Opin Pulm Med 2000; 6: 430‚Äì435.
7. Lee RW, D‚ÄôCruz DP. Pulmonary renal vasculitis syndromes. Autoimmun Rev 2010; 9: 657‚Äì660.
8. Collard HR, Schwarz MI. Diffuse alveolar hemorrhage. Clin Chest Med 2004; 25: 583‚Äì592.
9. Mark E, Ramirez J. Pulmonary capillaritis and hemorrhage in patients with systemic vasculitis. Arch PatholLab Med 1985; 109: 413‚Äì418.
10. Chung SA, Langford CA, Maz M, et al. 2021 American College of Rheumatology/Vasculitis Foundation guideline for the management of antineutrophil cytoplasmic antibody-associated vasculitis. Arthritis Rheumatol 2021; 73: 1366‚Äì1383.

PULMONARY RENAL SYNDROME

Definition

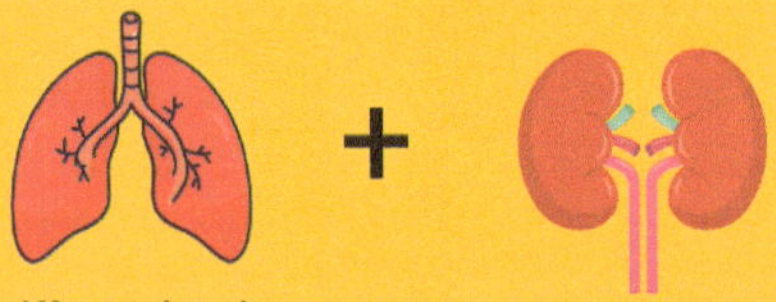

Diffuse alveolar hemorrhage + Glomerulonephritis

Presentation

Pulmonary and renal manifestations can occur weeks apart

- Cough
- Dyspnea
- Fever
- Hematuria
- Hemoptysis
- Peripheral edema
- Disease-specific symptomatology

DIFFERENTIAL DIAGNOSIS FOR PULMONARY RENAL SYNDROME

Pauci-Immune

- ***ANCA-positive vasculitis***
  - Eosinophilic granulomatosis with polyangiitis
  - Granulomatosis with polyangiitis
  - Microscopic polyangiitis
- ***ANCA-negative vasculitis***
  - IgA-associated vasculitis
  - Behcet disease
  - Cryoglobullinemia

Immune Complex

- ***Systemic Lupus Erythematous***
- ***Rheumatoid Arthritis***
- ***Cryoglobullinemia***

Anti-Glomerular Basement Membrane

- ***Goodpasture's Disease***

Investigations

- CBC, KFT and urinalysis (look for dysmorphic RBC, casts, proteinuria)
- Specific antibodies (ANA, ANCA, ANTI GBM Ab, APLA Ab)
- Microbiologic culture or specific staining
- Chest Xray
- Radiology
- Bronchoalveolar lavage
- Biopsy of lung, kidney or skin

Treatment

- Treatment of underlying cause
- Treatment of infection if present;
- Inflammatory causes of DAH (eg: rheumatic arthritis, SLE, ANCA ANTI GBM, are typically treated with systemic glucocorticoids, with additional immunosuppressive therapy

ANA : Antinuclear Antibody, **ANCA :** Antineutrophil cytoplasmic antibody, **ANTI GBM :** Anti-glomerular basement membrane, **APLA :** Antiphospholipid antibodies, **CBC :**Complete blood count, **DAH :** Diffuse alveolar hemorrhage, **IgA :** Immunoglobulin A, **KFT:** Kidney Function Test, **SLE :** Systemic lupus erythematosus

SECTION 6

Renal Replacement Therapy

20

HEMODIALYSIS

Garima Aggarwal, Umesh Khanna

As chronic kidney disease progresses, patients experience a gradual decline in the function of most organs; this constellation of symptoms associated with advanced kidney failure is known as Uremic Syndrome. This syndrome constitutes a myriad of functional disturbances such as anemia, mineral bone disease, inflammation, fluid overload, electrolyte disturbances, vascular calcification, cardiovascular disease, and hypertension. At this stage, the patient's survival and quality of life can only be ensured by starting the patient on renal replacement therapy (RRT) namely – Dialysis or Kidney Transplantation. Dialysis has made survival possible for millions of people throughout the world who have end-stage kidney disease (ESKD) with limited or no kidney function.

When to Start Dialysis:

In Chronic Kidney Disease (CKD)

For patients with CKD, the decision of starting chronic dialysis is taken together by the treating nephrologist and the patient. The 2015, KDOQI guidelines suggested that the decision to start dialysis should be based on uremic signs and symptoms, evidence of protein-energy wasting, and the inability to medically manage metabolic abnormalities and volume overload, and not based upon the level of kidney function.

Indications for initiating dialysis in CKD

Absolute indications:

- Uremic pericarditis or pleuritis
- Uremic encephalopathy

Other indications:

- Refractory metabolic acidosis
- Hyperkalemia
- Volume overload, not responding to diuretic management – presenting as frequent hospitalizations with refractory hypertension or pulmonary edema
- Hyperphosphatemia
- Poor nutritional status – presenting as anorexia, weight loss, or poor oral intake
- Worsening fatigue and malaise
- Cognitive impairment

In Acute Kidney Injury (AKI)

Large-scale randomized controlled trials (RCTs) have compared early versus late initiation of hemodialysis/RRT in critically ill patients with AKI (without absolute indications), with a majority of the trials not showing any difference in patient or renal outcomes.

Indications for initiating dialysis in AKI

Absolute indications:

- Hyperkalemia ($K \geq 6.5$)
- Metabolic acidosis ($pH < 7.1$)
- Uremic pericarditis or encephalopathy

- Fluid overload (in liguric or anuric patients)
- Certain poisonings – especially methanol, lithium, metformin, ethylene glycol

RRT is indicated in AKI with persistent hyperkalemia, metabolic acidosis, and volume overload, despite medical management and aggressive diuresis.

Principles of Hemodialysis

Hemodialysis performs two main functions of solute and fluid removal. Solute removal happens via two major mechanisms – diffusion and convection. Fluid removal happens via ultrafiltration.

Diffusion is defined as the movement of solutes from a higher concentration to a lower concentration via a semi-permeable membrane. This is the primary method of solute removal in hemodialysis. Diffusion of solutes from the blood into the dialysate depends on the solute concentration and molecular weight. The process relies on the interaction between the patient's blood and the dialysate liquid, facilitated by its passage through the openings present in every strand of the dialysis membrane. The concentration gradient is maximized and maintained throughout the length of the membrane by running the dialysate in a flow that is counter-current to the blood flow. Small molecules diffuse quickly, whereas larger molecules diffuse much more slowly.

There are 3 main groups of uremic solutes:

1. Small molecules (< 500 Da), which are removed during the diffusion process;
2. Middle and large molecules (500–15,000 Da); and
3. Molecules bound with proteins weighing 500 Da, which are hard to remove and the dissociation process is time-consuming (Table 20.1).

Table 20.1: Classification of Solutes Based on Molecular Weight

Molecular Weight Range of Solutes (in Daltons, Da)	Classification of Uremic Solutes
< 500	SMALL MOLECULES E.g. Urea, creatinine, phosphate, potassium
500–15,000	MIDDLE MOLECULES E.g. Vitamin B12, vancomycin, insulin, endotoxin fragments, parathyroid hormone, beta2 microglobulin
> 15,000	LARGE MOLECULES E.g. Myoglobin, erythropoietin, albumin, transferrin
Protein-bound solutes	p-cresy sulfate, homocysteine, other pro-inflammatory compounds

Convection or "solute drag" is the movement of molecules within fluids. This occurs when transmembrane pressure is applied on the blood side of the membrane forcing large amounts of plasma water through the pores of the membrane that drags solutes with it. Convection is better for the removal of middle molecules.

Ultrafiltration is plasma water forced across a semipermeable membrane by a hydrostatic pressure gradient (called transmembrane pressure – TMP), which is created by the dialysis machine. The primary purpose of ultrafiltration is the removal of excess total body water by movement of fluid from the side of high hydrostatic pressure (blood) to the side of low pressure (dialysate). The TMP (positive pressure on the blood compartment and negative pressure on the dialysate compartment) is adjusted by the dialysis machine at each session to allow for desirable fluid removal from the patient.

Hemodialysis Procedure:

Hemodialysis (HD) is a procedure in which the blood flows outside the body through vascular access via an extracorporeal circuit, and passes through a semi-permeable membrane called the dialysis membrane, which removes uremic toxins from it and is then returned to the body. In Hemodialysis, the dialysis membrane separates the blood from a solution with a specified electrolyte composition called the dialysate. Hemodialysis relies on mechanical methods to remove uremic toxins, balance fluid and electrolyte levels, and correct acid-base disturbances.

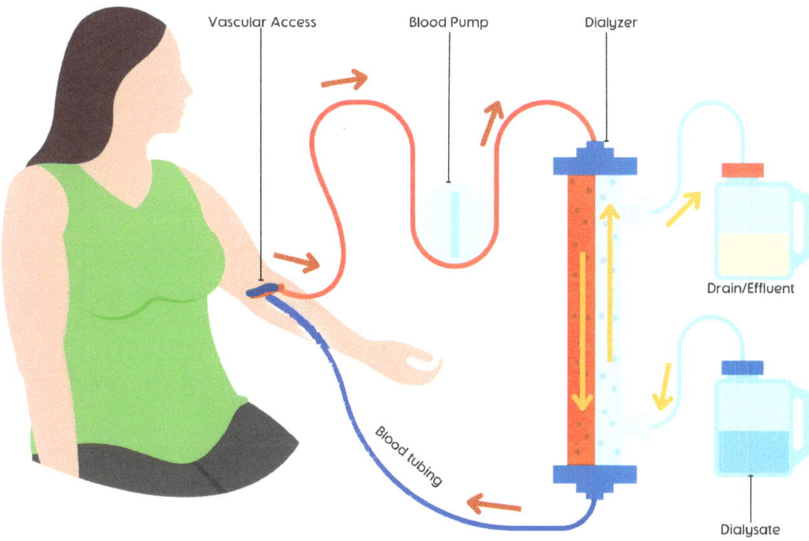

Figure 20.1: Hemodialysis Circuit

- **Blood circuit**

This consists of tubing, which begins at the vascular access; from here the blood is pumped through an inflow, "arterial" blood line, to the filter called the dialyzer. The filtered blood is returned from the dialyzer via an outflow, "venous" blood line, back to the vascular access. All the blood passing through the blood circuit is essentially venous, but "arterial" and "venous" blood lines are the traditional names for inflow and outflow lines, to and from the dialyzer, respectively. The blood circuit consists of a sampling port, infusion lines for saline and heparin, pumps, and pressure monitors.

- **Dialyzer**

The dialyzer is where the blood and the dialysis solution circuits interact. Here, the movement of fluid and solutes takes place across a semi-permeable membrane. The dialyzers currently in use are called hollow-fiber dialyzers. This dialyzer is a cylindrical module filled with hollow polymeric fibers. The hollow fiber acts as a semi-permeable membrane and is the site of diffusion and convection as each of the hollow fibers contains pores that allow the passage of molecules. The movement of solutes takes place when blood inside each hollow strand encounters the dialysate solution surrounding the strands. The solutes move based on a concentration difference, either transitioning from the blood to the dialysate or vice versa (in both directions). Blood and dialysate flows are typically run in opposite directions (counter-current) to improve clearance but can be run in the same direction (co-current) if less solute clearance is desired.

Dialysis membranes are made up of four types of biomaterials: cellulose, substituted cellulose, mixed cellulose synthetic, and pure synthetic. Pure synthetic membranes do not contain cellulose materials and are the most commonly used membranes today. They are highly biocompatible, have increased middle molecular clearance, are hydrophobic and expensive. Examples include polysulphone, polyamide, and polyacrylonitrate.

Characteristics of Dialyzers

- **Flux** – This depends on the thickness and pore sizes of the membranes. High flux membranes have larger pores and are thereby more permeable to larger molecules.

Flux is the ability of a dialyzer to remove middle or larger molecules. Most centers in India currently use low-flux dialyzers. Flux can be divided as:

- Low-flux < 10 mL/min
- Medium flux 10 to 20 mL/min
- High flux > 20 mL/min

- **Efficiency** – The efficiency of a dialyzer refers to its ability to remove small molecular solutes such as urea. This is usually denoted by the **mass transfer-area coefficient (KoA)** of urea. The KoA is related to the clearance of a dialyzer (Ko) and the surface area of the dialyzer (A). The dialyzer's efficiency depends on membrane porosity and thickness, solute size, and the flow rate of blood and dialysate. The manufacturer provides clearance values for different dialyzers at different blood flows, which can be useful to help compare performance.
- **Ultrafiltration coefficient (KUf)** – The permeability of a dialyzer to water is measured by this. The KUf is the volume of fluid (in mL/hour) transferred across the dialyzer membrane per mmHg of transmembrane pressure (TMP). A dialyzer with a low KUf would have a low permeability to water and would require a higher TMP to achieve ultrafiltration.

Dialyzer properties are all provided by the manufacturers in dialyzer specification sheets.

Dialysate Solution

The dialysate is a dilute solution of electrolytes and, sometimes, glucose. To reduce bulk and transport costs, the dialysis fluid is manufactured commercially as a concentrate and the dialysis machine mixes it with water, in defined proportions, to form the final dialysate. The commercially available concentrates are the "acid" concentrate and the "bicarbonate" concentrate. A typical dialysate contains sodium, magnesium, and chloride ions at the same concentration as in normal plasma; additionally, it also contains bicarbonate (or acetate) to buffer the pH of the solution, and potassium, calcium, and glucose in low concentrations. Sometimes a fine-tuning of the dialysate composition is performed to calibrate the treatment on the patient.

Hemodialysis Prescription:

The hemodialysis prescription for each patient has to be individualized based on their specific status at the time. The important components of HD prescription are the choice of dialyzer, dialysis session duration and frequency, blood flow rate, dialysate composition and temperature, ultrafiltration (UF), anticoagulation, and any intradialytic drugs to be administered (Table 20.2).

Table 20.2: Components of Hemodialysis Prescription

Component	
Dialyzer	• Synthetic, hollow fiber dialyzers • High flux vs low flux • Low/conventional efficiency vs high efficiency • Dialyzer surface area to be selected based on the patient's surface area. Larger patients may require larger (surface area) dialyzers.
Dialysis duration	• Usually 4 hours • Longer treatment times are used in hemodynamically unstable patients (during SLED) or when excessive ultrafiltration is desired.
Dialysis frequency	• Usually 3 times per week • 2 times per week may be suitable for some patients with residual renal function or preserved urine output • > 3 times a week maybe be desired in patients to improve solute and fluid removal.

Component	
Blood flow rate (Qb)	• 200–400 ml/min • Achievable blood flow depends on vascular access • Lower blood flows are used in hemodynamically unstable patients or when excessive solute removal is not desired (e.g. first dialysis).
Dialysate flow rate (Qd)	• Usually kept at twice the blood flow rate
Fluid removal/ Ultrafiltration	• As per weight gain from dry weight* • Should be < 10 ml/kg body weight/ hour • Higher ultrafiltration rates increase the risk of intradialytic hypotension.
Dialysate composition	• Usually standard dialysate is used (mentioned above) • In hyperkalemia – low or zero (0–1 mEq/L) potassium dialysate solutions may be used • In Hypercalcemia – a low calcium dialysate solution may be used.
Dialysate temperature	• Normal temperature ranges between 35–37°C • Low dialysate temperature is used in patients with hypotension.
Anticoagulation	• Unfractionated heparin (most common) 1000–2000 IU bolus followed by 500 IU/hour infusion • Heparin-free dialysis – the circuit is flushed with 100–200ml saline every 30–60 minutes to avoid clotting • Low molecular weight heparins • Citrate anticoagulation – a continuous infusion of isosmotic trisodium citrate into the arterial blood line and calcium infusion into the venous blood line.
Medications	• Common medications given during dialysis include erythropoietin or analogs, IV iron, and sometimes, antibiotics.

*Dry weight is the lowest tolerated post-dialysis weight at which the patient is euvolemic and has no signs or symptoms of either hypovolemia or hypervolemia.

Dialysis adequacy or dose is calculated based on the clearance of urea during dialysis, which can be readily and accurately measured. The amount of urea to be removed is usually calculated according to the patient's body size with the use of Kt/V, which relates the clearance of urea to its volume of distribution in the patient: Kt/Vurea, where 'K' is the urea clearance of the dialyzer, 't' is the duration of dialysis in minutes, and 'Vurea' is the patient's volume of urea distribution (total body water corrected for ultrafiltration).

Types of Hemodialysis Therapies:

Refer to Table 20.3

Table 20.3: Types of Hemodialysis

Type of RRT	Principle	Indications	Comments
Intermittent Therapies			
Hemodialysis (HD)	Diffusion > Convection	• Conventional dialysis	• Cheap and most commonly available
Hemofiltration (HF)	Convection	• Hemodynamic instability – Cardiovascular diseases	• Fluid is removed by the dialysis machine, replacement solution is infused intravenously
Hemodiafiltration (HDF)	Convection > Diffusion	• Hemodynamic instability – Cardiovascular diseases • Hyperphosphatemia	• Combination of hemodialysis and hemofiltration Pros • Better middle molecular clearance Cons • High cost • Low availability
Slow Low Efficiency Dialysis (SLED)	Diffusion + Convection	• Hemodynamic instability • Transition from CRRT to Intermitted HD	• Extended duration dialysis 6–18 hours

Type of RRT	Principle	Indications	Comments
Intermittent Therapies			
Continuous Therapies			
Slow Continuous Ultrafiltration (SCUF)	Ultrafiltration	• Refractory congestive heart failure • Excessive fluid overload	• Not for patients with uremia or hyperkalemia • No diffusive solute clearance
Continuous Renal Replacement Therapy (CRRT)		• Hemodynamic instability/shock • Fulminant hepatic failure • Raised intracranial pressure – e.g. Acute traumatic brain injury • Sepsis • Burns • Heart failure	• Indicated in acute kidney injury • Continuous for 24–48 hours

*Qb: Blood flow rate; **Qd: Dialysate flow rate

References:

1. Cooper BA, Branley P, Bulfone L, Collins JF, Craig JC, Fraenkel MB, et al. A randomized, controlled trial of early versus late initiation of dialysis. N Engl J Med [Internet]. 2010;363(7):609–19. Available from: http://dx.doi.org/10.1056/NEJMoa1000552.
2. KDOQI Clinical Practice Guideline for Hemodialysis Adequacy: 2015 update. National Kidney Foundation. Am J Kidney Dis. 2015;66(5).
3. UpToDate[Internet].Uptodate.com.[cited2023Jan18].Available from: https://www.uptodate.com/contents/indications-for-initiation-of-dialysis-in-chronic-kidney-disease?search=2.%09Uptodate%20Indications%20for%20initiation%20of%20dialysis%20in%20chronic%20kidney%20disease&source=search_result&selectedTitle=1~150&usage_type=default&display_rank=1.
4. Tolwani A. Continuous renal-replacement therapy for acute kidney injury. N Engl J Med [Internet]. 2012;367(26):2505–14. Available from: http://dx.doi.org/10.1056/NEJMct1206045.
5. Olczyk P, Małyszczak A, Kusztal M. Dialysis membranes: A 2018 update. Polim Med [Internet]. 2018;48(1):57–63. Available from: http://dx.doi.org/10.17219/pim/102974.
6. Daugirdas JT, Ing TS, Blake PG. Handbook of dialysis. 5th ed. Philadelphia, PA: Lippincott Williams and Wilkins; 2015.
7. A randomized, controlled trial of early versus late initiation of dialysis. Cooper BA, Branley P, et al; N Engl J Med. 2010;363(7):609.

HEMODIALYSIS

INDICATIONS

- Usually eGFR <10ml/min in CKD
- Serositis
- Pericarditis/ Pleuritis
- Very High Blood Pressure
- Refractory Acidosis
- Hyperkalemia
- Hyperphosphatemia
- Other eletrolyte disorders
- Pre emptive transplants
- Fluid overload despite maximum diuretics
- Recurrent admissions with Pulmonary edema
- Decreased urine output
- Progressive deterioration in nutritional status
- Anorexia
- Chronic Fatigue
- Coginitive impairment
- Intractable itching
- Nausea, vomiting-persistent

PRINCIPLES OF HEMODIALYSIS

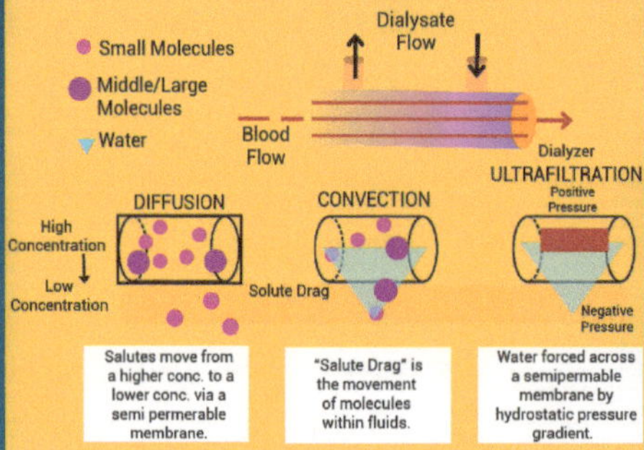

HEMODIALYSIS CIRCUIT

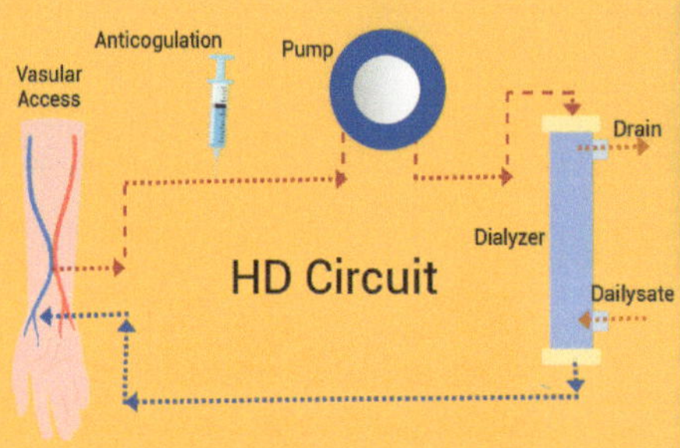

HEMODIALYSIS MODALITIES

- Intermittent Dialysis
  - Intermittent Hemodialysis (HD)
  - Hemofiltration (HF)
  - Hemodia Filtration (HDF)
  - Sustained low efficiency dialysis (SLED)
  - Extended dialy dialysis (EDD)
- Continous Dialysis
  - Continuous Renal Replacement Therapies (CRRT)
    - Slow Continuous ultrafiltration (SCUF)
    - Continuous AV/veno Venous Hemofiltration (CAVH/CVVH)
    - Continuous AV/veno-venous Hemo-dialysis (CAVHD/ CVVHD)
    - Continuous AV/veno-venous Hemodia Filtration (CAVHDF/ CVVHDF

CKD : Chronic Kidney Disease, ***Conc. :*** Concentration, ***eGFR :*** Estimated glomerular filtration rate, ***HD :*** Hemodialysis

21

VASCULAR ACCESS IN HEMODIALYSIS

Gireesh Reddy, Vinant Bhargava

Vascular access, as the name defines, is an access that is meant to convey the blood flow from the patient's body to the dialysis machine and from the dialysis machine back to the patient. As dialysis is a life-sustaining treatment for patients with End stage kidney diseases (ESKD), vascular access is the most important component of renal replacement therapy. Vascular access is also considered as the Achilles heel of ESKD patients.

Types of Vascular Access:

The three primary categories of access are native arteriovenous fistula (AVF), arteriovenous graft, and central venous catheter (CVC). The AVF technique, as originally proposed by Brescia and Cimino, continues to be the preferred option for patients requiring long-term hemodialysis. AVF is widely regarded as the most optimal means of achieving longevity with the least morbidity and mortality. As a result, guidelines from various nations strongly advocate the utilization of AVF. The utilization of CVCs has emerged as an adjuvant supplement in the management of patients undergoing hemodialysis. The internal jugular and femoral veins are the preferred sites for insertion. An ArterioVenous access is a continuous circuit, which begins at the left ventricle and ends at the right atrium, thereby completing the circuit.

In order of longevity and preference, the following dialysis access is preferred:

- Arteriovenous fistula
- ArterioVenous graft
- Tunneled Catheter

The arteriovenous fistula, being the natural conduit, has the highest duration of longevity.

AV Fistula:

The ideal time for vascular access creation is when the patient's estimated glomerular filtration rate is less than 20 ml/min/1.73m^2 or within six months of the anticipated initiation of dialysis. As the CKD progresses, the vessels become more and more rigid, thereby making it difficult for the creation of vascular access. All the possible sites for the creation of vascular access are preserved by avoiding IV cannula insertions and blood pressure measurements.

As per the guidelines outlined by the National Kidney Foundation (NKF-K/DOQI), the recommended sequence for the surgical procedure of AVF for hemodialysis (HD) is as follows: first, the forearm (radio-cephalic or distal AVF) is preferred, followed by the elbow (brachio-cephalic or proximal AVF), and finally, the arm (brachial-basilic AVF with transposition or proximal AVF).

The AVF located on the wrist is widely regarded as the optimal method for vascular access.

Once the access is created, good physical examination and monitoring/surveillance of the access continuously helps in ensuring the longevity of the access.

The goal of monitoring/surveillance is to periodically assess the integrity of this circuit and detect any abnormalities in the circuit early, thereby managing them cost-effectively in our country with challenging resources.

Once the diagnosis of dysfunctional vascular access is made, then the findings are confirmed with ultrasonography of the vascular access. Like any other blood vessel, arterial-venous access is prone to multiple complications. These include:

Management of Dysfunctional Vascular Access

There are two modalities of managing dysfunctional vascular access:

- Surgical modality
- Endovascular modality

Endovascular modality can further be divided into fluoroscopy-assisted or ultrasound-assisted. Each modality has its own advantages and disadvantages, and based on the lesion, expertise, and availability of resources, every modality is employed interchangeably. The ultimate goal of any vascular access salvage process is to restore the functionality of the access and avoid missing a dialysis session due to dysfunctional access and avoid catheter insertions. The aim is to prevent catheter-associated complications.

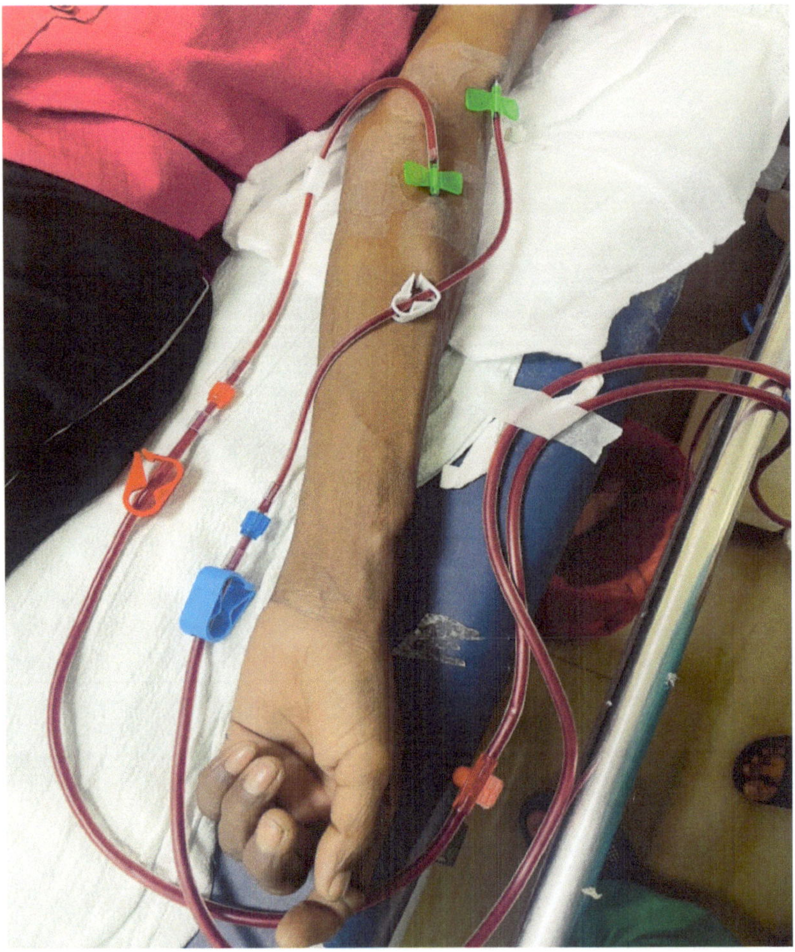

Figure 21.1: A Patient Receiving Hemodialysis via Radiocephalic Arteriovenous Fistula, Both Arterial (red color) and Venous Lines (blue color) Are Shown

Central Venous Catheter

The use of a CVC is a favorable option, particularly in cases where immediate or critical hemodialysis is necessary, either during the commencement of renal replacement therapy or when a long-term access site is non-functional. These are widely accessible, capable of being implanted in various bodily locations, and do not necessitate a maturation period, thereby enabling prompt HD.

The internal jugular and femoral veins are the preferred locations for insertion, followed by the subclavian vein as a third option. Ultrasonography is a valuable method for identifying the specific location of a target vein, while also offering valuable insights into venous pressure and the potential existence of intravascular thrombi. Incorporating its usage is thus imperative in the process of central venous catheterization.

Central venous catheters utilized for hemodialysis can be classified into two main categories: acute catheters, which are non-tunneled, and chronic catheters, which are tunneled. The selection of whether to place an acute/temporary or a chronic/permanent catheter should be predicated upon a variety of factors, including but not limited to the length of time the catheter will be utilized, the presence of bacteremia, and the overall health status of the patient.

Acute dialysis catheters refer to non-cuffed and non-tunneled catheters that are utilized for prompt vascular access. The predominant application of these medical devices is in the management of acute kidney injury, as well as for the temporary utilization in patients with impaired functionality of permanent access. The extended utilization of acute catheters is not advisable; however, it is observed in dialysis facilities where tunneled, cuffed catheters are not accessible, and the infection rates are acceptable. Polyurethane is the material of choice for a majority of acute catheters due to its favorable properties. These catheters are typically available in larger lumen sizes and are capable of delivering blood flow rates exceeding 300 mL/min, as per the guidelines established by the National Kidney Foundation's Kidney Disease Outcomes Quality Initiative (NKF-K/DOQI).

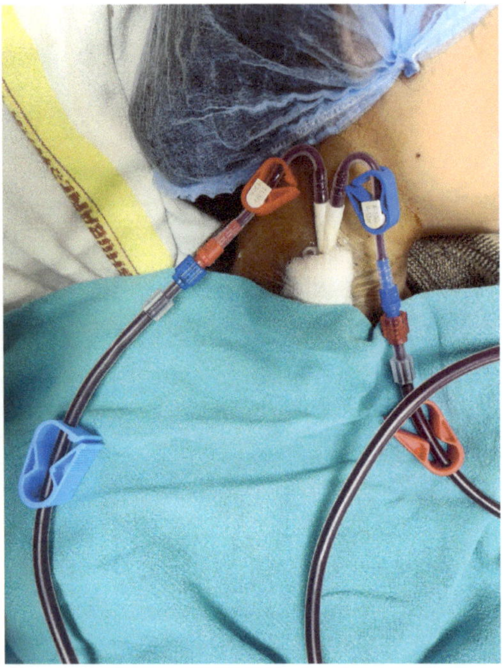

Figure 21.2: A Patient Receiving Hemodialysis via a Temporary, Non-cuffed Double Lumen Internal Jugular Vein Hemodialysis Catheter. Both Arterial (red color) and Venous Lines (blue color) Are Shown

Regarding the duration of catheter access indwelling, it is noteworthy that the acute catheter, which lacks a subcutaneous cuff, should be limited to the initial 2–3 weeks of hemodialysis. It is important to note that beyond the first week, the incidence of infection increases exponentially. Additionally, it is recommended by guidelines that temporary catheters be retained for a maximum of 5-7 days at the femoral vein.

The subcutaneous cuff of a chronic catheter is positioned in the subcutaneous tissue, adjacent to the insertion site of a tunneled catheter. The cuff facilitates the fibrous sealing of the skin entry, thereby creating a barrier against infection by impeding the migration of bacteria along the outer surface of the catheter. This design allows for prolonged use of the catheter, ranging from months to years. It is advisable to perform the placement of a cuffed, tunneled catheter expeditiously upon determination of the necessity for extended renal replacement therapy, specifically exceeding a duration of two weeks of hemodialysis.

Table 21.1: Complications of Vascular Access for Hemodialysis

ArterioVenous Access	Central Venous Catheters
Stenosis	Insertion complications include vascular injury (arterial puncture andpseudoaneurysm), hematoma, air embolism, pneumothorax, and malposition
Rupture	Infection
Thrombosis	Thrombosis
Infection	Stenosis of vessel
Aneurysmal dilatation	
Vascular steal syndrome	
Ischemic monomelic neuropathy	

References:

1. Lok CE, Huber TS, Lee T, et al. KDOQI vascular access guideline work group. KDOQI clinical practice guideline for vascular access: 2019 update. Am JKidney Dis. 2020; 75(4): S1- S164. doi:10.1053/j.ajkd.2019.12.001.
2. Murea M, Woo K. New Frontiers in vascular access practice: from standardized to patient-tailored care and shared decision making. Kidney360. 2021; 2(8): 1380-1389. doi:10.34067/KID.0002882021.
3. Allon M. Vascular Access for Hemodialysis Patients: New Data Should Guide Decision Making. Clin J Am Soc Nephrol. 2019 Jun 7;14(6):954-961. doi: 10.2215/CJN.00490119. Epub 2019 Apr 11. PMID: 30975657; PMCID: PMC6556719.
4. Brown RS. Barriers to optimal vascular access for hemodialysis. Semin Dial. 2020 Nov;33(6):457-463. doi: 10.1111/sdi.12922. Epub 2020 Oct 8. PMID: 33030298.

VASCULAR ACCESS FOR HEMODIALYSIS

ARTERIOVENOUS FISTULA (AVF)

Surgical connection made between an artery and vein

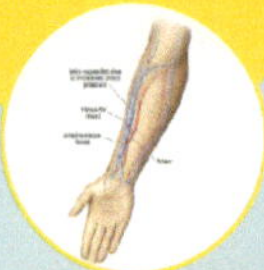

Maturation time is 4-6 weeks

Best access for longevity and has the lowest association with morbidity and mortality in chronic HD patients.

COMMON SITES

Forearm (RC AVF), elbow (BC-AVF), arm (brachial-basilic AVF with transposition

COMPLICATIONS

Immediate Complications:

At surgical site : Hematoma, bleeding, edema, acute thrombosis

Early Complications:

Stenosis, thrombosis, infection, failure to mature venous hypertension, ischemic steal syndrome

Late Complications:

Aneurysm, stenosis, thrombosis, infection, ischemic neuropathy, central venous stenosis, high cardiac output failure

ARTERIOVENOUS GRAFT

AV grafts are constructed by interposing a graft between an artery and a vein

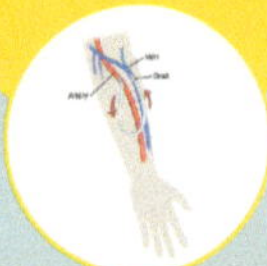

Can be used with 72hrs of placements

COMMON GRAFT SITES

Forearm (brachial artery to cephalic vein, radial artery to cephalic vein), upper arm (axillary artery to axillary vein and brachial artery to axillary vein)

Lower extremity grafts

Looped chest grafts

Axillary- axillary (necklace grafts)

COMPLICATIONS

Bleeding, seroma formation, Aneurysms, stenosis, thromboisis, steal syndrome, lesser patency rates than AVF

CENTRAL VENOUS CATHETER (CVC)

Types: Acute (non-tunneled) catheters and chronic (tunneled) catheters

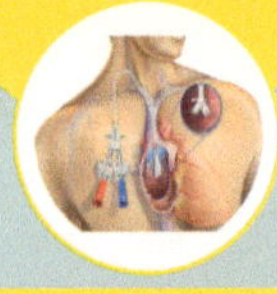

Allows immediate Hemodialysis

Used when urgent HD is required either at the time of initiation of dialysis or when permanent access becomes dysfunctional.

COMMON SITES

Internal jugular and femoral veins, and subclavian vein

COMPLICATIONS

Insertion Complications:

Vascular injury (arterial puncture, pseudoaneurysm and AVF), hematoma, air embolism, pneumothorax and malposition

Thromobosis

Central Vein Stenosis

AVF : Arteriovenous Fistula, ***CVC :*** Central Venous Catheter,

22

PERITONEAL DIALYSIS

Vineet Behera, Manisha Sahay

Introduction:

Peritoneal dialysis (PD) is a modality for renal replacement therapy (RRT) used in renal failure patients in acute settings, as well as for maintenance therapy. In this form of dialysis, the peritoneal membrane acts as the dialyzer. PD has the advantage of being more physiologic, as it is a slow and continuous process with no requirement of vascular access as compared to hemodialysis.

Principle of Peritoneal Dialysis:

The peritoneal barrier is made up of tissue cellular-interstitial matrix and blood vessels, covered with a single layer of mesothelial cells, which acts as an endogenous dialyzing membrane. The peritoneal membrane has multiple pores, including specialized water channels (Aquaporin-1), small pores of 40 to 50 Å, and large pores of 150 Å, through which the exchange of solutes, electrolytes, and water occurs.

The major principles of dialysis through the peritoneal membrane are diffusion (which is driven by concentration gradients), and convection (which is driven by osmotic or hydrostatic pressure gradients). During the diffusion process, the solute concentration gradient between the capillary blood and PD solution permits the solute to move from a higher to a lower concentration compartment. The glucose present in dialysis fluid generates ultrafiltration, which is in proportion to the overall osmotic gradient.

Peritoneal Dialysis Procedure:

The main component of peritoneal dialysis is the PD catheter, which has one end in the peritoneum (open end with multiple pores) while another end exits out of the skin to lie outside, as shown in Figure 22.1. In CAPD, nearly 2 to 2.5 liters of dialysis fluid is instilled into the peritoneal cavity for up to three to four times per day. This is done using a double bag system with a Y-set tubing system, as shown in Figure 22.1.

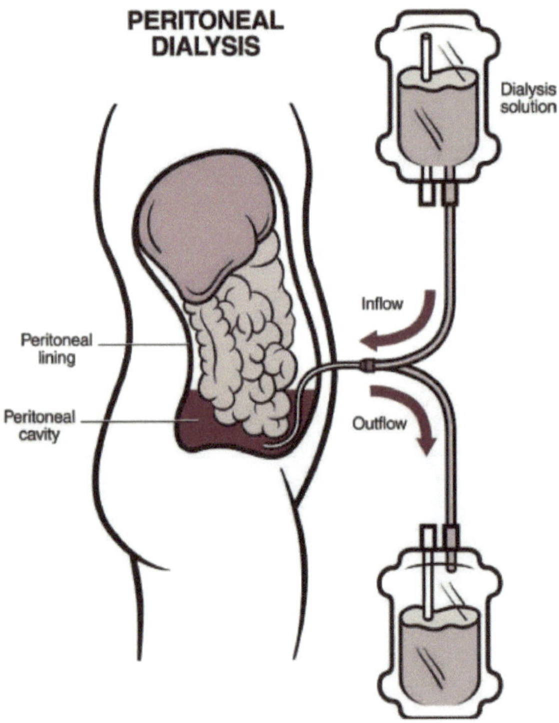

Figure 22.1: Shows the Basic Functioning of PD with the Catheter In Situ and the Double Bag System with Y-set Tubing

Peritoneal Dialysis Catheter and Insertion:

The commonly used PD catheter is a silastic or polyurethane tube, which has side pores present along its intraperitoneal part. It usually has one or two dacron cuffs along its length that allow tissue ingrowth and fibrosis in the connective tissue. This helps to fix the catheter, prevents leakage around the catheter, and prevents infection. The most commonly used types of catheters are straight, swan neck, and coiled catheters as given in Figure 22.2.

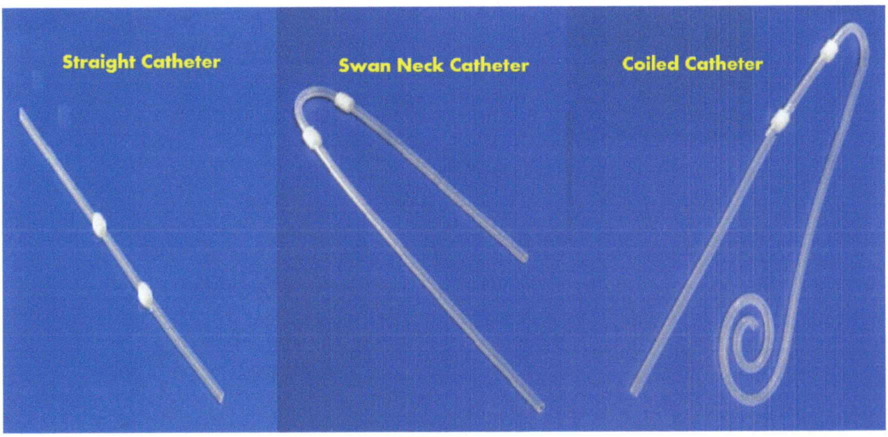

Figure 22.2: Common Types of Peritoneal Dialysis Catheters

Catheters can be inserted by a percutaneous method, laparoscopically, or via an open surgical technique as shown in Figure 22.3. Open surgical technique involves an open surgical laparotomy to expose the peritoneum, and inserting the catheter into the peritoneal cavity under vision. Laparoscopic/peritoneoscopic is a less invasive technique, which is done using laparoscopic ports or peritoneoscope as shown in Figure 22.3. The percutaneous technique is a minimally invasive technique that involves a percutaneous puncture after which the insertion is done by a modified Seldinger technique.

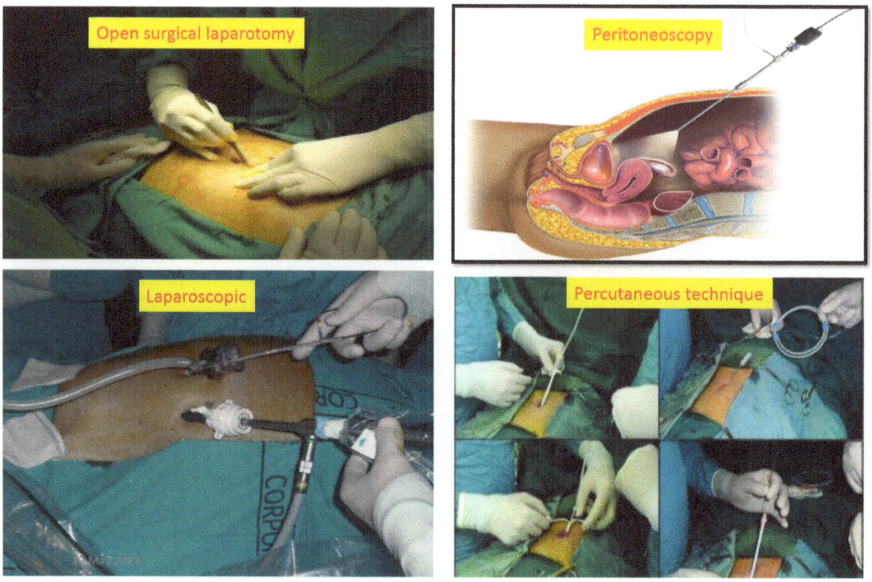

Figure 22.3: Showing Various Types of PD Catheter Insertions

Types of Peritoneal Dialysis and Prescription:

There are two broad types of PD, which are given below.

Continuous Ambulatory Peritoneal Dialysis (CAPD) – The peritoneal exchanges are performed manually 3–4 times a day, by the patient or his attendant, using 2–2.5L bags as shown in Figure 22.4. These bags contain PD fluid that is a lactate buffered, balanced salt solution containing glucose (1.5%, 2.5%, or 4.5%) as the osmotic agent (e.g. 04 x cycles of 2L PD fluid 1.5% dextrose with a dwell time of 4 hours). Other alternative osmotic agents include icodextrin, which is available as a 7.5% solution and is generally used for long dwell exchanges.

Automated Peritoneal Dialysis (APD) or Continuous Cyclical PD (CCPD) – The manual fluid exchanges, as done in CAPD, are replaced by the use of a cycler or an APD machine, with fluid bags of generally 5L size of different concentrations. It is advantageous for patients with active daytime routines, as most of the exchanges are done during nighttime.

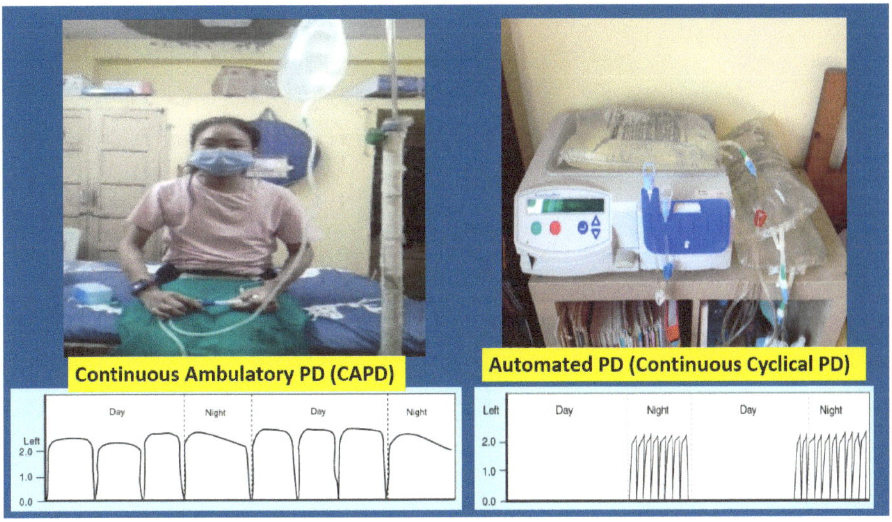

Figure 22.4: Showing a Patient Doing Continuous Ambulatory Peritoneal Dialysis (left) and a Automated Peritoneal Dialysis Machine (right)

The choice between APD and CAPD should be guided by the patient's and physician's preference, membrane transport status, and resource availability. The common prescriptions and modalities used for PD are given in Figure 22.5.

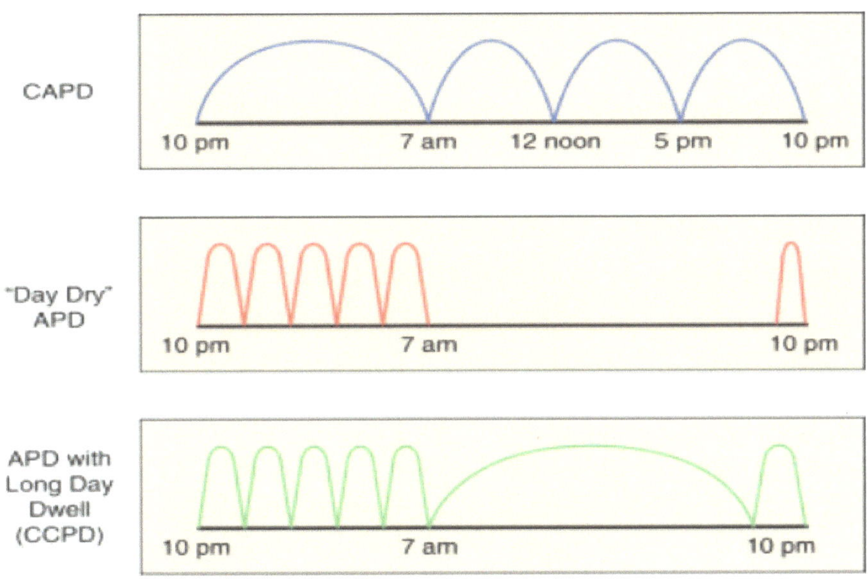

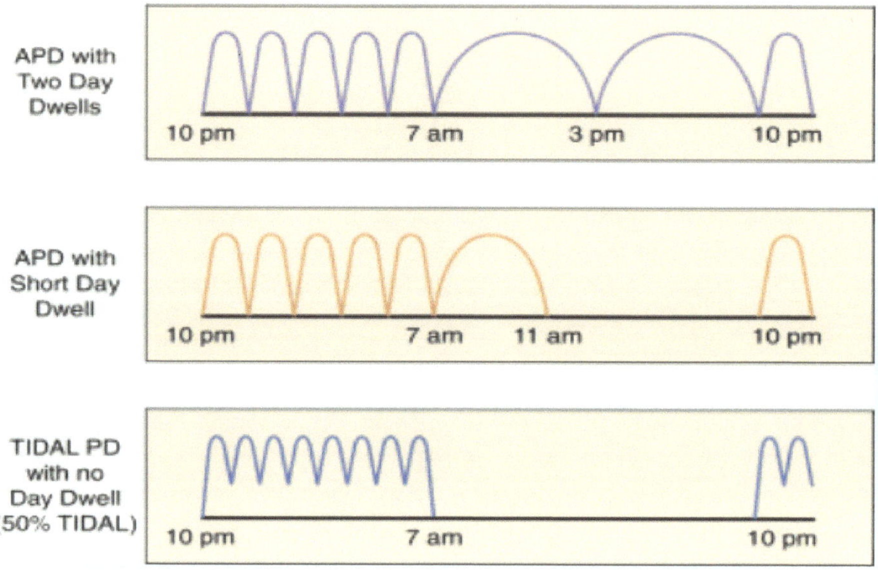

Figure 22.5: Showing the Common Peritoneal Dialysis Modalities

Acute Peritoneal Dialysis:

Peritoneal dialysis may be done in an acute setup in patients with acute kidney injury or CKD, without any vascular access. A stiff rigid polyurethane catheter (without cuff) may be inserted in the midline infra-umbilical area, or the abovementioned soft-cuffed PD catheter may also be used. Acute PD bottles of 1 L (1.5% dextrose) may be used for this process. Acute PD catheters can be used for 3–5 days, after which they may either be removed or exchanged with a regular soft PD catheter. The use of this technique has steadily declined over the years in view of better availability of hemodialysis. However, it is an important modality for children with AKI, especially in the government sector. Acute PD is also used in adults with hemodynamic instability or with bleeding diathesis in resource-limited settings.

Acute PD showed good results, especially in children as compared to adults. Data from a high-volume Indian center

(Chetan V, Sahay M, et al.; WCN 2023) compared acute PD in acute kidney injury in children (n=447) and adults (n=398), and they found that death and complete recovery were seen in 126 (28%) and 156 (34.9%) in children, while it was seen in 174 (43.3%) and 57 (14.37%) in adults, respectively ($p < 0.01$). Interestingly, the predominant etiologies in children were sepsis, acute glomerulonephritis, and acute gastroenteritis; while it was septic shock, tropical AKI, and poisoning in adults. Repeat PD was done more frequently in children vs adults (46% vs 9.8%), however, mechanical complications were more in children (19.5% vs 3%).

Complications of Peritoneal Dialysis:

Peritonitis:

PD peritonitis is diagnosed when at least 2 of these 3 features are present: typical clinical features of peritonitis that include fever, pain abdominal, and turbid PD fluid; PD fluid effluent WBC count > 100/µL (with > 50% PMN leucocytes); and a positive culture from dialysis effluent. For diagnosing peritonitis in APD, a percentage of PMN exceeding 50 is strong evidence suggestive of PD peritonitis. The common organisms causing PD peritonitis are gram-positive organisms like staphylococcus aureus, coagulase-neg staphylococcus; gram-negative organisms like pseudomonas, E coli, and other rarer organisms like fungi or mycobacteria.

Most patients present with abdominal pain during a peritonitis episode are associated with complaints of nausea, vomiting, fever, and constipation or diarrhea. Classically, the dialysate fluid will appear "cloudy" due to an increase in the cellular components as shown in Figure 22.6. Physical examination may reveal generalized abdominal tenderness.

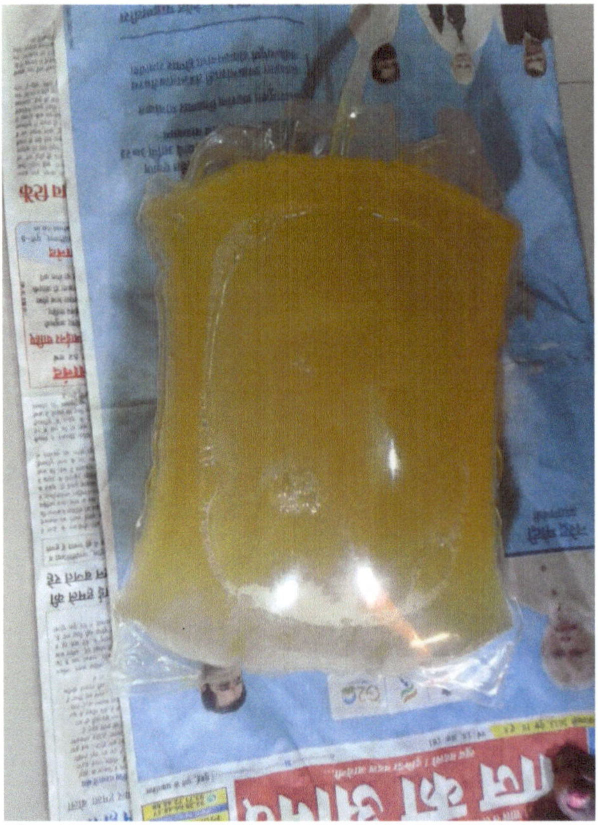

Figure 22.6: Shows Cloudy Peritoneal Dialysis Fluid in Peritonitis

The treatment of peritonitis involves early administration of antibiotics. Use of intraperitoneal (IP) antibiotics is the preferred route of administration, except in cases of severe sepsis or shock, where intravenous antibiotics are preferred. Empirical antibiotic therapy should be initiated as soon as possible, which can further be modified after the culture reports.

Gram-positive organisms are treated by a first-generation cephalosporin or vancomycin (15–30 mg/kg every 5–7 days) and gram-negative organisms by a third-generation cephalosporin (ceftazidime 1000–1500 mg daily) or an aminoglycoside (amikacin 2 mg/kg/daily). Penems (meropenem 1000 mg daily) and antifungals may be used in refractory cases. The recommended duration of therapy is 2–4 weeks, depending on the type of organism.

PD catheter should be removed for refractory peritonitis (defined by the failure of resolution of peritonitis after 5 days of appropriate antibiotics), relapsing peritonitis (infection caused by the same organism as the original infection occurring within 4 weeks), tubercular and fungal peritonitis.

Exit Site Infection:

Exit site infection is identified by erythema or discharge coming from the exit site, as seen in Figure 22.7. Staphylococcus aureus is the most prevalent infection-causing agent. A minimum of 2 weeks of treatment with gram-positive covering antibiotics is advised, with 3 weeks being advised in case of pseudomonas infections.

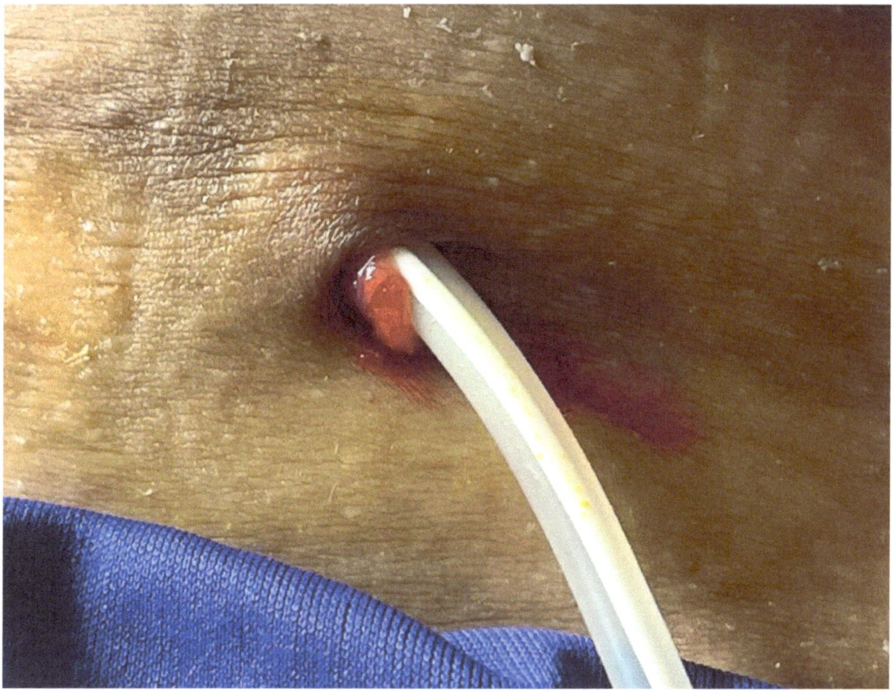

Figure 22.7: Shows Exit Site Infection of Peritoneal Dialysis Catheter

Ultrafiltration Failure:

Ultrafiltration failure (UFF) is defined as fluid overload in a patient on PD associated with ultrafiltration volume < 400 mL after a PD cycle, using a modified peritoneal equilibrium test. This leads to reduced ultrafiltration after PD cycles.

Type 1 UFF occurs due to a hyper-permeable peritoneum causing a high solute transport, bringing about a more rapid diffusion of small solutes across the membrane, while type 2 UFF occurs due to aquaporin dysfunction, leading to high average transport. In patients with long-term PD, the peritoneum undergoes both structural and functional changes with time, owing to the exposure of hyperosmolar glucose solution. This leads to type 3 UFF, causing low solute transport. Management of UFF consists of an alteration of PD prescriptions, the use of APD cyclers, or ultimately shifting the patient to hemodialysis.

Encapsulating Peritoneal Sclerosis is a rare but serious PD complication, in which the bowel and intraperitoneal contents are covered by a thick cocoon of fibrous tissue, causing intestinal obstruction. This requires stopping PD and surgical modalities like adhesiolysis.

Mechanical Problems

Mechanical complications of PD include peri-catheter leaks and hernias, infusion and drain pain, flow failure, catheter tip migration, and superficial cuff extrusion. Catheter tip migration leads to the movement of the tip to the right or left upper quadrants of the abdomen, leading to a poor inflow or outflow, as shown in Figure 22.8. In rare cases, especially in children, the omentum may wrap the CAPD catheter, leading to mechanical obstruction and floor CAPD flow. These mechanical problems often require surgical management by open or laparoscopic repair, and repositioning of the PD catheter.

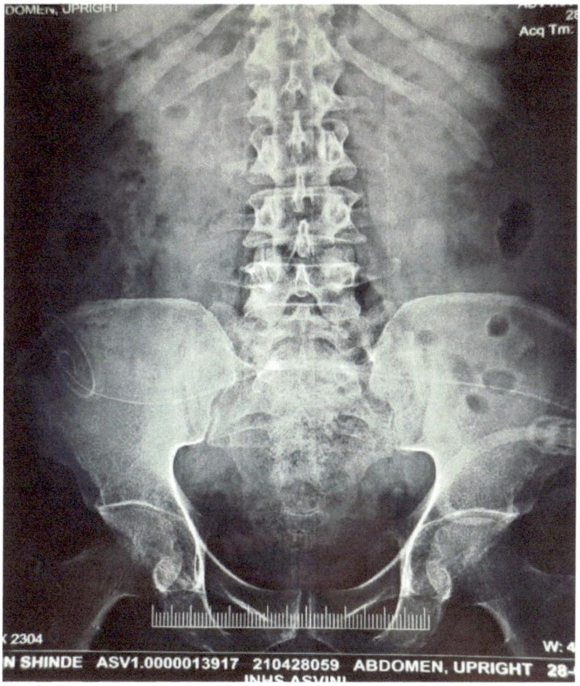

Figure 22.8: Shows Migration of Peritoneal Dialysis Catheter to the Right Upper Quadrant (white arrow)

Metabolic Complications

Peritoneal dialysis using glucose-based solution leads to significant daily glucose absorption causing weight gain, and deranged glycemic and lipid profile. Dialysis exchanges lead to protein loss via peritoneum, almost up to 7–8 gm/day, which gets compounded during episodes of peritonitis, leading to hypoalbuminemia and protein malnutrition. Therefore, it has been recommended that PD patients should consume at least 1.2 to 1.3 g of protein per kilogram of body weight daily.

Advantages of Peritoneal Dialysis

Peritoneal dialysis offers a "home-based" renal replacement therapy. There is no requirement for permanent vascular access. It avoids any chances of blood borne or cross infections. It is particularly useful in infants and young children, as well as patients with cardiac comorbidities and hypotension, or those having inadequate access to hemo-dialysis facilities. Even though the overall mortality of patients on PD compared with hemo-dialysis is not significantly different, but the risk of death in patients treated with PD is lower when compared with those treated with hemo-dialysis.

References:

1. Blake PG, Daugirdas JT. Physiology of Peritoneal Dialysis. In: Handbook of Dialysis, 5th edition, edited by Daugirdas JT, Blake PG, Ing TS, Lippincott Williams & Wilkins, Philadelphia. 2015:392-407.
2. Figueiredo A, Goh BL, Jenkins S, Johnson DW, Mactier R, Ramalakshmi S, et al. Clinical practice guidelines for peritoneal access. Perit Dial Int. 2010;30(4):424-9.
3. Bansal S, Teitelbaum I. Causes, Diagnosis, and Treatment of Peritoneal Membrane Failure. In: Principles and Practice of Dialysis, 5th edition, edited by Lerma EV, Weir MR, Lippincott Williams & Wilkins, Philadelphia.2017:194-219.
4. Figueiredo AE, Bernardini J, Bowes E, Hiramatsu M, Price V, Su C, Walker R, Brunier G. A Syllabus for Teaching Peritoneal Dialysis to Patients and Caregivers. Perit Dial Int. 2016 11-12;36(6):592-605.
5. Peritoneal Dialysis Adequacy Work Group. National Kidney Foundation Kidney Disease Outcomes Quality Initiative: NKF-K/DOQI Clinical practice guidelines for peritoneal dialysis adequacy. Am J Kidney Dis. 2006;48(Suppl 1):S98–129.
6. Li PKT, Chow KM, Cho Y, Fan S, Figueiredo AE, Harris T, et al. ISPD peritonitis guideline recommendations: 2022 update on prevention and treatment. Peritoneal Dialysis Int. 2022;42(2):110–53.

PERITONEAL DIALYSIS

DIALYSER
- Peritoneal membrane

PRINCIPLES
- Diffusion
- Convection

OSMOTIC GRADIENT
- Dextrose concentration

PD Bags
- 1.5% Dextrose
- 2.5% Dextrose
- 4.5% Dextrose
- 7.5% Dextrose

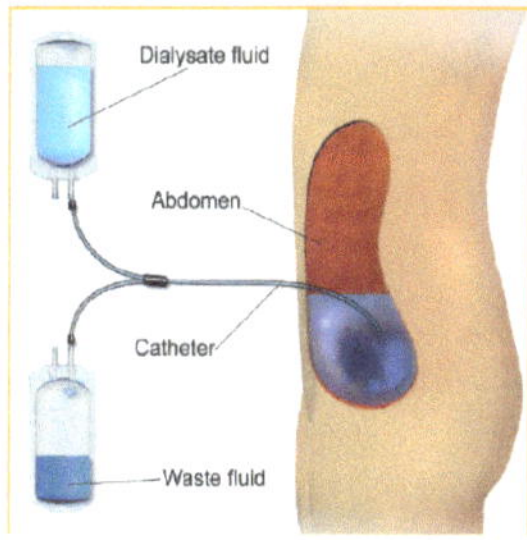

PD Types
- CAPD
- CCPD/APD

PD Catheter features
- Pores intraperitoneal
- 2 Dacron cuffs

Catheter Types

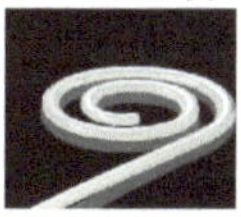

- Straight
- Coiled
- Swan neck

Insertion By
- Open Surgery
- Laparoscopic
- Peritoneoscopy
- Percutaneous

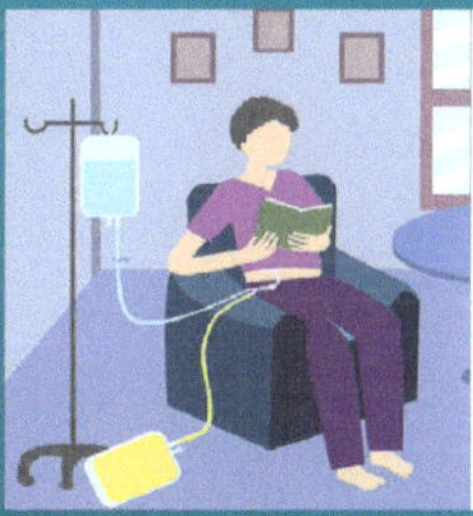

CAPD
- 3-4 exchanges/day
- Done manually
- Dwell time 4-12hrs
- Dwell volume 1-2.5L

CCPD
- Done by cycler
- 4-6 rapid cycles
- Fluid bags 5L
- During night

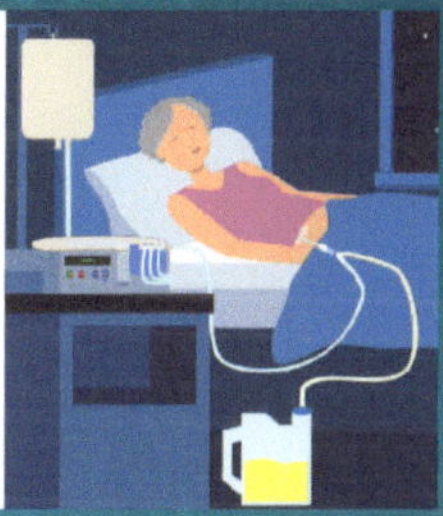

PREFER PD IN

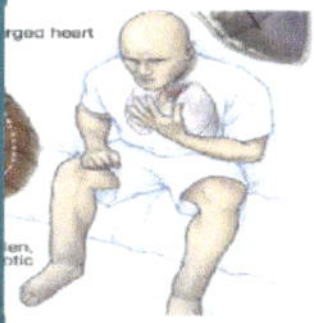

POOR CARDIAC FUNCTION

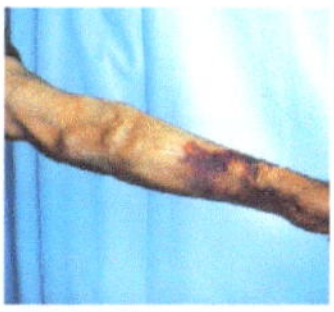

FAILED AV FISTULA

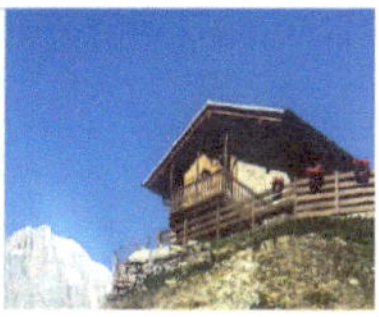

STAYING REMOTE AREAS

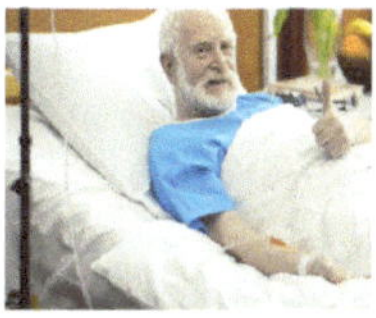

BEDRIDDEN/NON AMBULANT

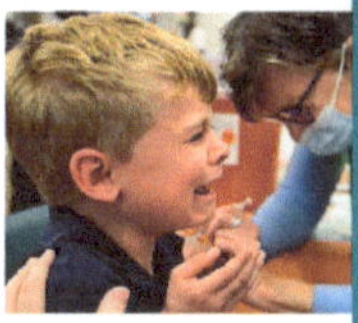

SCARED OF NEEDLES/CHILDREN

COMPLICATIONS
- Peritonitis
- Exit site infection
- Ultra-filtrate failure
- Malposition, Migration
- Hyperglycemia

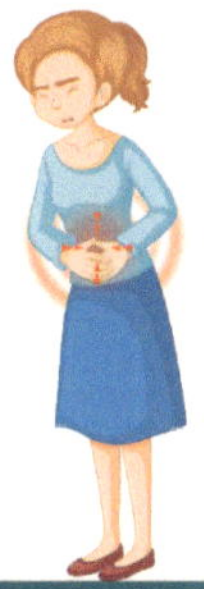

PERITONITIS
- Pain abdomen, cloudy fluid
- Diagnosis - cells > 100 (50% PMN)
- Culture - Staph, CONS, E Coli, GNB
- Rx - Empirical Intraperitoneal antibiotics
- Catheter removal if Refractory/ Recurrent

APD: Automated Peritoneal Dialysis, ***AV :*** Arteriovenous, ***CAPD:*** Continuous ambulatory peritoneal dailysis, ***CCPD:*** Continuous cyclic peritoneal dialysis, ***CONS:*** Coagulase negative staphylococci ***E Coli:*** Escherichia coli, ***GNB:*** Gram negative bacteria, ***PD:*** Peritoneal Dialysis ***PMNs:*** Polymorphonuclear Leukocytes, ***Rx:*** Prescription, ***Staph:*** Staphylococcus aureus

23

KIDNEY TRANSPLANTATION

Sandip Panda, Priti Meena

Kidney transplantation (KT) is the best treatment modality for end-stage kidney disease patients (ESKD). Those placed on the waiting list and eventually receive a transplant have a higher chance of long-term survival than those who remain on dialysis. Furthermore, those who undergo the procedure often experience better quality of life and a projected survival benefit of 10 years, compared to those who stay on dialysis. This is largely due to the advancements in transplantation and immunology, surgical technology, and availability of better drugs since the first successful transplant was performed by Dr Joseph Murray in 1954.

Types of KT

KT can be of two types—living donor KT and deceased donor KT—with the majority of renal transplants in India being from living donors. Deceased donors are either donation after Brainstem Death (DBD) or Donation after Circulatory Death (DCD).

Donor and Recipient Evaluation:

The most important aspect of renal transplant evaluation is a written informed consent from the donor as well as the recipient. Donors should possess the ability to make decisions voluntarily, without being forced, should be medically and psychologically capable, completely aware of associated risks and benefits, and informed of other possible treatments that the recipient may receive. The recipients should be informed of all the possible treatment options including renal transplantation along with their advantages and disadvantages. Contraindications of KT in prospective recipients are provided in Box 23.1.

Immunological Evaluation:

- **Blood typing –** It is preferred to get a kidney from a donor whose blood type is compatible. However, ABO incompatible KT is possible, but extra medical care will be needed before and after the procedure to reduce the risk of organ rejection.
- **Tissue typing –** Human leukocyte antigen (HLA) typing: HLA-A,B and DR typing of both donor and recipient is done to determine the major mismatches prior to transplantation.
- **HLA Crossmatch –** A crossmatching test is implemented by mixing a sample of the recipient's blood with the donor's blood to determine if the recipient's blood has any antibodies that might react to the donor's antigens.

Donor Evaluation

The primary goal of the donor evaluation process is to ensure the suitability of the donor as well as ruling out any evidence of progressive kidney or endorgan damage in the future. A thorough medical evaluation with clinical history and examination, along with a psychosocial evaluation, should be done.

- Apart from immunological work, other work-up of the donor includes complete blood count, urine test, measurement of protein excretion rate, renal function assessment, measurement of functional GFR, liver function tests, coagulation screen (PT and APTT), evaluation for diabetes, hypertension, thyroid abnormalities, virology (HIV, Hepatitis B, and C), and infection screen.
- A thorough evaluation to rule out cardio, pulmonary, and gastrointestinal diseases is also done.
- Psychiatric evaluation is a must.
- Donors should be screened for malignancies (as per age-appropriate risk profile).
- Well-controlled diabetes and hypertension are not absolute contraindications for KT but need to be carefully evaluated by a transplant physician for the presence of end-organ damage.

Recipient Evaluation:

Prospective organ transplant recipients must go through a psychological evaluation to determine any social, financial, or behavioral issues that could affect their adherence to the post-transplant management and follow up.

- The first assessment should include a comprehensive medical history, physical exam, psychological exam, and laboratory and imaging tests.
- Specialized tests for any accompanying medical conditions such as cardiovascular disease, lung disease, peripheral vascular disease, neurological, hematological, and gastrointestinal problems, and urological issues must also be done.
- Before a transplant, the recipient must have no active infections, and any active tumor is an absolute reason to deny the transplant.

- The cause of the end-stage kidney disease should also be determined in the initial evaluation.

BOX 1 : Contraindications of KT in recipient:

Absolute contraindications for KT include:

- Severe cardiac or pulmonary disease
- Active malignancy
- Active infection
- Reversible kidney failure
- Uncontrolled psychiatric disease

Relative contraindications:

- limited life expectancy

Box 23.1: Contraindications for Kidney Transplantation

BOX 2 : Basics of Kidney transplant surgery

The kidney is usually transplanted in a different location, usually into the iliac fossa, and the original kidneys are not usually taken out. The renal vein is connected side-by-side to the external iliac vein, and the renal artery is connected side-by-side to the external or internal iliac artery. The kidney from the living donor is kept cool by using cold saline for irrigation. After the kidney is reperfused, any bleeding vessels are either tied off, stitched up, or cauterized. The ureter is then typically implanted into the bladder in an extravesical technique. Depending on the preference, a stent may be used, generally a double J stent, and it is kept in place for four to six weeks before being removed during the hospital discharge

Box 23.2: Basics of KT Surgery

Medications:

The risk of acute rejection is the highest in the first few months after transplantation (induction phase) and diminishes afterward (maintenance phase).

- Induction agents: At the time of transplantation, patients are typically treated with induction therapy, either a T-lymphocyte–depleting agent (anti-thymocyte globulin [Thymoglobulin]) or an interleukin 2 (IL-2) inhibitor (basiliximab).
- Maintenance immunosuppression: All KTRs receive immunosuppressant therapy to prevent acute rejection and loss of the graft. It is essential to reduce the immune response to the transplant, but the level of continuous immunosuppression must be decreased over time, when the risk of acute rejection is low, to reduce the risk of infection and cancer; these risks are directly connected to the level of immunosuppression.
- Commonly used immunosuppressive agents in KTR include steroids, azathioprine, mycophenolate mofetil (MMF), cyclosporine (in non-modified or modified [microemulsion] form), tacrolimus, everolimus, and belatacept. The most widely used immunosuppressive therapy across the country is a triple-drug regimen comprising a calcineurin inhibitor (mostly tacrolimus) antiproliferative drugs (MMF or MPS) and corticosteroids. The dose of calcineurin inhibitor is adjusted as per the levels of the drug in the blood.

Common Drug Interactions

Most drug interactions are due to drugs that are inducers or inhibitors of the hepatic cytochrome P450 system. Common examples of P450 system inducers are rifampin/rifabutin, barbiturates, phenytoin, and carbamazepine, and inhibitors are non-dihydropyridine calcium channel blockers (verapamil and diltiazem), azole antifungals, and macrolide antibiotics and protease inhibitors.

Causes of Graft Dysfunction:

A general rule in monitoring transplant recipients is that a 20 to 25% increase in serum creatinine concentration above baseline warrants attention.

Causes of early post-transplant period graft dysfunction are:

- Surgical and vascular causes (for example bleeding and thrombosis of vessels)
- Acute tubular necrosis
- Acute rejections
- Calcineurin inhibitor nephrotoxicity
- Infections (UTI, sepsis)
- Recurrent primary disease (Rare)
- Dehydration
- Urinary tract obstruction (post renal)

Rejections

Rejections can be of 3 types – hyperacute, acute, and chronic.

- Hyperacute rejection is an exceptionally uncommon event that occurs immediately after a transplant, due to the presence of large amounts of antibodies in recipient's blood against the antigens on the glomeruli and microvasculature of the donor kidney.
- Cellular rejections are usually seen during the early transplant period, but they can also occur at a later stage, especially when immunosuppression is reduced
- Acute antibody-mediated rejection (AMR), which is an acute form of rejection, can happen shortly after a transplant or may take several years. The most frequent

cause of this is previous exposure to antigens, including those from pregnancy, blood transfusions, or prior transplantation, which triggers an immune response.

Infections

KTRs are particularly vulnerable to infections due to the immunosuppressed state. Urinary tract infection is the most common infection seen in KTRs. Community-acquired infections such as common cold, influenza, pneumococcal pneumonia, and diarrheal syndromes can also all affect KTR. Opportunistic infections can occur at any time following transplantation but tend to occur after the first month when the immunosuppressive effect is at its peak. The degree of immunosuppression is clearly linked to the development of opportunistic infections. Cytomegalovirus (CMV) is one of the most common infections encountered in renal transplants followed by Pneumocystis, Epstein Barr virus, and Herpes simplex virus. Mycobacterial infection (tuberculosis) and fungal infections are also common in post-transplant patients.

Long Term Complications:

The short term graft survival has improved significantly with time and at present the 1 year graft survival in more than 90 % whereas the long term graft survival is still not that satisfactory with the 10 year graft survival is around 65% only. Similarly, the patient survival at 1 year is around 92% whereas it's only around 78% at 10 years. The causes of death following KT are cardiovascular disease and infections. Additional complications, over a longer period of time, usually involve recurrent infections, diabetes mellitus, or malignancy. Glomerulonephritis of transplanted kidneys, both existing and developing, is responsible for 18–22% of graft failures not ending in death. The likelihood of recurrent glomerulonephritis is contingent on the original state of the donor. In contrast to the general population, transplant recipients have a higher risk of squamous cell carcinoma rather than basal cell carcinoma being the most frequent type of skin cancer, followed by Post transplant lymphoproliferative disorders. The immunosuppression drugs also predispose to complications like infection, diabetes, hypertension, bone and mineral diseases, and cancer, particularly in the skin.

Managing immunosuppression for a prolonged period of time is a difficult task, as it requires finding the right balance between improving the patient and graft survival and minimizing toxicity. So far, no immunosuppression regimen has been proven to be without any shortcomings.

References:

1. Hariharan S, Israni AK, Danovitch G. Long-Term Survival after Kidney Transplantation. N Engl J Med. 2021 Aug 19;385(8):729-743. doi: 10.1056/NEJMra2014530. PMID: 34407344.
2. Lim MA, Kohli J, Bloom RD. Immunosuppression for kidney transplantation: where are we now and where are we going? Transplant Rev (Orlando). 2017;31(1):10-17.
3. Nankivell BJ, Alexander SI. Rejection of the kidney allograft. N Engl J Med. 2010;363(15):1451-1462.
4. Allen PJ, Chadban SJ, Craig JC, et a; Recurrent glomerulonephritis after kidney transplantation: risk factors and allograft outcomes. Kidney Int. 2017;92(2):461-469.
5. Sprangers B, Nair V, Launay-Vacher V, Riella LV, Jhaveri KD. Risk factors associated with post-kidney transplant malignancies: an article from the Cancer-Kidney International Network. Clin Kidney J. 2018;11(3):315-329.

KIDNEY TRANSPLANTATION

Best treatment modality for ESKD patients

MEDICATIONS

Induction agents (given before/at the time of surgery)

All ESKD patients should be referred to a transplantation program when the estimated glomercular filtration rate (eGFR) is <30 mL/min/1.73m2

MAINTENANCE THERAPY

Triple-drug regimen comprising a calcineurin inhibitor (mostly tacrolimus) antiproliferative drugs (MMF or MPS) and corticosteroids commonly used

Better long-term survival and quality of life than those who remain on dialysis

ABSOLUTE CONTRAINDICATIONS

1. Severe cardiac or pulmonary disease
2. Active malignancy
3. Active infection
4. Reversible kidney failure
5. Uncontrolled psychiatric disease

COMPLICATIONS OF KIDNEY TRANSPLANT

Early Complications

- Surgical and Vascular
- Acute tubular necrosis
- Acute rejections
- CNI nephrotoxicity
- Infections
- Dehydration

Long Term Complications

- Cardiovascular disease
- Malignancies
- Infections
- Graft failure
- Recurrent primary disease
- Complications of medications

eGFR : Estimated Glomercular Filtration Rate, ***ESKD :*** End Stage Kidney Disease, ***MMF :*** Mycophenolate Mofetil, ***MPS :*** Mucopolysaccharidoses

SECTION 7

Miscellaneous

24

RENAL CALCULUS DISEASE

Manoj Das, Kirti Singh, Swarnendu Mandal

Introduction:

Renal calculus disease refers to the formation of hard minerals and salt deposits within the kidneys. These stones are composed of various substances such as calcium, oxalate, uric acid, cystine, and struvite. The size of the kidney stones can vary from small grains to large ones, leading to urinary tract obstruction and even nephron loss.

Epidemiology:

The prevalence of renal calculus disease has been increasing worldwide. The exact prevalence rates vary across different regions and populations. Several studies have provided insights into the epidemiology of kidney stones:

1. Global Prevalence: Kidney stones affect approximately 1 in 11 people worldwide. The prevalence varies geographically, with higher rates reported in regions with hot climates and low water availability.
2. Gender and Age: Historically, kidney stones were more common in men than women. However, recent studies

suggest that the gender gap is narrowing. Kidney stones can occur at any age, but the highest incidence is observed between the ages of 30 and 60 years.

3. Ethnicity: Certain ethnic groups have a higher predisposition to kidney stone formation. For example, individuals of South Asian, Middle Eastern, and Hispanic descent have a higher prevalence compared to the other populations.
4. Recurrence Rates: Kidney stones have a high recurrence rate, with up to 50% of patients experiencing another stone within 5 to 10 years of their initial episode.

Types of Kidney Stones:

Kidney stones can be classified into different types, based on their composition. The most common types of kidney stones include:

1. **Calcium Oxalate Stones**: These are the most prevalent type of kidney stones, accounting for about 70–80% of the cases. They are formed when calcium combines with oxalate in the urine.
2. **Calcium Phosphate Stones:** These stones are less common and occur when calcium combines with phosphate in the urine.
3. **Uric Acid Stones:** They form when there are high levels of uric acid in the urine, which can be caused by factors such as a high-purine diet, gout, or certain genetic conditions.
4. **Struvite Stones:** They are also known as infection stones, and are typically formed in the presence of urinary tract infections. They can grow rapidly and may be associated with certain bacteria that produce urease.
5. **Cystine Stones:** They are rare and occur in individuals with a hereditary disorder called cystinuria. This condition causes increased levels of cystine in the urine, leading to stone formation.

Pathogenesis of Renal Calculus Disease:

The pathogenesis of renal calculus disease involves a complex interplay of several factors that contribute to the formation and growth of kidney stones. Understanding the underlying mechanisms is crucial for effective management and prevention strategies. The key components of pathogenesis include supersaturation and nucleation, crystal growth and aggregation, and modifying factors.

1. **Supersaturation and Nucleation**

Supersaturation: Supersaturation refers to the presence of dissolved solutes in urine at concentrations higher than their solubility limits. When the concentration of certain substances such as calcium, oxalate, uric acid, or cystine exceeds their saturation points, it promotes stone formation.

Nucleation: Nucleation is the initial step in stone formation, where solutes aggregate to form microscopic crystals. These crystals act as nuclei for further stone growth.

2. **Crystal Growth and Aggregation**

Crystal Growth: Once nucleation occurs, crystals grow by accretion of solutes from urine. The growth of crystals depends on factors such as supersaturation levels, pH, and the presence of inhibitors or promoters.

Crystal Aggregation: Crystals can aggregate together to form larger structures. Aggregation can occur due to physical forces such as crystal-cell interactions, urine flow dynamics, and organic matrix components.

3. **Modifying Factors – Promoters and Inhibitors**

Promoters: Various factors can promote stone formation by enhancing crystal nucleation, growth, or aggregation. These include urinary pH imbalances, low urine volume, high concentrations of stone-forming substances, and certain genetic or metabolic disorders.

Inhibitors: The urinary system has natural defense mechanisms to prevent stone formation. Inhibitors such as citrate, magnesium, glycosaminoglycans, and certain proteins help regulate crystal growth and aggregation. Deficiencies in these inhibitors can contribute to stone formation.

Risk Factors and Predisposing Conditions for Renal Calculus Disease:

The formation of kidney stones can be influenced by various risk factors and predisposing conditions. Understanding these factors is important for identifying individuals at higher risk and implementing preventive measures.

Following are some of the commonly recognized risk factors and predisposing conditions associated with renal calculus disease:

1. **Genetic Factors and Family History**
    1. Genetic predisposition: Certain genetic disorders such as cystinuria and primary hyperoxaluria increase the risk of kidney stone formation.
    2. Family history: Individuals with a family history of kidney stones have a higher likelihood of developing stones themselves.
2. **Metabolic Disorders and Systemic Conditions**
    1. Hypercalciuria: Increased urinary calcium excretion can result from metabolic disorders such as primary hyperparathyroidism or renal tubular acidosis.
    2. Hyperoxaluria: Elevated levels of urinary oxalate can be caused by genetic disorders, malabsorption syndromes, or excessive intake of oxalate-rich foods.

3. Hyperuricosuria: High urinary uric acid levels can be associated with gout, metabolic syndrome, or certain genetic conditions.
4. Cystinuria: A hereditary disorder characterized by increased urinary excretion of cystine.
5. Renal tubular acidosis: A condition that affects the acid-base balance in the kidneys, leading to stone formation.
6. Inflammatory bowel disease: Conditions such as Crohn's disease or ulcerative colitis can increase the risk of kidney stone formation.
7. Obesity and metabolic syndrome: These conditions are associated with changes in urinary composition and increased stone risk.

3. **Dietary Factors and Fluid Intake**

    1. Low fluid intake: Inadequate fluid intake can lead to concentrated urine, increasing the risk of stone formation.
    2. High sodium intake: Excessive sodium intake can result in increased urinary calcium excretion, promoting stone formation.
    3. High oxalate intake: Consuming foods rich in oxalate such as spinach, rhubarb, and chocolate can contribute to the formation of calcium oxalate stones.
    4. High purine intake: Purines are found in certain foods and their breakdown results in the production of uric acid, which can contribute to stone formation.

Diagnostic Evaluation of Renal Calculus Disease:

The diagnostic evaluation of renal calculus disease aims to confirm the presence of kidney stones, determine their location, size, and composition, and evaluate any associated complications. The following are commonly used diagnostic tools and tests in the evaluation of renal calculus disease:

1. **Imaging Studies:**

    1. Ultrasound: Ultrasound can detect larger stones and is helpful to rule out signs of obstruction or hydronephrosis. It is especially useful in pregnant women or individuals who should avoid radiation exposure.
    2. Non-contrast CT scan: Non-contrast computed tomography (CT) scan is considered the gold standard for diagnosing kidney stones. It provides detailed information about stone size, location, and composition. It also helps identify any associated complications such as obstruction or infection.
    3. Abdominal x-ray: X-ray imaging can detect radiopaque stones (calcium-based stones) and evaluate their size and location.

2. **Urine Analysis:** A urine sample is analyzed to check for the presence of blood, crystals, or infection. It can help identify the underlying causes of stone formation such as urinary tract infections or metabolic abnormalities.
3. **Stone Analysis:** If a stone is passed spontaneously or removed surgically, it can be sent for laboratory analysis. The stone analysis provides information about the stone's composition, which helps in guiding treatment and prevention strategies.
4. **Blood Tests:** To assess kidney function, electrolyte levels, and markers of stone-forming conditions (e.g., calcium, uric acid). Serum PTH levels may be measured to evaluate for hyperparathyroidism, a potential cause of kidney stone formation.
5. **Additional Tests:**

    1. Intravenous pyelogram (IVP): IVP involves the injection of a contrast dye followed by x-ray imaging to visualize the urinary tract, including the kidneys, ureters, and

bladder. It is less commonly used today but may be employed in specific cases.

2. 24-hour urine collection: A 24-hour urine collection can provide valuable information about urinary stone risk factors such as calcium, oxalate, citrate, or uric acid excretion.

Non-Surgical Management of Renal Calculus Disease:

The management of renal calculus disease depends on factors such as stone size, location, composition, and symptoms. In many cases, non-surgical approaches are employed to facilitate the passage of stones or prevent their recurrence. The following are common non-surgical management strategies for renal calculus disease:

1. **Observation and Supportive Care:**
    1. Small stone observation: Asymptomatic small stones (< 5 mm) located in the kidney or upper ureter may be observed without intervention, as they have a good chance of passing spontaneously.
    2. Analgesics and hydration: Adequate pain management using non-steroidal anti-inflammatory drugs (NSAIDs) and increased fluid intake to promote stone passage are often recommended.
2. **Medical Expulsive Therapy:**
    1. Alpha-blockers: Alpha-blocker medications such as tamsulosin can be prescribed to relax the ureter muscles and facilitate stone passage. They are commonly used for stones located in the distal ureter (< 10 mm) and have been shown to increase stone clearance rates.
    2. Calcium channel blockers: Nifedipine, a calcium channel blocker, has also been used to promote stone passage by relaxing the ureteral smooth muscles.

3. **Extracorporeal Shock Wave Lithotripsy (ESWL):**

   ESWL uses shock waves to fragment stones into smaller pieces that can pass more easily. It is typically employed for stones in the kidney or upper ureter. However, the efficacy of ESWL may depend on factors such as stone size, location, composition, and patient characteristics.

Surgical Management of Renal Calculus Disease:

In certain cases, surgical intervention may be necessary for the management of renal calculus disease. Surgical approaches are typically employed when stones are large, causing obstruction, or associated with complications that cannot be managed effectively through non-surgical means. The following are common surgical management options for renal calculus disease:

1. Percutaneous Nephrolithotomy (PCNL): PCNL involves the insertion of a nephroscope through a small incision in the back to access the kidney and remove or fragment the stone.

   It is typically employed for large or complex stones in the kidney or upper ureter. The procedure allows for direct visualization of the stones and enables their complete removal or fragmentation using various techniques such as ultrasonic or pneumatic lithotripsy.

2. Ureteroscopic Lithotripsy (URSL) and Retrograde Intrarenal Surgery (RIRS): Ureteroscopy involves the insertion of a thin, semi-rigid or flexible scope into the ureter/kidney (RIRS) to locate and remove or fragment the stone. Laser lithotripsy is commonly used during both techniques to break down stones into smaller fragments for easier passage.

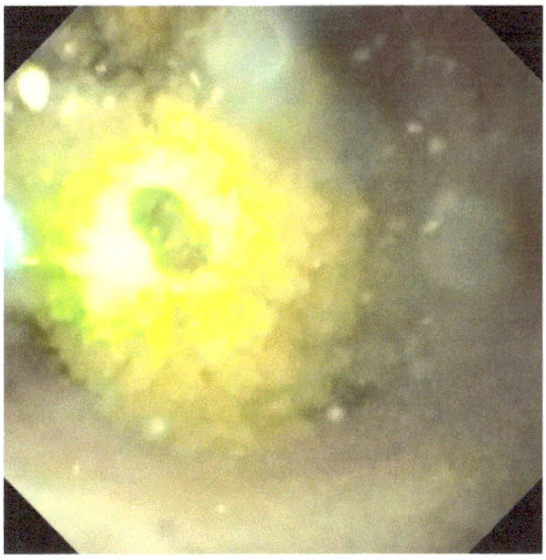

Figure 24.1: RIRS – Stone Visualized in Flexible URS Using Digital Ureterorenoscope

3. Open/Laparoscopic Surgery: Open surgery for kidney stones is now less common and is reserved for complex cases or when other approaches are not feasible. It involves making a larger incision in the abdomen or flank to directly access and remove the stones. However, in selected cases, laparoscopy can be warranted instead of a morbid open procedure.

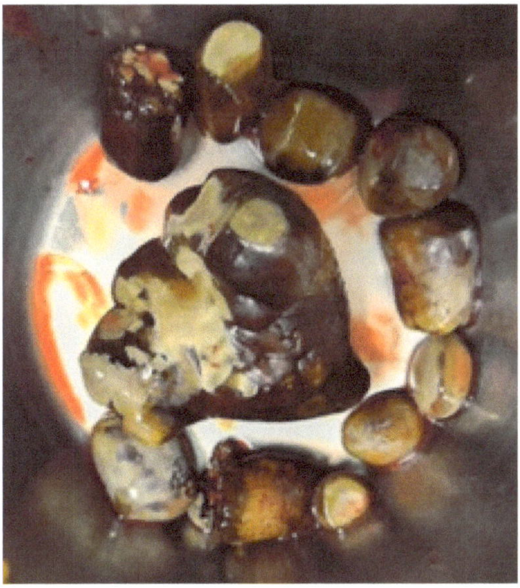

Figure 24.2: Stones Extracted Following Laparoscopic Pyelolithotomy of Ectopic Kidney

It is important to note that the choice of surgical management depends on several factors, including stone characteristics, patient anatomy, and the surgeon's expertise. The specific approach used will be determined based on the individual patient considerations.

Prevention and Follow-up of Renal Calculus Disease:

Prevention and long-term follow-up are crucial aspects of managing renal calculus disease. The primary goal is to prevent stone recurrence and minimize the risk of complications. The following are key strategies for prevention and follow-up:

1. **Lifestyle Modifications:**

    1. Hydration: Encouraging an adequate fluid intake to achieve a urine output of 2–2.5 liters per day helps maintain urine dilution and reduce the risk of stone formation.
    2. Weight management: Encouraging weight loss in overweight or obese individuals to reduce the risk of stone formation associated with metabolic syndrome.
    3. Dietary modifications: Promoting a balanced diet and making specific dietary adjustments based on stone composition and underlying risk factors. For example: Limiting sodium intake to reduce urinary calcium excretion. Moderating intake of oxalate-rich foods (e.g., spinach, rhubarb) in individuals prone to calcium oxalate stones. Adjusting purine intake (found in certain foods) to manage uric acid stones.

2. **Medications for Stone Prevention:**

    1. Thiazide diuretics: These medications reduce urinary calcium excretion and can be effective in preventing calcium-based stone formation.

2. Allopurinol: Allopurinol may be prescribed to individuals with hyperuricosuria or a history of uric acid stones to reduce uric acid levels and prevent stone recurrence.
3. Citrate supplementation: Citrate supplementation helps increase urinary citrate levels, which can inhibit stone formation.

3. **Regular Follow-up:**

1. Periodic imaging: Periodic imaging, such as low-dose non-contrast CT scans or ultrasounds, may be recommended to monitor stone size and assess for any changes or complications.
2. 24-hour urine collection: Periodic collection of a 24-hour urine sample can provide valuable information about urinary stone risk factors. This allows for tailored preventive strategies based on individual patient characteristics.
3. Blood tests: Monitoring blood chemistry, including electrolytes and markers of stone-forming conditions, to assess kidney function and manage any underlying metabolic abnormalities.

4. **Patient Education and Counseling:**

1. Patient education regarding stone prevention strategies, lifestyle modifications, and adherence to prescribed medications.
2. Counseling on dietary choices, fluid intake, and lifestyle habits can help reduce the risk of stone formation.

In conclusion, renal calculus disease, commonly known as kidney stones, is a prevalent condition that can cause significant discomfort and complications. Understanding the various aspects of this disease is essential for its effective management.

Procedure	Advantages	Disadvantages
X-ray KUB	Readily available; inexpensive; limited radiation; useful for follow-up.	Limited sensitivity
Ultrasound	Readily available; no radiation exposure (procedure of choice during pregnancy); high sensitivity for urinary tract obstruction; detects radiolucent stones	Moderately expensive; poor sensitivity for small stones
IVP	Useful in planning therapy and diagnosis of obstructing stones	Intravenous contrast is required; moderate X-ray exposure
NCCT scan	New gold standard; no intravenous contrast needed; high sensitivity and specificity; detects radiolucent stones; detects other causes of flank or abdominal pain	Expensive; moderate radiation exposure

Box 24.1: Diagnostic Imaging Techniques for Renal Calculus Disease

Table 24.1: Overview of Treatment Options for Renal Calculus Disease

Treatment Option	Description
Watchful Waiting	Monitoring small, asymptomatic stones, or stones causing mild symptoms without immediate intervention.
Medications	Prescribing medications to manage pain, or address underlying causes of stone formation.
Extracorporeal Shock Wave Lithotripsy (ESWL)	Non-invasive procedure that uses shock waves to break kidney stones into smaller fragments for easier passage.

Treatment Option	Description
Ureteroscopy	Inserting a thin tube (ureteroscope) through the urethra and bladder to remove or fragment stones in the ureter or kidney.
Percutaneous Nephrolithotomy (PCNL)	Surgical procedure involving the creation of a small incision in the back to access and remove larger kidney stones.
Surgical Stone Removal	Open/Laparoscopic surgery (nephrolithotomy) to remove larger or complex stones when other treatment options are not feasible.
Prevention and Lifestyle Modifications	Adopting preventive measures, such as increasing fluid intake, following a balanced diet, and managing underlying conditions.

Table 24.2: Risk Factors for Renal Calculus Disease

Risk Factors	Description
Genetic Predisposition	Family history of kidney stones or genetic disorders affecting urine composition.
Dietary Factors	High intake of oxalate-rich foods, sodium, or animal protein.
Dehydration	Inadequate fluid intake leads to concentrated urine.
Metabolic Disorders	Conditions such as hypercalciuria, hyperoxaluria, hyperuricosuria, and cystinuria.
Urinary Tract Infections	Recurrent or chronic urinary tract infections that promote stone formation.
Medications	Certain medications such as diuretics, antacids containing calcium, and protease inhibitors used in HIV treatment.

Table 24.3: Common Symptoms of Renal Calculus Disease

Symptoms	Description
Severe Pain	Renal colic, usually originating in the flank area and radiating to the groin or lower abdomen.
Hematuria	Blood in the urine, which can vary in severity and color.
Frequent urination	Increased urge to urinate more frequently than usual.
Urgency	A strong and sudden need to urinate.
Discomfort or Pressure	A persistent feeling of discomfort or pressure in the lower abdomen or back.
Nausea and Vomiting	Nausea, often accompanied by vomiting, due to intense pain or associated with urinary tract obstruction.
Cloudy or Foul-smelling urine	Urine that appears cloudy or has an unusual odor.

References:

1. Romero V, Akpinar H, Assimos DG. Kidney stones: A global picture of prevalence, incidence, and associated risk factors. Rev Urol. 2010;12(2-3):e86-96.
2. Khan SR. Kidney stones. Nat Rev Dis Primers. 2016 Dec 1;2:16008. doi: 10.1038/nrdp.2016.8.
3. Miller NL, Evan AP. Pathogenesis of urinary stone disease. Endocrinol Metab Clin North Am. 2012 Sep;41(3):585-viii. doi: 10.1016/j.ecl.2012.04.005.
4. Siener R, Hesse A. The influence of diet on stone risk. Urolithiasis. 2016 Apr;44(2):89-96. doi: 10.1007/s00240-015-0815-2.
5. EAU Guidelines. 2023 Edn. presented at the EAU Annual Congress Milan 2023. ISBN 978-94-92671-19-6. http://uroweb.org/guidelines/compilations-of-all-guidelines.

6. Pearle MS, Goldfarb DS, Assimos DG, et al. Medical Management of Kidney Stones: AUA/Endourology Society Guideline. J Urol. 2014 Aug;192(2):316-24. doi: 10.1016/j.juro.2014.05.006.
7. Pearle MS, Goldfarb DS, Assimos DG, et al. Surgical Management of Stones: American Urological Association/ Endourological Society Guideline. J Urol. 2016 May;195 (4 Pt 1):1153-63. doi: 10.1016/j.juro.2015.11.071.

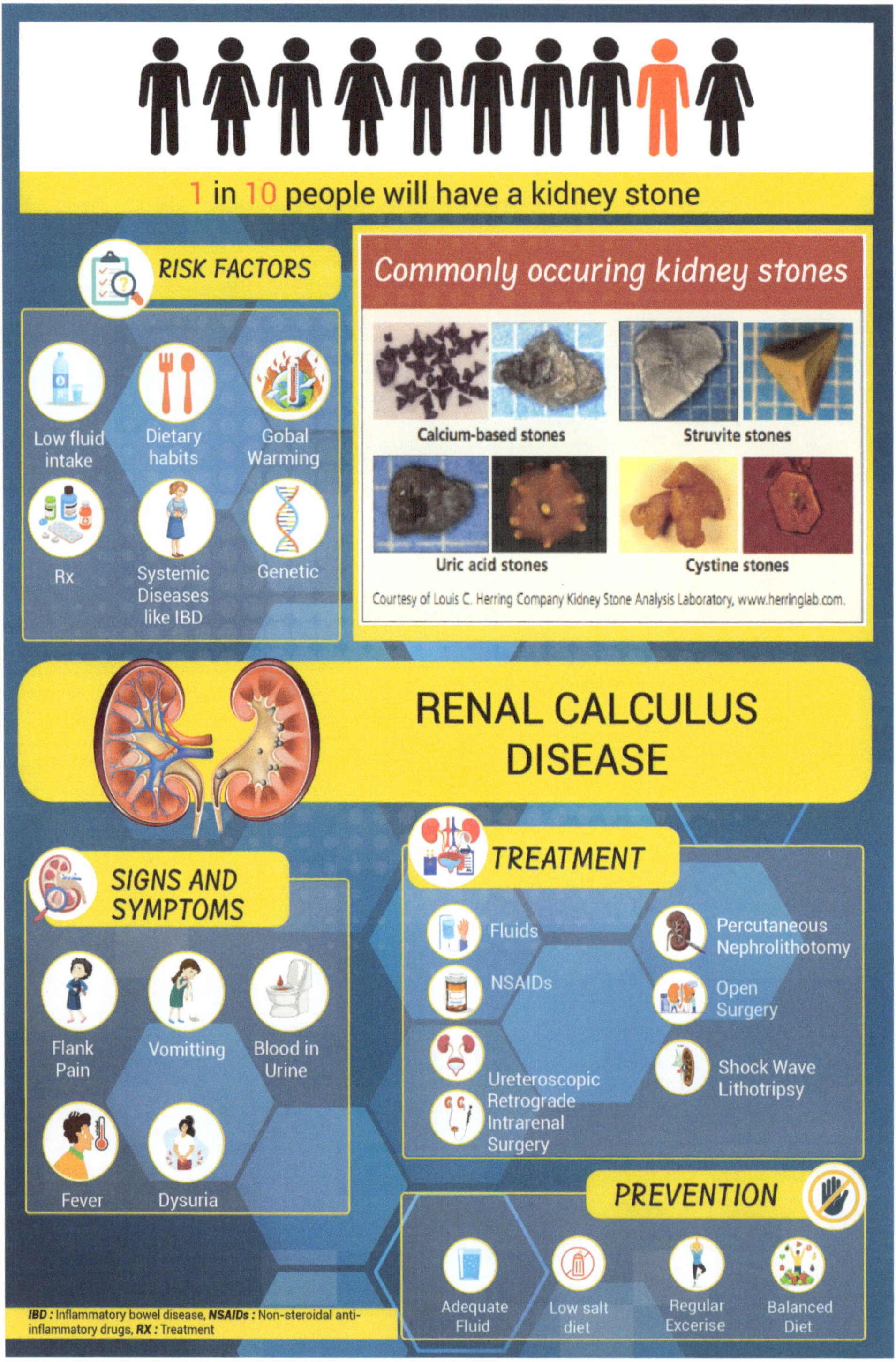
1 in 10 people will have a kidney stone
RISK FACTORS
Low fluid intake
Dietary habits
Gobal Warming
Rx
Systemic Diseases like IBD
Genetic
Commonly occuring kidney stones
Calcium-based stones
Struvite stones
Uric acid stones
Cystine stones
Courtesy of Louis C. Herring Company Kidney Stone Analysis Laboratory, www.herringlab.com.
RENAL CALCULUS DISEASE
SIGNS AND SYMPTOMS
Flank Pain
Vomitting
Blood in Urine
Fever
Dysuria
TREATMENT
Fluids
NSAIDs
Ureteroscopic Retrograde Intrarenal Surgery
Percutaneous Nephrolithotomy
Open Surgery
Shock Wave Lithotripsy
PREVENTION
Adequate Fluid
Low salt diet
Regular Excerise
Balanced Diet
IBD : Inflammatory bowel disease, NSAIDs : Non-steroidal anti-inflammatory drugs, RX : Treatment

25

PREGNANCY AND KIDNEY DISEASE

Garima Aggarwal, Swarnalatha

Pregnancy and Normal Kidney

Pregnancy is a physiological state associated with changes in body fluids and kidneys. In normal pregnancy, there is an increase in blood volume, a decrease in systemic vascular resistance, and an increase in cardiac output. Physiological changes seen in the kidneys of pregnant women are:

- Increase in glomerular filtration rate (GFR) by 40–60%,
- Lower normal serum creatinine in pregnancy, ranging between 0.4 and 0.6 mg/dl,
- Increase in proteinuria up to 300 mg/day due to renal hyperfiltration, returns to baseline by 3 months post-partum,
- Increase in kidney size,
- Fall in systemic blood pressure, which reaches nadir by 20 weeks of gestation, and
- Metabolic alkalosis.

Pregnancy-related Acute Kidney Injury

Pregnancy-related acute kidney injury (PrAKI) has variable definitions from a mild increase in creatinine during pregnancy to AKI requiring dialysis. PrAKI leads to poor pregnancy outcomes (maternal and fetal morbidity and mortality) as well as poor kidney outcomes like worsening of the mother's kidney functions, leading to chronic kidney disease and end-stage kidney disease. The causes of AKI during pregnancy vary based on the gestational period and are as follows:

Early pregnancy (usually in the first trimester) causes of AKI are:

- Hyperemesis Gravidarum
- Septic abortions

Late pregnancy (beyond 20 weeks of gestation) causes of AKI are:

- Preeclampsia/Eclampsia,
- Hemolysis, Elevated liver enzymes, Low Platelet Count (HELLP) Syndrome
- Acute fatty liver disease of pregnancy
- Thrombotic Thrombocytopenic Purpura (TTP), and atypical Hemolytic Uremic Syndrome (aHUS)
- Lupus Nephritis
- Obstructive Uropathy
- Urinary tract infections/Pyelonephritis
- Acute cortical necrosis secondary to placental abruption or hemorrhage
- Hydronephrosis due to uterine compression of the ureter/bladder
- Iatrogenic or spontaneous injury to ureter/bladder/urethra during cesarean section or vaginal delivery.

The various causes of PrAKI, its clinical features, diagnosis, and specific treatments are shown in Table 25.1.

Table 25.1: Causes of AKI in Pregnancy

Cause of PrAKI	Clinical Features	Etiopatho genesis	Diagnosis	Specific Treatments
Hyperemesis Gravidarum	• Seen in the first trimester • Symptoms – Intractable nausea and vomiting	AKI is due to severe dehydration leading to acute tubular necrosis	Clinical signs of severe dehydration, the absence of any other cause of AKI	– Oral or intravenous resuscitation
Septic abortions	• Seen in first trimester • Symptoms – Fever, chills, abdominal pain	AKI is due to sepsis-related acute tubulo interstitial nephritis	• Ultrasound scan suggestive of remaining products of conception	– Prompt antibiotics – Intravenous resuscitation – Removal of products of conception
Preeclampsia	• Known to occur in 2–8% of all pregnancies • New onset hypertension after 20 weeks of gestation • Symptoms – Headache, visual disturbances, pedal edema, seizures, abdominal pain	Preeclampsia is associated with reduced renal blood flow. AKI is multifactorial due to endothelial damage, coagulopathy, thrombotic microangiopathy, and acute tubular necrosis	• New onset of hypertension after 20 weeks of gestation in a previously normotensive woman, • Hypertension is defined by blood pressure ≥ 140/90 mm Hg on two occasions 4 hours apart, or ≥ 160/110 mm Hg single recording • Proteinuria ≥ 300mg/24-hour urine or spot urine protein creatinine ratio 0.3g (dipstick 1+). Or • Any signs of end-organ dysfunction ○ elevated serum creatinine > 1.1 mg/dl or doubling of serum creatinine in the absence of other kidney disease, ○ thrombocytopenia (< 100,000/microliter), ○ elevated liver transaminases ≥ two times normal, ○ pulmonary edema or, ○ cerebral/visual symptoms.	– Prompt delivery – IV Magnesium for prevention of eclampsia

Cause of PrAKI	Clinical Features	Etiopatho genesis	Diagnosis	Specific Treatments
HELLP Syndrome	• Hemolysis, • Elevated liver enzymes, • Low platelets • Hypertension and proteinuria are frequent	AKI is multifactorial and is a complication of preeclampsia, acute tubular necrosis is seen due to coagulopathy associated bleeding	• Hemolysis, • Elevated liver enzymes, • Low platelets • High LDH	– Prompt delivery
Acute fatty liver of pregnancy (AFLP)	• Seen in the third trimester of pregnancy, usually after 30 weeks of gestation • Symptoms – Nausea, vomiting abdominal pain, jaundice, ascites • Difficult to differentiate AFLP from HELLP syndrome/ preeclampsia	Fetal long-chain 3-hydroxyacyl CoA dehydrogenase (LCHAD) deficiency, - > excessive fetal free fatty acids accumulate - > cross placenta, - > Maternal Hepatotoxicity AKI is due to hepatorenal syndrome	Swanson Criteria • encephalopathy, • hyperbilirubinemia, • abdominal ascites, • hypoglycemia, • micro vesicular steatosis on liver biopsy • Maternal and fetal testing for LCHAD gene mutation	– Prompt delivery – Platelet transfusions prior to delivery if the platelet count is < 40,000, – liver transplant in severe cases. – Plasma exchange may be beneficial

Cause of PrAKI	Clinical Features	Etiopatho genesis	Diagnosis	Specific Treatments
Thrombotic Thrombocytopenic Purpura (TTP),	• Seen in the late second and third trimesters	ADAMTS13 (von Willebrand factor protease) deficiency, AKI is due to thrombotic microangiopathy (TMA)- disseminated occlusion of arterioles and capillaries with fibrin	Diagnostic criteria for TTP • thrombocytopenia, • schistocytosis, • neurologic manifestations and • absence of coagulation abnormalities • ADAMTS13 activity < 10%	– Plasma exchange – Rituximab may be tried
atypical Hemolytic Uremic Syndrome (aHUS)	• more common in the postpartum period	Complement dysregulation and activation - > causes complement induced endothelial damage AKI is due to TMA	• Thrombocytopenia • Evidence of Hemolysis • High LDH • AKI • Genetic testing for complement cascade gene mutations	– Plasma exchange – Eculizumab

Cause of PrAKI	Clinical Features	Etiopatho genesis	Diagnosis	Specific Treatments
Acute cortical necrosis	• Irreversible AKI	Results following • Obstetric hemorrhagic complications like abruptio placentae or uterine rupture • Puerperal sepsis or urosepsis	• Kidney Biopsy shows diffuse or patchy cortical necrosis	– Renal Replacement Therapy (RRT) when indicated
Lupus nephritis and/or Antiphospholipid antibody syndrome (APLA)	Differentiating between lupus nephritis flare and pre-eclampsia can be difficult • worsening proteinuria, • hypertension, • AKI • extrarenal lupus symptoms (ie, neutropenia, rash, photosensitivity, arthritis, or oral ulcers)	Autoimmune disease flare	• Low complements (may be normal in pregnancy) • Positive anti-dsDNA, anti-cardiolipin, or anti-β2 glycoprotein antibodies • Kidney Biopsy only if diagnosis unclear and will change management	– Steroids – Hydroxychloroquine – Immunosuppressive drugs – Azathioprine/ calcineurin inhibitors/Rituximab – SLE should be quiescent for ≥ 6 months before planning pregnancy – APLA – treated with aspirin and low molecular weight heparin

Management of Pregnancy induced AKI

Patients with suspected pregnancy-induced AKI should undergo detailed history taking about previous kidney diseases, miscarriages in the past, history suggestive of autoimmune disease, and a detailed physical examination, followed by evaluation in the form of urinalysis, kidney and liver function tests, coagulation profile, workup for hemolysis, placental growth factor, and the appropriate serological workup for ANA, APLA, etc. Serum complement levels can be elevated in pregnancy due to increased synthesis by the liver, hence, it is difficult to diagnose low complement states like lupus nephritis flares during pregnancy. An ultrasound scan of the kidneys should be performed for suspected post-obstructive causes of AKI. Special investigations like ADAMTS13 activity and genetic testing for complement gene mutations may be needed. Kidney biopsy should be considered only when the diagnosis is inconclusive, treatment benefits outweigh the risks of a kidney biopsy, and it is usually preferred to be done in the first or second trimester and contraindicated in the third trimester.

AKI in pregnancy should be managed in tertiary care centers with a multidisciplinary team consisting of nephrologists, obstetricians, and neonatologists. General measures to treat pregnancy-induced AKI include:

- Intravenous fluid resuscitation
- Prompt delivery, if needed
- Timely initiation of dialysis, if needed
- Blood products to be transfused as per need
- Identification and treatment of the specific cause of AKI in pregnancy (refer to Table 25.1).
- Glomerulonephritis is treated with steroids and immunosuppressive drugs. Azathioprine and calcineurin inhibitors (cyclosporine and tacrolimus) are not

teratogenic and are commonly used during pregnancy. Mycophenolate mofetil is contraindicated during pregnancy due to teratogenicity.

- Antibiotics that are safe to use in pregnancy include:
    - Oral Antibiotics – Amoxicillin, Ampicillin, Amoxicillin-clavulanate, Cephalexin, Cefpodoxime, Nitrofurantoin (avoid in the third trimester and G6PD deficiency)
    - IV Antibiotics – Piperacillin-tazobactam, Ceftriaxone, Meropenem, Imipenem/Cilastin, Aztreonams.

Pregnancy in Chronic Kidney Disease

Fertility is decreased in women with chronic kidney disease (CKD). There is a disruption of the hypothalamic gonadal axis in CKD that results in impairment of sexual function in both men and women. Uremia results in lower levels of estrogen, progesterone, and testosterone. There is a loss of luteinizing hormone (LH) surge that results in anovulation. In contrast, the pituitary hormones LH and prolactin are elevated due to impaired renal clearance and secondary hyperparathyroidism, which results in the loss of gonadotropin hormone (GH) surge from the hypothalamus, ultimately causing anovulation. For these reasons, infertility rates are very high in women with advanced CKD.

Pregnancy is safer and should be advised only in women who have early CKD with mild renal impairment (usually creatinine ≤ 1.5mg/dl), normal blood pressure, and/or minimal proteinuria.

Women with CKD are at high risk for maternal and fetal complications. In advanced stages of CKD, pregnancy is hazardous for both the mother and the baby. Pregnancy in women with CKD can lead to a progressive loss of kidney function, which may progress to requiring dialysis. Underlying

CKD in pregnant women results in an almost 10-fold increased risk of preeclampsia; increased risk for small for gestational age babies; pre-term deliveries; more cesarean deliveries and pregnancy losses.

Management of pregnancy in women with CKD includes:

- Blood pressure should be optimized to < 140/90 before conception. Pregnancy-safe anti-hypertensives include – labetalol, long-acting nifedipine, and methyldopa.
- Proteinuria should be minimized before conception. Angiotensin converting enzyme inhibitors (ACEIs) and angiotensin receptor blockers (ARBs), which are used for decreasing proteinuria, should be stopped safely before conception.
- Stopping all teratogenic medications.
- Supplementation with calcium and folic acid daily.
- Low-dose aspirin should be started after conception and continued till 34–36 weeks of gestation to prevent preeclampsia.
- Women with glomerulonephritis should plan pregnancy only after their disease is in remission for at least 6 months.
- Nephrotic syndrome during pregnancy should be managed with loop diuretics; IV albumin infusions; safe immunosuppressive drugs; anticoagulation with low molecular weight heparin should be considered in women with severe hypoalbuminemia, and severe proteinuria.
- Pregnancy in women on dialysis is exceedingly rare, but if present, should be managed by a multidisciplinary team of nephrologists, obstetricians, dieticians, and neonatologists. It requires diligent management with intensification of dialysis; vitamin, iron, and erythropoietin supplementation; calcium and phosphate balance;

dietary support and regular surveillance for fetal growth and placental sufficiency.

- Breastfeeding is encouraged. Labetalol and nifedipine can be safely used as anti-hypertensives during this period.

Pregnancy in Kidney Transplant Recipients

Women with end-stage renal disease (ESRD) have a functional disruption in their hypothalamic-pituitary-gonadal axis due to uremia. However, fertility improves after these women undergo kidney transplantation. Regular menses and ovulatory cycles are restored as early as 3 weeks after kidney transplantation, as well as a recovery of normal hormone levels occurs 6 months post the transplantation.

Pregnancy can be safely planned in kidney transplant recipients (KTRs) who are preferably ≥ 1–2 years post transplantation, have normal blood pressure, stable serum creatinine below < 1.5 mg/dL, proteinuria < 500 mg/24 h, have not had a rejection episode in the past year, are on stable immunosuppression doses, and are not on any fetotoxic drugs. Preconception counseling must be done for all pre-menopausal women KTRs regarding methods of contraception to prevent unplanned pregnancies; timely stoppage of fetotoxic drugs; the need for a multidisciplinary approach and to discuss the possible complications.

Steroids, azathioprine, calcineurin inhibitors (CNIs), and mTOR inhibitors are considered relatively safe during pregnancy. Rituximab and eculizumab may be used in pregnancy if the benefits outweigh the risks. Mycophenolate mofetil (MMF), bortezomib, cyclophosphamide, ACEIs, and ARBs are fetotoxic and should not be prescribed to pregnant women. MMF is a part of the triple immunosuppression regimen prescribed routinely to most KTRs, and current guidelines suggest that women who are planning pregnancy should discontinue MMF at least 6 weeks before conception. In our practice, we discontinue this drug at least 3 months before planned conception and replace it with azathioprine. Pregnancy in KTRs remains high risk and may be complicated by pregnancy-induced hypertension, preeclampsia, miscarriage, abortions, gestational diabetes, intrauterine deaths, ectopic pregnancies, cesarean section, and preterm delivery. KTRs are also at risk of urinary tract infections, acute rejection episodes, worsening of kidney allograft function, and lower CNI drug levels during pregnancy. Hence, regular monitoring is needed by nephrologists and obstetricians during pregnancy.

References:

1. Taber-Hight E, Shah S. Acute Kidney Injury in Pregnancy. Adv Chronic Kidney Dis. 2020 Nov;27(6):455–60.
2. Hladunewich MA. Chronic Kidney Disease and Pregnancy. Semin Nephrol. 2017 Jul;37(4):337–46.
3. Gonzalez Suarez ML, Parker AS, Cheungpasitporn W. Pregnancy in Kidney Transplant Recipients. Adv Chronic Kidney Dis. 2020 Nov;27(6):486–98.
4. Ponticelli C, Zaina B, Moroni G. Planned Pregnancy in Kidney Transplantation. A Calculated Risk. J Pers Med. 2021 Sep 26;11(10):956.

PREGNANCY AND KIDNEY

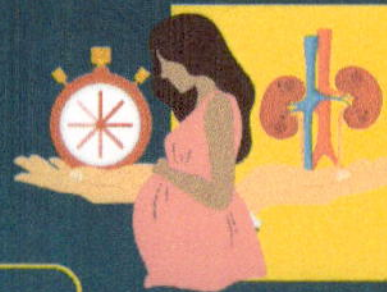

PHYSIOLOGICAL CHANGES

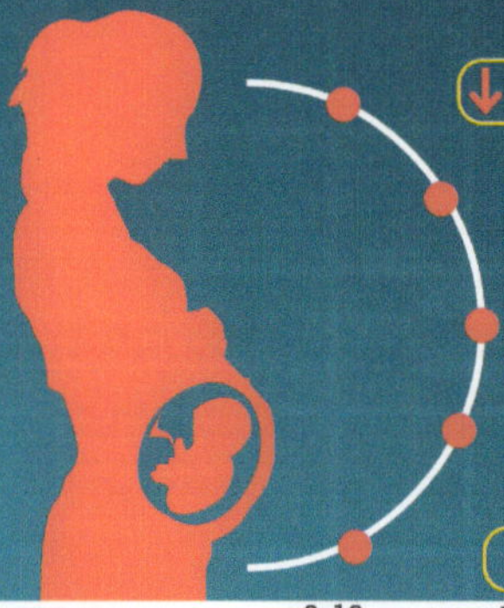

- ↓ Blood Pressure
- ↑ GFR 40-60%
- ↓ Normal creatinine- 0.4-0.6
- ↑ Proteinuria upto 300-500mg/day
- ↑ Kidney Size

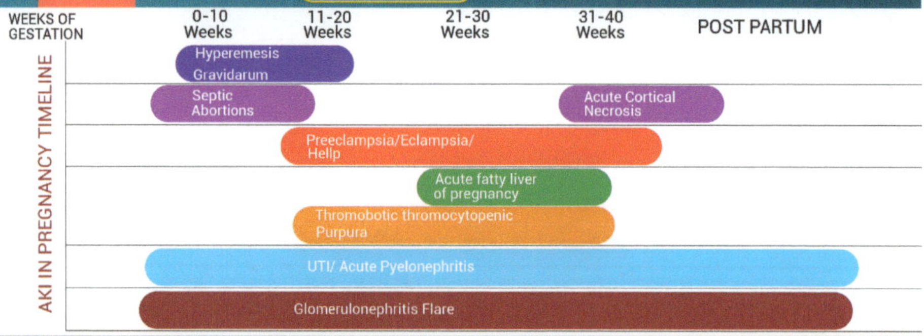

DRUGS IN PREGNANCY

DRUGS	SAFE in pregnancy	UNSAFE in pregnancy
IMMUNOSUPRESSIVE DRUGS	Steroids, CNI (Tacrolimus, Cyclosporine), Azathioprine, Eculizumab - if essential to use	MMF, Cyclophosphamide, Bortezomib, mTor Inhibitors (Sirolimus, Everolimus)
ANTIHYPERTENSIVES	Labetalol, Nifedipine-long acting, Methyldopa, other calcium channel blockers	Angiotensin converting enzyme inhibitors (ACEIs), Angiotensin receptor blockers (ARB)
ANTIBIOTICS (oral)	Amoxicillin, Ampicillin, Cefpodoxime, Cephalexin, Nitrofurantoin	

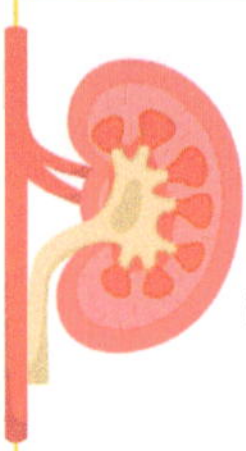

PREGNANCY in CKD and Kidney Transplant Recipients is safer in women with

- ✓ Creatinine <1.5mg/dl
- ✓ Normal Blood Pressure
- ✓ Minimal proteinuria <500mg/24h
- ✓ >1-2yrs post transplantation
- ✓ No rejection episodes in last 1 year
- ✓ Stable immunosupression
- ✓ Not on any fetotoxic drugs

ACEI : Angiotensin-converting enzyme inhibitors, ***AKI :*** Acute Kidney Injury, ***ARB :*** Angiotension receptor blockers, ***CKD :*** Chronic Kidney Disease, ***CNI :*** Calcineurin inhibitors, ***GFR :*** Glomerular filtration rate, ***MMF :*** Maxillomandibular fixation, ***UTI :*** Urinary Tract Infection

26

CYSTIC KIDNEY DISEASES

Manisha Dassi, Manjusha Yadla

Introduction:

Cystic kidney diseases are a heterogeneous group of disorders, characterized by the presence of cysts in the kidneys. They can affect patients of all age groups and may have an onset anywhere from intrauterine life to late adulthood. They may be hereditary or developmental in nature and may be associated with systemic diseases or the presence of extra-renal cysts.

The various cystic kidney diseases are classified into the following categories (Table 26.1).

1. Developmental
2. Genetic
3. Associated with systemic disease
4. Acquired
5. Neoplastic/Malignant

Autosomal Dominant Polycystic Kidney Disease (ADPKD) is the most common hereditary cystic kidney disease in children as well as adults.

Table 26.1: Classification of Cystic Kidney Diseases

Classification
Developmental 1. Multicystic Dysplastic Kidney Disease 2. Medullary Sponge Kidney
Genetic 1. Autosomal Dominant Polycystic Kidney Disease 2. Autosomal Recessive Polycystic Kidney Disease 3. Glomerulocystic Kidney Disease 4. Juvenile Nephronophthisis 5. Autosomal Dominant Tubulo-interstitial Kidney Disease
Cysts Associated with Systemic Diseases 1. Tuberous Sclerosis Complex 2. Von Hippel Lindau Syndrome 3. Meckel Gruber Syndrome 4. Bardet-Biedl Syndrome 5. Beckwith-Wiedemann Syndrome
Acquired 1. Simple Cysts 2. Acquired Cystic Renal Disease 3. Hypokalemic Renal Cystic Disease
Malignancy 1. Cystic Renal Cell Carcinoma

Developmental

1) Multicystic Dysplastic Kidney Disease

It is a congenital developmental disorder, characterized by the presence of multiple cysts of variable sizes in the kidney. Dysplastic renal parenchyma anchors the cysts, the arrangement of which resembles a bunch of grapes. Usually, it is unilateral; bilateral involvement is not compatible with life. It is associated with other abnormalities of the urinary tract like pelvi-ureteric junction obstruction and vesico-ureteric reflux.

2) Medullary Sponge Kidney (MSK)

MSK is characterized by dilated medullary and papillary collecting ducts that give the renal medulla a spongy appearance. In addition, patients may also have:

1. Nephrocalcinosis
2. Renal tubular acidification and concentrating defects
3. Bone mineralization defects
4. Nephrolithiasis
5. Recurrent UTIs

It is usually sporadic. Hereditary cases with autosomal dominant inheritance patterns have also been reported. Patients are mostly asymptomatic and the condition is detected as an incidental finding on radiological investigations. Progression to chronic kidney disease is uncommon.

Genetic

1) Autosomal Dominant Polycystic Kidney Disease (ADPKD)

ADPKD is a multisystemic disease, characterized by the presence of cysts in the kidneys along with various other organs, including the liver, pancreas, spleen, arachnoid mater, inguinal cord, round ligament, and has various non-cyst related disease associations. It is a genetic disease that is inherited in an autosomal dominant fashion with variable expression. There are two mutations in ADPKD: PKD1 (85% of cases), whose clinical manifestations occur early and progress rapidly; and PKD2 (15% of cases).

Clinical Manifestations:

Renal Manifestations:

The various renal manifestations of ADPKD include:

- Hypertension
- Enlarged palpable kidneys due to the presence of multiple bilateral cysts

- Hematuria
- Cyst infection
- Cyst hemorrhage
- Recurrent urinary tract infections
- Nephrolithiasis
- End-stage renal disease. The kidney and cyst volume are the strongest predictors of a decline in kidney functions.

Extra Renal Manifestations:

ADPKD has myriad extra-renal manifestations and may involve different organ systems (Tables 26.2 & 26.3).

Table 26.2: Extra-renal Manifestations of ADPKD

Gastro Intestinal	1. Polycystic Liver Disease 2. Intestinal Diverticulae 3. Cysts in Pancreas, Spleen
Vascular Abnormalities	1. Arterial Aneurysms a. Intracranial b. Coronary Artery c. Abdominal Aortic 2. Arterial Dissection a. Thoracic Aortic b. Cervico-cephalic 3. Vascular Occlusion a. Retinal Artery b. Retinal Vein
Cardiac	1. Mitral Valve Prolapse (25% of pts) 2. Mitral Regurgitation 3. Tricuspid Regurgitation 4. Tricuspid Prolapse 5. Aortic Regurgitation
Others	1. Cysts in Arachnoid Mater 2. Cysts in Prostate, Seminal Vesicle, Epididymis 3. Cysts in Round Ligament of Uterus 4. Inguinal Hernia

Table 26.3: Polycystic Liver Disease – Clinical Manifestations

Asymptomatic – most common	
Symptoms due to cysts' mass effect: a. Orthopnea, b. Early satiety c. Gastroesophageal reflux d. Mechanical low back pain e. Uterine prolapse f. Rib fracture g. Hepatic venous outflow obstruction h. IVC compression i. Portal vein compression j. Bile duct compression	Other cyst-related complications: a. Hemorrhage b. Infection c. Torsion d. Rupture

Diagnosis

Ultrasound KUB is useful in the pre-symptomatic screening of patients. Specific ultrasound criteria for diagnosis have been defined (Table 26.4). Other radiological techniques such as MRI or CT KUB may help better in evaluating kidney and cyst volume. For people with a positive family history of ADPKD, aged between 16–40 years, MRI criteria have been described to diagnose or exclude ADPKD, this is particularly useful when selecting kidney donors (Table 26.5). Genetic testing may be offered to patients where radiological tests are indeterminate and precise diagnosis is needed; or in the setting of a negative or unknown family history; and for selection of living related renal donor. Preimplantation genetic diagnosis (PGD) may be offered to patients considering pregnancy.

Table 26.4: Ultrasound Criteria for the Diagnosis of Autosomal Dominant Polycystic Kidney Disease

Revised Unified Diagnostic Criteria for ADPKD when there is a positive family history			
Age	Criteria	Positive Predictive Value (PPV)	Negative Predictive Value (NPV)
15-29	≥ 3 cysts, unilateral or bilateral	100	86
30-39	≥ 3 cysts, unilateral or bilateral	100	86
40-59	≥ 2 cysts in each kidney	100	95
≥ 60	≥ 4 cysts in each kidney	100	100
Revised Diagnostic criteria when diagnosis needs to be excluded in patients with a positive family history			
15-29	≥ 1 cyst	97	91
30-39	≥ 1 cyst	94	98
40-59	≥ 2 cysts	97	100
≥ 60	≥ 3 cysts in each kidney	100	100

Table 26.5: MRI Criteria to Diagnose or Exclude ADPKD (aged 16–40 years; positive family history)

Number of cysts on MRI	Diagnosis
> 10 cysts total	Sufficient for diagnosis (PPV & sensitivity 100)
< 5 cysts total	Sufficient for exclusion (NPV & specificity 100)

Treatment

At present, available treatment options are directed toward medical or surgical management of complications or associations of ADPKD. As the cyst and kidney volume have been found to be associated with a functional decline in renal functions, various drugs targeting a reduction in cyst size/volume are under clinical trials. Of the various trial drugs, Tolvaptan (V2 receptor antagonist) is being used in clinical practice in adults (aged 18–55 years) with an estimated GFR ≥ 25 ml/min/1.73 m^2 for those at risk of a rapidly progressive disease. People with ADPKD should be treated with the same recommendations as those with CKD from any other cause.

2) Autosomal Recessive Polycystic Kidney Disease (ARPKD)

ARPKD is an autosomal recessive disease caused by a mutation in the PKHD1 gene and is characterized by enlarged cystic kidneys and congenital hepatic fibrosis. Majority of the cases are identified at birth or in-utero. The affected fetuses may have enlarged echogenic kidneys and oligohydramnios. These fetuses may also have pulmonary hypoplasia and spine with limb deformities. Affected neonates may develop other progressive complications like severe systemic hypertension, renal impairment, and portal hypertension, secondary to congenital hepatic fibrosis. The estimated perinatal mortality rate is around 30%. Of those infants who survive the first month of life, the estimated 5-year mortality rate is 85 to 90%. The disease can be diagnosed on an ultrasound or CT KUB, in an appropriate clinical setting. Genetic testing for detection of the mutation in the PKHD1 gene is available. Kidney transplantation may be offered to patients with end-stage renal disease. In patients with portal hypertension, secondary to congenital hepatic fibrosis, liver and kidney transplants may be needed.

3) Glomerulocystic Kidney Disease (GCKD)

Glomerulocystic disease is a rare disease, characterized by cystic dilatation of the Bowman's capsule, with or without a dilation of adjacent tubules. It may be familial, sporadic, acquired, or associated with various heritable syndromes like tuberous sclerosis. Radiological studies like MRI or CT help in differentiating it from other cystic disorders.

4) Juvenile Nephronophthiasis

Juvenile nephronophthiasis is an autosomal recessive hereditary disease, caused due to a mutation in the NPHP gene. It is characterized by a decrease in renal tubular concentrating ability, chronic tubulointerstitial nephritis, renal cysts, and end-stage renal disease. It may be associated with other systemic abnormalities such as situs inversus, cardiac abnormalities, and congenital hepatic fibrosis, and may also occur with systemic hereditary syndromes such as Joubert syndrome. Diagnostic ultrasonography shows bilateral small kidneys with loss of corticomedullary junction and multiple cysts in the medulla. Renal transplant is offered in case of end-stage renal disease.

5) Autosomal Dominant Tubulo-interstitial Kidney Disease (ADTKD)

ADTKD was previously known as medullary cystic kidney disease, UMOD-related kidney disease, familial juvenile hyperuricemic nephropathy, or familial glomerulocystic disease with hyperuricemia. It is hereditary with an autosomal dominant pattern of inheritance and has variable penetrance. Patients have bland urine sediments, normal or small size kidneys in the radiological examination, hyperuricemia with gout, and a slowly progressive chronic kidney disease that reaches dialysis dependency in the fourth to seventh decade of life.

Cysts Associated with Systemic Disorders

Renal cysts may occur in association with various systemic hereditary syndromes, of which tuberous sclerosis and Von Hippel Lindou disease have been best characterized, including genetic mutations (TSC1, TSC2, VHL). They may be associated with both neoplastic or non-neoplastic cysts in the kidney.

A small subset of patients with tuberous sclerosis may show overlap with ADPKD.

Acquired

1) Simple Cysts

Simple cysts are the most commonly acquired benign renal cysts. They occur more frequently in men, are usually unilateral, may be either solitary or multiple, incidence increases with age, and are commonly asymptomatic. They are detected incidentally in abdominal imaging studies. The ultrasound features of simple cysts include smooth walls, lack of septae, and lack of intracystic debris. CT scanning should be performed in indeterminate cases. Bosniak classification based on the CT appearance of the cysts may help in further characterization and management (Table 26.6).

Table 26.6: Bosniak Classification of Renal Cysts

Bosniak Classification	
BOSNIAK I	Benign simple cyst • hairline-thin wall of ≤ 2 mm • no septa, calcifications, or solid components • no enhancement • work-up: none • percentage malignant: ~0%
BOSNIAK II	Benign cyst – "minimally complex" • few hairlines thin < 1 mm septa or thin calcifications (thickness not measurable) • non-enhancing high-attenuation (due to proteinaceous or hemorrhagic contents) renal lesions < 3 cm • generally well marginated • work-up: none • percentage malignant: ~0–6%

Bosniak Classification	
BOSNIAK IIF	Minimally complex • multiple hairline thin septa, or minimally smooth thickened walls, or septa • calcification can be present and may be thick and nodular • generally well marginated • high-attenuation lesion > 3 cm diameter, totally intrarenal (< 25% of wall visible); no enhancement • requiring follow-up (F for follow-up): needs ultrasound/CT/MRI follow-up at 6 months, 12 months, then annually for 5 years • percentage malignant: ~5–26%
BOSNIAK III	Indeterminate cystic mass • thickened irregular, or smooth walls, or septa with measurable enhancement • treatment: partial nephrectomy • percentage malignant: ~55–72%
BOSNIAK IV	Clearly malignant cystic mass • Bosniak III criteria + enhancing soft tissue components adjacent to but independent of wall or septum • treatment: partial or total nephrectomy • percentage malignant: ~91–100%

2) Acquired Cystic Kidney Disease (ACKD)

Acquired cystic kidney disease is characterized by the development of renal cysts in patients with long-standing end-stage renal disease. These patients do not have a history of any other cystic kidney disease. Incidence has been estimated at 44% after three years of dialysis and 90% after ten years of dialysis. The kidneys are small in size with more than 3 to 5 cysts in each kidney, on radiological examination. Patients are mostly asymptomatic or may rarely present with flank pain due to cyst hemorrhage. Patients with advanced ACKD may present with erythrocytosis.

Hyperplastic cysts may lead to renal cell carcinoma, the incidence of which is reported at 1 to 7%.

3) Hypokalemic Cystic Kidney Disease

Renal cysts may be seen with chronic hypokalemia. Nearly 50% of the patients with idiopathic adrenal hyperplasia and 60% of the patients with adrenal tumors have renal medullary cysts.

Neoplastic Cysts

Cysts may be seen in neoplastic conditions like cystic renal cell carcinoma and sarcoma. Benign tumors like renal lymphangioma and cystic nephroma may also present with complex renal cysts. These lesions require definitive surgical treatment.

Cystic renal diseases share a common feature of the presence of cysts in the kidneys. However, they have unique clinical presentations, genetics, inheritance patterns, complications, and outcomes. It is important to identify these diseases appropriately so that the management options can be tailormade as per specific clinical settings, with the ultimate goal being prevention or delay of end-stage renal disease.

References:

1. Cramer MT, Guay-Woodford LM. Cystic kidney disease: a primer. Adv Chronic Kidney Dis. 2015;22(4):297–305.
2. Guay-Woodford L. Other cystic diseases. In: Feehally RJaJ ed. Comprehensive Clinical Nephrology. 6th ed. London, UK: Mosby; 2019:545-559.
3. Kurschat, C., Müller, RU., Franke, M. et al. An approach to cystic kidney diseases: the clinician's view. Nat Rev Nephrol 10, 687–699 (2014).
4. Shivani Kwatra, Vinod Krishnappa, Christiane Mhanna, Taryn Murray, Robert Novak, Siddharth Kumar Sethi, Deepak Kumar, Rupesh Raina. Cystic Diseases of Childhood: a

Review, Urology(2017), http://dx.doi.org/doi:10.1016/j.urology.2017.07.040.

5. Katabathina VS, Kota G, Dasyam AK et al. Adult renal cystic disease: a genetic, biological, and developmental primer. Radiographics. 2010; 30: 1509-1523.
6. Kurschat, C. E. et al. An approach to cystic kidney diseases: the clinician's view. Nat. Rev. Nephrol. Advance online publication 30 September 2014; doi:10.1038/nrneph.2014.173.
7. Gupta I, Bitzan M. Cystic Renal Diseases. In: Phadke K, Goodyer P, Bitzan M. (eds) Manual of Pediatric Nephrology, Springer, Berlin, Heidelberg; 2014: 249-262. https://doi.org/10.1007/978-3-642-12483-9_5.

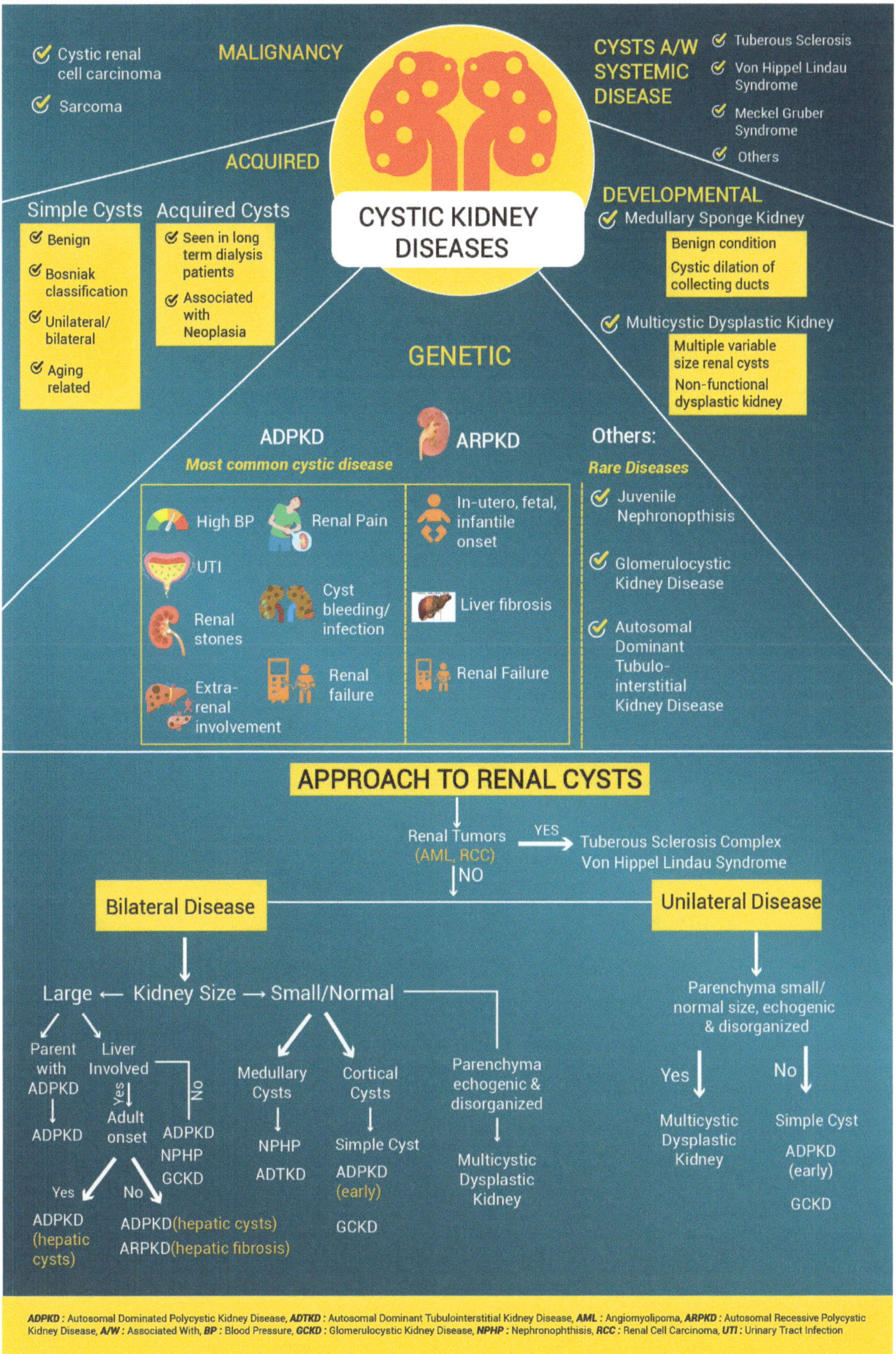

CYSTIC KIDNEY DISEASES
MALIGNANCY
Cystic renal cell carcinoma
Sarcoma
CYSTS A/W SYSTEMIC DISEASE
Tuberous Sclerosis
Von Hippel Lindau Syndrome
Meckel Gruber Syndrome
Others
ACQUIRED
Simple Cysts
Benign
Bosniak classification
Unilateral/ bilateral
Aging related
Acquired Cysts
Seen in long term dialysis patients
Associated with Neoplasia
DEVELOPMENTAL
Medullary Sponge Kidney
Benign condition
Cystic dilation of collecting ducts
Multicystic Dysplastic Kidney
Multiple variable size renal cysts
Non-functional dysplastic kidney
GENETIC
ADPKD
Most common cystic disease
High BP
Renal Pain
UTI
Cyst bleeding/ infection
Renal stones
Extra-renal involvement
Renal failure
ARPKD
In-utero, fetal, infantile onset
Liver fibrosis
Renal Failure
Others:
Rare Diseases
Juvenile Nephronopthisis
Glomerulocystic Kidney Disease
Autosomal Dominant Tubulo-interstitial Kidney Disease
APPROACH TO RENAL CYSTS
Renal Tumors (AML, RCC)
YES
Tuberous Sclerosis Complex
Von Hippel Lindau Syndrome
NO
Bilateral Disease
Unilateral Disease
Large
Kidney Size
Small/Normal
Parent with ADPKD
ADPKD
Liver Involved
Yes
No
Adult onset
ADPKD
NPHP
GCKD
Yes
ADPKD (hepatic cysts)
No
ADPKD(hepatic cysts)
ARPKD(hepatic fibrosis)
Medullary Cysts
NPHP
ADTKD
Cortical Cysts
Simple Cyst
ADPKD (early)
GCKD
Parenchyma echogenic & disorganized
Multicystic Dysplastic Kidney
Parenchyma small/ normal size, echogenic & disorganized
Yes
Multicystic Dysplastic Kidney
No
Simple Cyst
ADPKD (early)
GCKD
ADPKD : Autosomal Dominated Polycystic Kidney Disease, ADTKD : Autosomal Dominant Tubulointerstitial Kidney Disease, AML : Angiomyolipoma, ARPKD : Autosomal Recessive Polycystic Kidney Disease, A/W : Associated With, BP : Blood Pressure, GCKD : Glomerulocystic Kidney Disease, NPHP : Nephronophthisis, RCC : Renal Cell Carcinoma, UTI : Urinary Tract Infection

27

URINARY TRACT INFECTIONS

Garima Aggarwal, Vishwanath S

More than 50% of all women have had at least one urinary tract infection in their lifetime. Distinguishing between complicated versus uncomplicated urinary tract infections (UTI) is important, as it influences the investigations, treatment, and duration of the antibiotic therapy.

Uncomplicated UTI

Lower (cystitis) and/or upper urinary tract (pyelonephritis) infections, limited to non-pregnant women, with no known relevant structural or functional urinary tract abnormalities or any comorbidities, are called uncomplicated infections(1). These may be acute, sporadic, or recurrent. Most UTIs encountered in clinical practice are uncomplicated infections, occurring in young women, which do not require detailed evaluation and can be safely managed on an outpatient basis with oral antibiotics.

Complicated UTI

This refers to UTIs in individuals in whom risk factors related to the patient or anatomical or functional abnormalities of the urinary tract, result in an infection that is more difficult to eradicate than an uncomplicated infection. These patients are more likely to have treatment failure or recurrences and include the following conditions:

- Male sex
- Pregnancy
- Poorly controlled diabetes mellitus
- Obstruction or other structural factor in the urinary tract: urolithiasis, malignancies, ureteral and urethral strictures, bladder diverticula, renal cysts, fistulas, ileal conduits, other urinary diversions
- Functional abnormality: incomplete voiding, neurogenic bladder, vesicoureteral reflux
- Foreign body: indwelling catheter, ureteral stent, nephrostomy tube
- Other conditions: kidney failure, kidney transplantation, immunosuppression, multidrug-resistant uropathogens, and healthcare-associated.

Table 27.1: The Classification of Different Types of Urinary Tract Infections

Description	Clinical Features	Diagnosis	
		Pyuria (in unspun urine)	Urine culture (midstream, clean catch urine sample)*
Asymptomatic bacteriuria	No urinary symptoms	≥ 10 WBC/mm^3	≥ 10^5 CFU/ml in two consecutive cultures ≥ 24 hours apart in women, single sample in men

Description	Clinical Features	Diagnosis	
		Pyuria (in unspun urine)	**Urine culture (midstream, clean catch urine sample)***
Acute uncomplicated cystitis in women	Dysuria, urgency, frequency, suprapubic pain,	≥ 10 WBC/mm^3	≥ 10^3 CFU/ml
Acute uncomplicated pyelonephritis	Fever, chills, flank pain; other diagnoses excluded; no history or clinical evidence of urological abnormalities (ultrasonography, radiography)	≥ 10 WBC/mm^3	≥ 10^4 CFU/ml
Complicated UTI	Upper or lower urinary tract symptoms with one or more factors associated with a complicated UTI	≥ 10 WBC/mm^3	≥ 10^5 CFU/ml* in women ≥ 10^4 CFU/ ml* in men or in straight-catheter urine sample
Recurrent UTI	At least three episodes of uncomplicated infection: women only; no structural/ functional abnormalities		≥ 10^3 CFU/ml during episodes
*In a suprapubic bladder puncture specimen, any count of bacteria is considered diagnostic			

Asymptomatic Bacteriuria

The presence of bacteria in the urine that causes no illness or symptoms to the patient is referred to as asymptomatic bacteriuria (ABU). Bacterial growth in the urinary tract in patients without any symptoms is common and is due to the growth of commensal bacteria.

ABU in an individual without urinary tract symptoms is defined by a mid-stream sample of urine showing bacterial growth > 10^5 cfu/mL in two consecutive samples in women or one single sample in men (Refer Table 27.1).

Digital rectal examination should be done in all men to rule out prostatic abscesses/diseases. Imaging of the upper tract/ cystoscopy is not needed.

Treatment

Treatment of ABU in females with recurrent symptomatic UTIs and without identifiable risk factors, leads to an increased risk of developing a subsequent symptomatic UTI in studies. In patients without risk factors for complicated UTI, screening, surveillance urine cultures, or treatment of ABU is not recommended. Treatment of asymptomatic candiduria is also not found to be of any benefit.

Screening or treatment of ABU is not found to be of any benefit for the following groups of patients:

- women without risk factors;
- patients with well-controlled diabetes mellitus;
- post-menopausal women;
- elderly institutionalized patients;
- patients with dysfunctional and/or reconstructed lower urinary tracts;
- patients with urinary catheters;
- patients with renal transplants; and
- patients prior to arthroplasty surgeries.

Screening and treatment of ABU are recommended only in:

- Pregnant women – ABU in pregnant women is associated with a high risk of developing pyelonephritis, preterm labor, and low birth weight infants. Screen and treat with a short course of antibiotics (2–7 days). In general, safe antibiotics in pregnancy include penicillin, cephalosporin, fosfomycin, nitrofurantoin (not in case of G6PD deficiency and during the end of pregnancy), trimethoprim (not in the first trimester), and sulphonamides (not in the last trimester).
- Prior to urological surgeries – Urine culture must be taken prior to such interventions, and in the case of ABU, pre-operative treatment is given.

Cystitis

Acute uncomplicated cystitis presents with typical lower urinary tract symptoms like dysuria, suprapubic pain, urinary frequency, and urgency of acute onset (< 1 week) in non-pregnant, pre-menopausal women. Sometimes, women present with gross hematuria. Cystitis in men is usually associated with prostate involvement and is classified as a complicated infection.

The primary causative organism of uncomplicated cystitis is typically Escherichia coli (E. coli), seen in 75 to 90% of the cases & Staphylococcus saprophyticus in 5 to 15%.

The diagnosis of uncomplicated cystitis can be made in women with classical history and the absence of vaginal discharge or irritation. Urine analysis is only needed if the diagnosis is not clear. Urinalysis may reveal:

- Pyuria
- Bacteria seen on urine microscopy
- Urinary dipstick with nitrite or leukocyte esterase positivity.

Urine culture is not needed for treating patients with classical symptoms or positive urinalysis, and is only recommended in patients with suspected acute pyelonephritis, pregnant women, women with atypical symptoms, those who fail to respond to appropriate antibiotics, or when symptoms recur within 2–4 weeks of treatment.

Treatment

Antibiotic choice in treating cystitis has to be decided by keeping in mind the antibiotic susceptibility patterns of causative bacteria in your region of practice, tolerability of the patient, adverse drug reactions, costs, and availability, among others. Most women get symptomatic relief within 72 hours of starting antibiotics. Some common regimens include:

Table 27.2: Empirical Oral Antimicrobial Therapy in Uncomplicated Cystitis

Drug	Dose	Frequency	Duration	Comments
Fosfomycin trometamol	3 g	Single dose		– Cause significant GI side effects like nausea, vomiting, diarrhea, vaginitis
Nitrofurantoin	100 mg	Twice daily	5– 7 days	– Inactive against proteus and pseudomonas species – Causes GI upset
Trimethoprim-sulphamethoxazole/ Co-trimoxazole	160/ 800 mg (Double strength)	Twice daily	3 days	– When antibiotic resistance rates for E. coli of < 20%
Trimethoprim	200 mg	Twice daily	5 days	
Levofloxacin	500 mg	Once daily	3 days	– Moxifloxacin is not preferred due to inadequate urinary concentrations
Ciprofloxacin	500 mg	Twice daily	3 days	
Norfloxacin	400 mg	Twice daily	3 days	
Gatifloxacin	400mg	Once daily	3 days	
Cefpodoxime proxetil	100 mg	Twice daily	5–7 days	
Cephalexin	250 mg	Once daily	7 days	
Amoxicillin/ clavulanate	500/ 125 mg	Twice daily	7 days	

Cystitis in men requires treatment for at least 7 days, with antibiotics penetrating into the prostate tissue, preferably trimethoprim-sulphamethoxazole or a fluoroquinolone, according to susceptibility testing,

It is important to note that ampicillin/sulbactam or amoxicillin/clavulanic acid and oral cephalosporins are not recommended for empirical therapy in cystitis due to ecological collateral damage, high resistance rates, and the need to use them for extended spectrum beta-lactamase (ESBL)-producing bacteria, but may be used in selected cases.

For dysuria, phenazopyridine (200 mg) or flavoxate (200 mg) can be used for 1 or 2 days to reduce symptoms.

Post-treatment urinalysis or urine cultures are not needed and should only be performed for women whose symptoms persist or recur within 2 weeks. In such cases, it is advisable to assume that the causing organism is resistant to the initially prescribed medication. Consideration should be given to retreatment, using a different agent, typically at least a 7-day course of antibiotics.

Pyelonephritis

Uncomplicated pyelonephritis is seen in non-pregnant, pre-menopausal women with no known relevant urological abnormalities or comorbidities. Patients present with fever with chills, flank pain, nausea, vomiting, or costovertebral angle tenderness, with or without the symptoms of cystitis. Pregnant women with acute pyelonephritis need special attention, as this can have an adverse effect on the mother (anemia, renal, and respiratory insufficiency), as well as the fetus (pre-term labor and birth).

Urinalysis and urine culture sensitivity testing should be performed in all cases. A blood culture is usually not needed unless a complicated infection is suspected or the patient is already on antibiotics or has signs of severe sepsis.

Imaging should be done to rule out obstructive pyelonephritis if symptoms persist after 3 days of antibiotic treatment or when the diagnosis is doubtful. Imaging studies include:

- Ultrasound (US) whole abdomen or plain computed tomography (CT) KUB – For evaluation of the upper urinary tract to rule out urinary tract obstruction or renal calculus disease in patients with a history of urolithiasis, altered renal functions, or high urine pH.
- Contrast-enhanced CT scan or excretory urography – To be considered if the patient remains febrile after 72 hours of treatment, or immediately, if there is deterioration in the clinical status.
- In pregnant women, US or magnetic resonance imaging (MRI) is preferred for diagnosis of complicating factors.

Treatment

Oral Antibiotics

In clinically stable patients with uncomplicated infections, outpatient treatment with oral antibiotics is sufficient. Shorter courses of antibiotics are associated with a higher recurrence rate within 4 to 6 weeks, hence, the treatment should be done for at least 14 days. Choice of antibiotics includes:

Table 27.3: Empirical Oral Antimicrobial Therapy in Uncomplicated Pyelonephritis

Drug	Dose	Frequency	Duration	Comments
Ciprofloxacin	500–750 mg	Twice daily	14 days	Local flouroquinolone resistance should be less than 10%
Levofloxacin	750 mg	Once daily	14 days	
Trimethoprim-sulphamethoxazole/ Co-trimoxazole	160/800 mg (Double strength)	Twice daily	10–14 days	
Cefpodoxime	200 mg	Twice daily	10 days	
Ceftibuten	400 mg	Twice daily	10 days	

Intravenous (IV) Antibiotics

- Preferred first-line drugs are aminoglycoside (with or without ampicillin), or extended-spectrum cephalosporin, or penicillin.
- Carbapenems should only be considered in patients with early culture results, indicating the presence of multi-drug resistant organisms.
- If a patient starts showing clinical improvement, IV can be switched to oral antibiotics for a total duration of 7 to 10 days.
- In men with febrile UTI, pyelonephritis, or recurrent infection, or whenever a complicating factor is suspected, a minimum treatment duration of 2 weeks is recommended, preferably with fluoroquinolone since prostatic involvement is frequent.

Table 27.4: Empirical IV Antibiotic Therapy in Uncomplicated Pyelonephritis

Drug	Dose	Frequency	Duration	Comments
Ciprofloxacin	400 mg	Twice a day	7–10 days In Men – at least 14 days	
Levofloxacin	750 mg q.d	Once a day		
Cefotaxime	2 g	Thrice a day		
Ceftriaxone	1–2 g	Once a day		
Cefepime	1–2 g	Twice a day		
Piperacillin/ tazobactam	2.5–4.5 g	Thrice a day		
Gentamicin	5 mg/kg	Once a day		
Amikacin	15 mg/kg	Once a day		
Imipenem/ cilastatin	0.5 g	Thrice a day		Consider only if culture suggestive of multi-drug Resistance (MDR) organisms
Meropenem	1 g	Thrice a day		
Ceftolozane/ tazobactam	1.5 g	Thrice a day		
Ceftazidime/ avibactam	2.5 g	Thrice a day		

Complicated UTIs

A complicated urinary tract infection (cUTI) is characterized by typical features of cystitis or pyelonephritis in high-risk individuals. However, in certain clinical scenarios, the symptoms may be atypical, especially in patients with neurogenic bladders, urinary diversion surgeries, nephrostomy, or catheter-associated UTIs (CAUTI). Clinicians must be aware that symptoms, particularly lower urinary tract symptoms (LUTS), can be caused not only by UTIs but also by other urological disorders (for example benign prostatic hyperplasia, bladder outlet obstructions, obstructive uropathy, autonomic dysfunction in patients with spinal lesions and neurogenic bladders), and these should be ruled out.

Urine culture and blood cultures should be performed. Imaging studies are often needed to rule out other anatomical defects.

Causative bacteria usually consist of multi-drug resistant organisms, which commonly include E. coli, Proteus spp., Klebsiella spp., Pseudomonas spp., Serratia spp., and Enterococcus spp. Enterobacterales predominate (60–75%) with E. coli as the most common pathogen; particularly if the UTI is a first infection.

Treatment

cUTI with systemic symptoms usually requires hospitalization; initial treatment should be with an intravenous (IV) antimicrobial regimen. The choice of the IV antibiotic should be based on local resistance data, patient factors, and previous urine culture reports, if available, and later adjusted according to the culture susceptibility results. Antibiotics should be continued for a duration of 7 to 14 days (14 days when prostatitis cannot be excluded). In cases where the patient is stable hemodynamically and afebrile for at least 48 hours, a shorter treatment duration (e.g., 7 days) may be considered. Urological abnormality and/or underlying complicating factors must also be managed. Choice of antibiotics may include:

- Aminoglycoside with or without amoxicillin,
- Third-generation cephalosporin,
- Second-generation cephalosporin plus an aminoglycoside,
- An extended-spectrum penicillin with or without an aminoglycoside,
- Carbepenems.

Alternative treatment regimens, particularly for multidrug-resistant pathogens, include:

- Imipenem/cilastatin,
- Ceftazidime/avibactam,
- Aztreonam.

Due to the high levels of resistance, fluoroquinolones are no longer recommended as suitable empirical antimicrobial therapy for cUTI. This is particularly important when the patient has used them within the past 6 months. Fluoroquinolones can only be used for empirical therapy for cUTI in patients whose condition is not severe, are fit for oral treatment, whose local resistance to flouroquinolones is <10%, or have contraindications to third-generation cephalosporins, aminoglycosides, and other beta-lactam antimicrobials.

Antibiotic combinations like Ceftolozane/tazobactam; Cefiderocol; Plazomicin; Imipenem/cilastatin plus relebactam; Meropenem vadorbactam are recommended in European and American guidelines but are not yet available in India.

Recurrent UTI

Patients presenting with UTIs at a frequency of at least 3 UTIs per year or 2 UTIs in the last 6 months are said to have recurrent urinary tract infections (rUTI).

After the first UTI, most women will have occasional recurrences and 25–50% develop another UTI within one year. 3 to 5% develop rUTIs.

Risk factors for recurrent UTI include:

- Sexual intercourse
- Use of spermicide
- A new sexual partner
- A mother with a history of UTI during childhood
- Blood group antigen secretory status
- History of UTI before menopause
- Urinary incontinence
- Atrophic vaginitis due to oestrogen deficiency
- Cystocele
- Increased post-void urine volume
- Urine catheterization and functional status deterioration in elderly institutionalized women.

Prevention of recurrent UTIs can be achieved in the following ways:

- Avoidance of Risk Factors
    - Adequate hydration (at least > 1.5 L/day water),
    - Avoid post-coital delayed urination,
    - Never wiping from back to front after defecation,
    - Avoid douching with commercially available vaginal washes,
    - Avoid wearing occlusive underwear,
    - Avoid using spermicides or spermicide-coated condoms or diaphragms.
- Conservative Methods
    - Vaginal Estrogen Therapy – Vaginal estrogen replacement is known to prevent rUTIs in peri- and post-menopausal women. Vaginal creams are most commonly used, recommended doses are:
        - 17β-estradiol vaginal cream – 2 g daily for 2 weeks, then 1 g 2–3 times per week.

        - Conjugate equine vaginal estrogen – 0.5g daily for 2 weeks, then 0.5 g twice weekly.
    - Oral Probiotics that promote healthy vaginal flora
    - Cranberry extract
    - D mannose
    - Vaccine – Oral, intranasal, or sublingual vaccines made from uropathogenic bacterial extracts may be effective in preventing UTI.
- Antibiotic Prophylaxis
    - Continuous low-dose antibiotic prophylaxis – From 3 up to 12 months. This should not be started until active infection is eradicated, which is confirmed by a negative urine culture test at least 1–2 weeks after completion of treatment.
        - Nitrofurantoin 50 mg or 100 mg once daily,
        - Fosfomycin trometamol 3 g every 10 days,
        - Trimethoprim-sulfamethoxazole (SS-80/400 mg), half tablet every night or 3 times/week,
        - Trimethoprim 100 mg once daily,
        - Cephalexin 125 mg or 250 mg once daily.
    - Post-coital prophylaxis – Especially in women who get recurrent cystitis after sexual intercourse.
        - Trimethoprim-sulfamethoxazole (80/400 mg, Single strength) – half tablet or one tablet,
        - Nitrofurantoin 50 or 100 mg single dose,
        - Levofloxacin 250 mg single dose,
        - Ciprofloxacin 250 mg since dose.
    - Self-diagnosis and self-administration of a short course of antibiotics for 3 days may be considered in people with good adherence and compliance, if they develop symptoms. However, women should be guided to get medical help if symptoms don't resolve after 48–72 hours of completing the antibiotic course.

References:

1. EAU-Guidelines-on-Urological-infections-2023.pdf [Internet]. [cited 2023 Jun 14]. Available from: https://d56bochluxqnz.cloudfront.net/documents/full-guideline/EAU-Guidelines-on-Urological-infections-2023.pdf.
2. Grabe M, Bartoletti R, Cai T, Köves B, Tenke P, Wagenlehner F, et al. Guidelines on Urological Infections. In 2009 [cited 2023 Jun 18]. Available from: https://www.semanticscholar.org/paper/Guidelines-on-Urological-Infections-Grabe-Bartoletti/bb0622f0c4fabec2e5636ced6b2693c78b5e4a1e.
3. Fihn SD. Clinical practice. Acute uncomplicated urinary tract infection in women. N Engl J Med. 2003 Jul 17;349(3):259–66.
4. Hooton TM. Recurrent urinary tract infection in women. Int J Antimicrob Agents. 2001 Apr;17(4):259–68.
5. De Cueto M, Aliaga L, Alós JI, Canut A, Los-Arcos I, Martínez JA, et al. Executive summary of the diagnosis and treatment of urinary tract infection: Guidelines of the Spanish Society of Clinical Microbiology and Infectious Diseases (SEIMC). Enfermedades Infecc Microbiol Clínica. 2017 May;35(5):314–20.
6. van Nieuwkoop C, Hoppe BPC, Bonten TN, Van't Wout JW, Aarts NJM, Mertens BJ, et al. Predicting the need for radiologic imaging in adults with febrile urinary tract infection. Clin Infect Dis Off Publ Infect Dis Soc Am. 2010 Dec 1;51(11):1266–72.
7. Berti F, Attardo TM, Piras S, Tesei L, Tirotta D, Tonani M, et al. Short versus long course antibiotic therapy for acute pyelonephritis in adults: a systematic review and meta-analysis. Ital J Med. 2018 Mar 20;12(1):39–50.
8. Rudrabhatla P, Deepanjali S, Mandal J, Swaminathan RP, Kadhiravan T. Stopping the effective non-fluoroquinolone antibiotics at day 7 vs continuing until day 14 in adults with acute pyelonephritis requiring hospitalization: A randomized non-inferiority trial. PloS One. 2018;13(5):e0197302.
9. van der Starre WE, van Nieuwkoop C, Paltansing S, van't Wout JW, Groeneveld GH, Becker MJ, et al. Risk factors for fluoroquinolone-resistant Escherichia coli in adults with

community-onset febrile urinary tract infection. J Antimicrob Chemother. 2011 Mar;66(3):650–6.

10. Cai T, Mazzoli S, Mondaini N, Meacci F, Nesi G, D'Elia C, et al. The Role of Asymptomatic Bacteriuria in Young Women With Recurrent Urinary Tract Infections: To Treat or Not to Treat? Clin Infect Dis. 2012 Sep 15;55(6):771–7.
11. Anger J, Lee U, Ackerman AL, Chou R, Chughtai B, Clemens JQ, et al. Recurrent Uncomplicated Urinary Tract Infections in Women: AUA/CUA/SUFU Guideline. J Urol. 2019 Aug;202(2):282–9.

URINARY TRACT INFECTION

ASYMPTOMATIC BACTERURIA

No Urinary Symptoms

Urine c/s $\geq 10^5$ CFU/ml in two consecutive cultures > 24 hours apart in women, single sample in men

RECURRENT UTI

$\geq$ 3 UTI episodes/year OR $\geq$2 UTIs in last 6 months

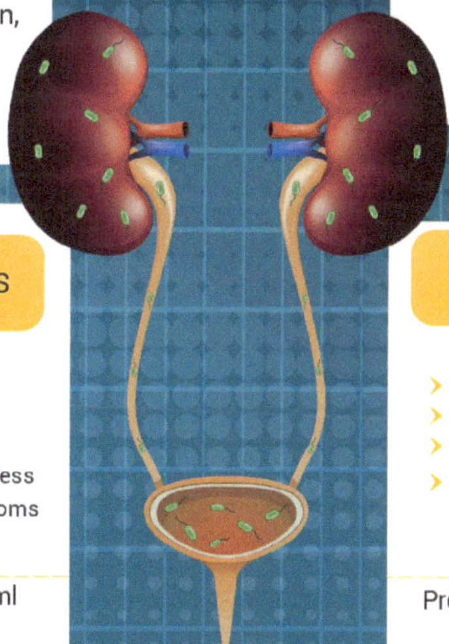

PYELONEPHRITIS

- Fever with chills
- Flank Pain
- Nausea/Vommiting
- Costoverbal angle tenderness
- With or without the symptoms of cystitis

Urine c/s with $\geq 10^4$ CFU/ml imaging evidence of pyelonephritis

CYSTITIS

- Dysuria
- Suprapubic Pain
- Urinary frequency
- Urgency of acute onset (<1week)

Presence of Pyuria/ Leucocyte esterase positive/Nitrite positive/Bacteria in urine

COMPLICATED UTI

- Male sex
- Pregnancy
- Poorly controlled diabetes mellitus
- **Sturctural:** Urolithiasis, malignancies, Ureteric and Urethral Strictures, Bladder outlet obstruction
- **Functional:** Incomplete voiding, neurogenic bladder, Vesicoureteric reflux
- **Foreign body:** Indwelling catheter, ureteral stent, nephrostomy tube
- **Other conditions:** kidney failure, kidney transplatation, immunosuppression, multidrug-resistant uropathogens, and health care-associated

UNCOMPLICATED UTI

Limited to non-pregnant women with no known relevant structural or functional urinary tract abnormalities or any comorbidities

C/s **:** Culture and sensitivity, ***CFU*** **:** Colony Forming Unit, ***UTI*** **:** Urinary Tract Infection

28

NEWER ADVANCES IN NEPHROLOGY

Narinder Pal Singh, Dinesh Khullar

Introduction:

Chronic kidney disease (CKD) and end-stage renal disease (ESRD) pose substantial global health challenges, with a soaring prevalence over the past two decades. Data from GBD 2017 revealed 697.5 million documented CKD cases worldwide, with a global prevalence of 9.1%, which is expected to rise. CKD's global mortality rate increased by 41.5% from 1990 to 2017, making it the 12th leading cause of death, projected to potentially become the 5th leading cause by 2040.

India significantly contributes to this burden, accounting for 17% of the global CKD cases. Mortality from CKD in India doubled from 1990 to 2016, highlighting room for improvement with existing resources.

CKD management includes supportive care and kidney replacement therapy (KRT) through dialysis or transplantation. However, the current dialysis methods are inadequate and inaccessible. In 2010, a substantial gap existed in providing dialysis to ESRD patients, projected to widen to 9 million by

2030. Patients on dialysis often experience a reduced health-related quality of life and a shortened life expectancy, primarily due to limited access and high costs.

The growing prevalence of kidney diseases and limited treatment options necessitate advances in nephrology. Inadequate funding and misconceptions about existing treatments have hindered advancement. Yet, there's a burgeoning wave of innovation in nephrology. This review explores recent developments, focusing on evidence-based practices and emerging trends in nephrology, which are crucial for improving patient outcomes, reducing economic burdens, and enhancing the quality of life for those affected by these conditions.

Novel Diagnostic Methods:

There's an urgent need for innovative diagnostic methods in CKD to enable early detection. Currently, CKD is often diagnosed in its advanced stages, with over 50% of kidney function already compromised, leading to a higher risk of disease progression and premature mortality. Existing interventions are less effective at this late stage. While elevated urine albumin levels can signal CKD, a significant number of patients still progress to severe stages (G3) despite having normal albumin levels. Detecting the subclinical phase of CKD, which can persist for decades without symptoms, presents a considerable challenge for timely diagnosis. To bridge this diagnostic gap, various approaches, including imaging and biomarker assessment in biological fluids, are under exploration (see Table 28.1). The field of nephrology is also witnessing a revolution through artificial intelligence (AI) and machine learning. AI algorithms can analyze extensive datasets, identify patterns, and predict outcomes, aiding nephrologists in diagnosing kidney diseases and optimizing treatment plans, ultimately improving patient care.

Table 28.1: Advances in Diagnostic Methods

Imaging: • **Assessing nephron number**: CFE-MRI, RadioCF-PET, Sodium MRI (currently not used in clinical practice) • **Assessing kidney fibrosis**: CNA35-CT, ESMA-based MRI • **Functional MRI** (measure kidney volumes, renal arteries blood flow, and tissue oxygenation): DW-MRI, BOLD-MRI, and HP-13C MRI • **Contrast enhanced ultrasound**: Imaging for renal lesions.
Biological fluid biomarkers: • **CKD biomarkers:** PCX, KIM-1, TNF-alfa, 8-OHdG • **AKI Biomarkers:** KIM-1, NGAL, L-FABP, IGFBP-7, TIMP-2 • **Drug Induced Kidney Injury Biomarkers:** miRNAs: miR-192-5p
Proteomic and metabolomic analysis: • CKD273 (urinary peptides), KRIS (a protein involved in the inflammatory process), THSD7A (detection in primary MN), NAD metabolites (involved in AKI risk prediction), FAT1 (In MN after HST), Anti-nephrin ab (In minimal change disease).
Cell-free DNA: Used in the detection of renal cell carcinoma, evaluation of acute rejection, detection of AKI after cardiac surgery (cardiorenal syndrome), prognosis in ESRD, and assessment of acute rejection in kidney transplant.

Novel Therapeutic Alternatives

Emerging ESRD treatments, such as wearable artificial kidneys, xenotransplantation, stem cell therapy, and bioengineered kidneys, aim to enable at-home care, reducing reliance on dialysis centers. Advanced CKD medications nearing approval, seek early intervention to potentially reverse or prevent CKD progression. Improved diagnostics complement these new therapeutic approaches.

Table 28.2: Novel Therapeutic Strategies

Wearable Artificial Kidneys: • Allow greater mobility and flexibility compared to traditional dialysis techniques. • Allow continuous toxin clearance and provide good hemodynamic stability. • Reusable dialysate solutions (without the requirement of a large amount of water). Complications: Clotting at the vascular site, infection risk, variation in blood/dialysate flow rates, and toxin clearance.
Online Hemodiafiltration (OL-HDF): • The inclusion of both convection and diffusion methods for efficient removal of intermediate-sized molecules and has been demonstrated to have a significant and positive influence on long-term survival outcomes.
Peritoneal Dialysis (PD) Advancements: • Innovations in PD solutions, catheter design, and remote monitoring have made this modality more accessible and effective, offering greater flexibility to patients
Xenotransplantation: • It is the process of transplanting organs/tissues from animals of different species, commonly pigs, into humans. • Less hyperacute rejection and stable urine output for a shorter duration is the favorable outcome of transplant. • Transplanted kidneys are unable to excrete creatinine at a physiological level and cause TMA.
Stem Cell-based Therapy: • Mesenchymal stem cell therapy holds promise for kidney diseases. • Mechanisms include upregulating autophagy, antiapoptotic effects, paracrine signaling, and anti-inflammatory properties. • Stem cell-derived extracellular vesicles may combat vascular calcification and prevent fibrosis.

- Kidney organoids are in vitro kidney models generated from stem cells and exhibit a remarkable degree of similarities with native tissue, in terms of cell type, morphology, and function.
- These organoids mimic the structure and function of the kidney, enabling researchers to study kidney development, disease modeling, drug screening, and regenerative medicine applications.

Bioengineered/Bio-artificial Kidneys

Renal Assist Device (RAD):

- The bio-artificial RAD combines synthetic hollow fibers with porcine kidney cells, enhancing hemodialysis.
- Clinical trials showed improved outcomes, with most patients experiencing positive results.
- Cell sourcing, manufacturing time and cost, storage, and distribution limit its widespread use.
- Bioartificial Renal Epithelial Cell System (BRECS), is promising but has not undergone human trials since 2017.

Implantable Bioartificial Kidney (iBK):

- Similar to wearable artificial kidneys, iBK offers continuous daily dialysis.
- It comprises a silicon membrane blood filter and a bioreactor with engineered renal cells, enhancing toxin removal, cardiovascular stability, and quality of life.
- Durability and blood filter clotting are potential issues, but iBK shows promise as a RRT alternative.

Glomerulus/Organ-on-a-chip:

- Organ-on-a-chip technology replicates human organ activities and physiology.
- It supports long-term cell culture while maintaining natural cell characteristics.
- Microfluidic platforms enable advanced 3D structures for disease modeling, drug screening, and regenerative medicine.
- Additionally, bioengineering seeks to develop complete kidney scaffolds with 3D geometry and vasculature.

Newer Medications:

- Non-steroidal selective MRA: Finerenone.
- Reno-protection by Sodium-glucose cotransporter-2 (SGLT2) inhibitors.
- Aldosterone synthase/CYP11B2 inhibitors: fadrozole.
- Endothelin receptor antagonists: Sparsentan, sitaxentan.
- HIF prolyl hydroxylase inhibitor: Daprodustat.
- Calcineurin inhibitor: Voclosporin.

Xenotransplantation, particularly in light of recent advancements such as the successful pig kidney transplant performed in Boston, represents a burgeoning frontier in medical science. This technique involves transplanting organs or tissues from one species to another, typically from animals to humans, to address the acute shortage of human organ donations. With the advent of CRISPR and other gene-editing technologies, scientists can modify animal organs to be more compatible with the human immune system, potentially reducing the risk of rejection. Despite genetic modifications, the human body may still recognize the transplanted organ as foreign and mount an immune response, leading to organ rejection. There is also a risk of transmitting animal viruses to humans, potentially leading to new infectious diseases. The recent success at Massachusetts General Hospital signals a positive step forward, but xenotransplantation remains a complex field with many challenges to overcome. Ethical debates, the technical complexity of making animal organs compatible with humans, and the long-term effects of such transplants on human health are crucial areas for ongoing research and discussion.

Novel Therapies for Vascular Access in Hemodialysis:

The selection of vascular access for HD has remained largely unchanged for an extended period and is linked to significant health complications, mortality, and substantial healthcare expenditures. A major challenge in the placement of arteriovenous (AV) fistulas is the frequent failure of fistula maturation, influenced by factors like patient age, blood vessel size, blood flow, vessel remodeling, and underlying health conditions. Innovations in this domain primarily concentrate on new external support devices, biological therapies, and novel techniques for improving HD vascular access. These innovations aim to introduce fresh approaches to control the structure and biology of fistulas, and manipulate blood flow through unique molecular and cellular pathways involved in vascular endothelium remodeling, ultimately affecting fistula maturation and formation.

For instance, the straight-line onlay technique (SLOT) for radiocephalic fistula placement has displayed the potential to reduce stenosis, compared to conventional methods. Devices such as VasQ and Optiflow are designed to aid surgical fistula placement. A sirolimus-eluting collagen implant (SeCI) is in development to enhance fistula maturation. Balloon-assisted maturation (BAM), involving angioplasty to improve maturation success, is widely adopted, and drug-coated balloons like paclitaxel-sirolimus show promise in reducing stenosis. Ongoing efforts explore endovascular techniques and novel graft materials to address patency concerns. While BAM is prevalent, the field of vascular access continues to welcome innovative interventions, aimed at improving patient care.

Innovations in Peritoneal Dialysis

In the field of PD, there has been a noticeable lack of significant innovation for quite some time. However, recent breakthroughs are aimed at not only improving the efficiency of PD but also addressing its environmental impact. For instance, Ellen Medical Devices has introduced a groundbreaking solar-powered PD device designed to purify water from various sources. This innovation carries the potential to reduce the overall costs associated with PD and tackle the environmental concerns tied to its practices. Another noteworthy advancement comes from Baxter, which has developed an on-demand solution that leverages tap water to generate dialysate. This revolutionary approach eliminates the need for transporting and storing dialysate, subsequently reducing the associated costs and logistical complexities. Furthermore, enhancements in packaging and connectivity, exemplified by systems like the Y-tubing set, have emerged as promising developments in reducing the risk of peritonitis, a serious complication of PD. In the realm of wearable PD, technologies like the Vicenza Wearable Artificial Kidney (ViWAK) and the Automated Wearable Artificial Kidney (AWAK) have introduced mobility and improved the quality of life for patients. However, it is crucial to emphasize that these wearable PD methods require further testing and refinement to ensure their safety and effectiveness.

Challenges and Future Directions:

In nephrology, despite significant progress, several challenges persist. Early detection and prevention methods for chronic kidney disease (CKD) need to be more accurate and cost-effective, targeting high-risk groups. Personalized treatment approaches, such as tailored therapies and regenerative medicine, are necessary to expand beyond dialysis and transplantation. Managing concurrent conditions like diabetes and hypertension alongside kidney disease is crucial. Telemedicine and remote monitoring, as highlighted by the COVID-19 pandemic, can enhance nephrology care accessibility, especially in underserved areas. Reliable biomarkers for early diagnosis and treatment response are needed, utilizing genomics and proteomics advancements. Patient education, lifestyle changes, and addressing healthcare disparities are essential. Cost-efficient solutions are imperative and global collaboration is key. Future nephrology directions include bioengineered kidneys, stem cell therapies, health equity promotion, and patient-centered care.

Conclusion:

In summary, advancements in the battle against kidney disease hold promise for earlier detection and intervention, improving long-term outcomes, and offering more patient-friendly kidney replacement options. These developments may also help delay the progression of CKD and enhance its management. Diagnostic markers may enable earlier disease detection when it's still reversible. Additionally, novel therapies could slow disease progression, reduce CKD complications, and decrease the need for RRT or transplants. However, large-scale clinical studies with reliable results are necessary before the widespread use of these therapies and diagnostics, making it challenging to predict when these developments will become available.

References:

1. Copur S, Tanriover C, Yavuz F, Soler MJ, Ortiz A, Covic A et al. Novel strategies in nephrology: what to expect from the future? Clin Kidney J. 2022 Sep 20;16(2):230-244.
2. Ibi Y, Nishinakamura R. Kidney Bioengineering for Transplantation. Transplantation. 2023 Sep 1;107(9):1883-1894.
3. Singh NP, Gupta AK, Ahmed S. Novel Innovation in Dialysis Modalities. In: Upadhyay R, Prakash A, Pangtey G (eds.). Progress in medicine, An official publication of ICP, an academic wing of API. New Delhi, India: Evangel Publication Ltd; 2022. p. 540-547.
4. GBD Chronic Kidney Disease Collaboration and Singh N P. Global, regional, and national burden of chronic kidney disease, 1990–2017: a systematic analysis for the Global Burden of Disease Study 2017. Lancet 2020;395:709–33.

NEWER ADVANCES IN NEPHROLOGY

Advances in VASCULAR ACCESS

- External devices implants
- Balloon assisted maturation: Drug coated baloon
- Endovascular approach: Anastomoses by thermal/ radiofrequency methods
- Manipulation in graft material
- Bioengineered tissue vessels (graft materials)

Advances in DIAGNOSTICS

IMAGING

- Assessing nephron numbers/kidney fibrosis-by Functional MRI/USG

BIOMARKERS

- KIM-1, NGAL, L-FABP, IGFB-7, TIMP-2, miRNAs:miR-192-5p, PCX, KIM-1, TNF-alfa, 8-OHdG

PROTEOMIC & METABOLOMIC

- KRIS, NAD metabolities, FAT1, Anti-nephrin ab, urinary peptides

CELL FREE DNA

Advances in MEDICATIONS

- Non-steroidal selective MRA
- SGLT2 inhibitors
- Aldosterone synthase/ CYP11B2 inhibitors
- Endothelin receptor antogonists
- HIF prolyl hydroxylase inhibitor
- Newer Calcineurin inhibitor

Advances in THERAPEUTICS

- Wearable artificial kidneys
- Online Hemodiafiltration (OL-HDF)
- Xenotransplantation
- Stem cell-based therapy
- Bioengineered/bio-artificial kidneys
  - Renal assist device (RAD)
  - Implantable bioartificial kidney (iBK)
  - Glomerulus/organ-on-a-chip

AB : Antibody, ***DNA :*** Deoxyribonucleic acid, ***FABP :*** Fatty acid binding proteins, ***HIF :*** Hpyoxia-inducible factor, ***KIM :*** Kidney Injury Molecule, ***KRIS :*** Kidney risk inflammatory, ***MRA*** :Mineralocorticoid Receptor Antagonist ***NGAL :*** Neutrophil gelatinase-associated l ipocalin, ***NAD :*** Nicotinamide adenine dinucleotide, ***SGLT2 :*** Sodium-Glucose Cotransporter-2 , ***USG :*** Ultrasound Sonography

SECTION 8

Electrolyte Disorders

HYPONATREMIA

Ajay Kher, Priti Meena

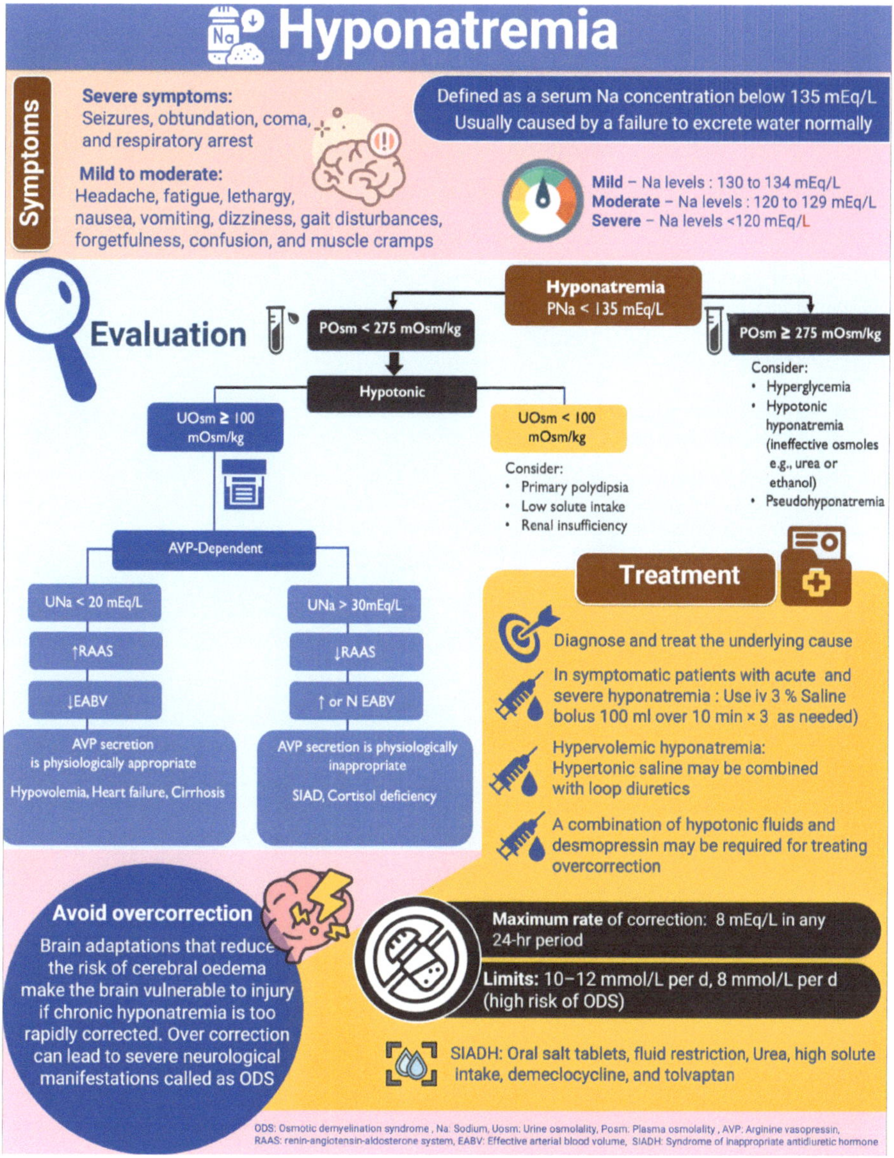

HYPERNATREMIA

Anish Garg, Priti Meena

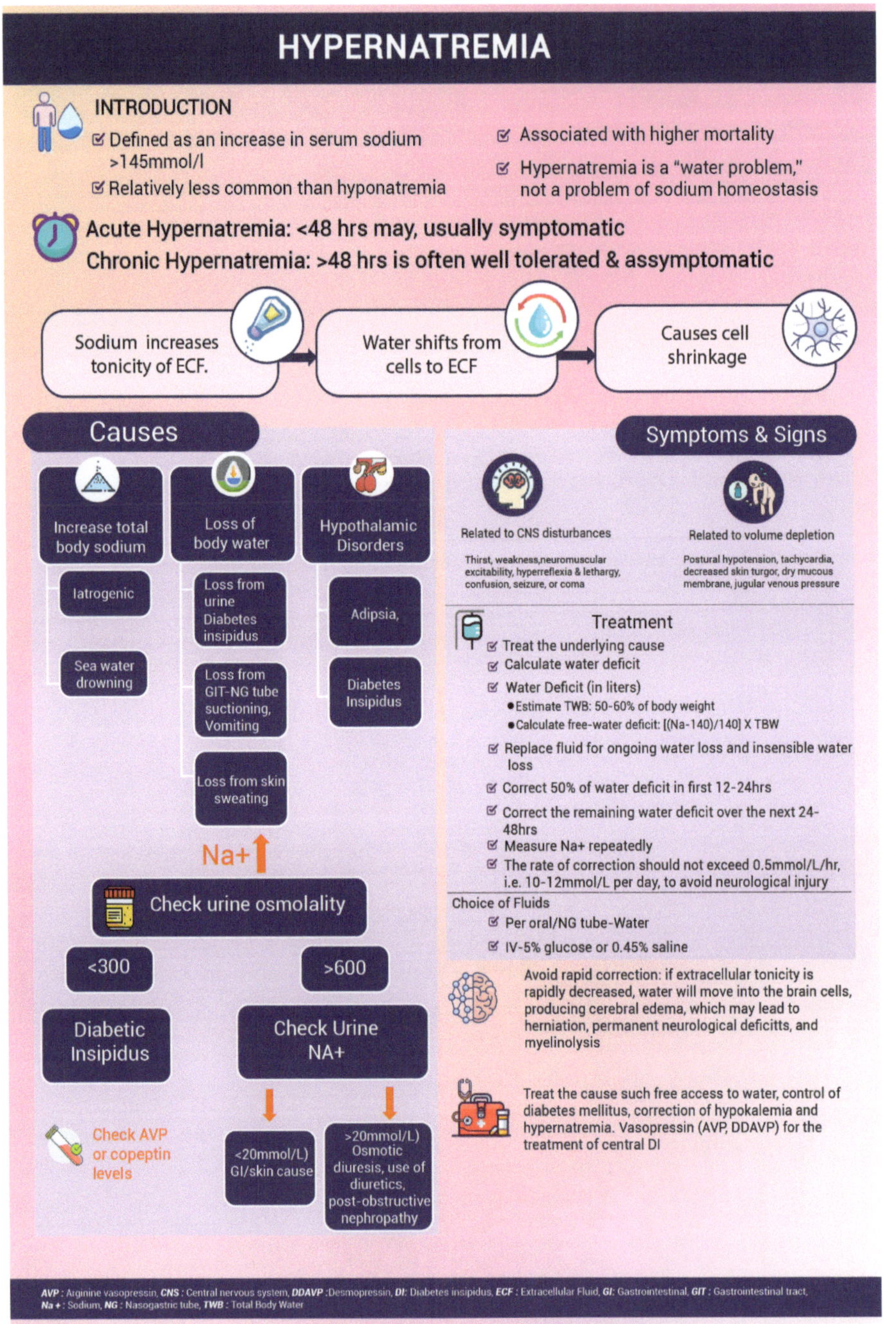

HYPOKALEMIA

Priti Meena

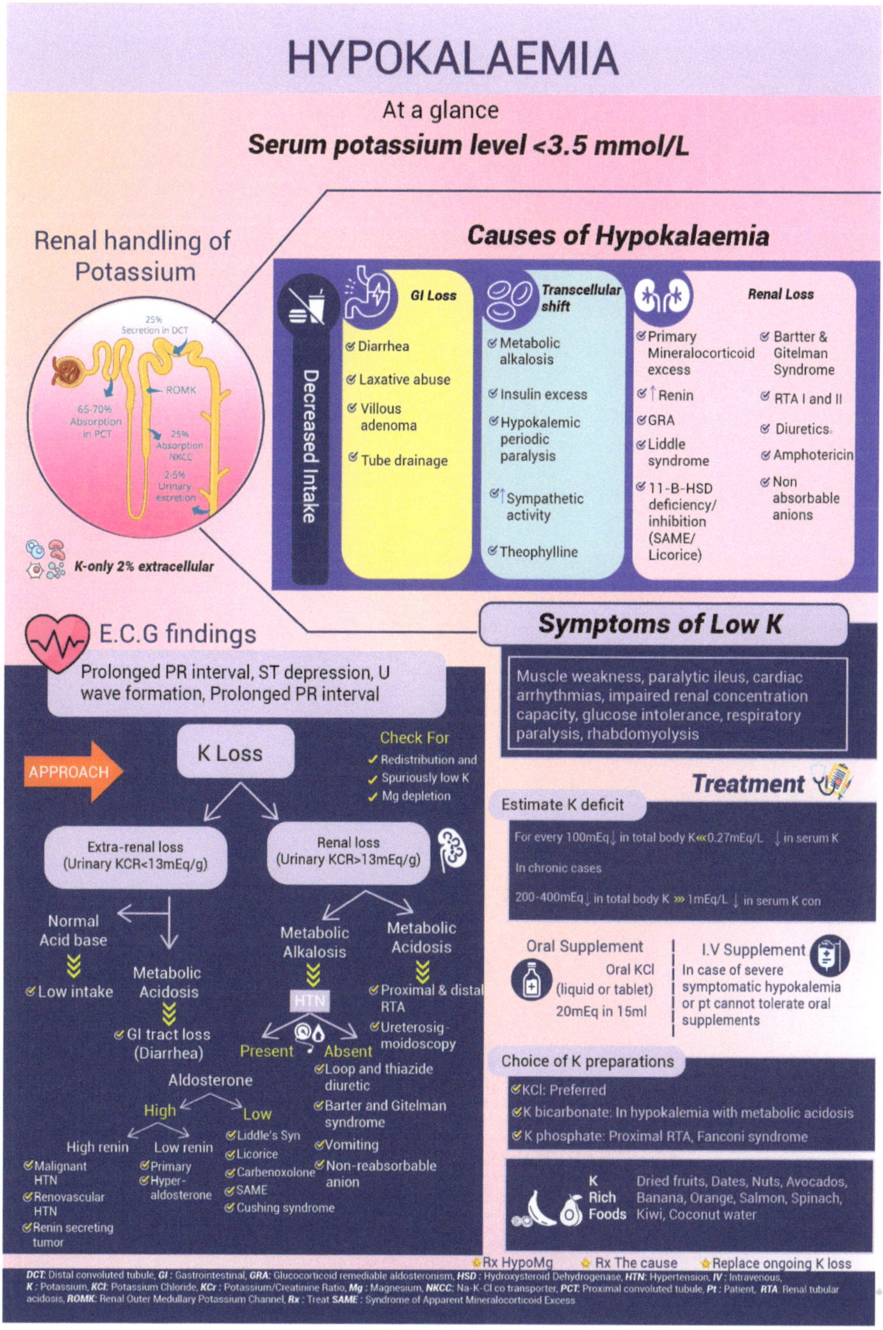

HYPERKALEMIA

Garima Aggarwal

HYPERKALEMIA

NORMAL K 3.5-5.5 | K > 5.5 - 6.0 | K > 6.5-7.5 | K > 8.0

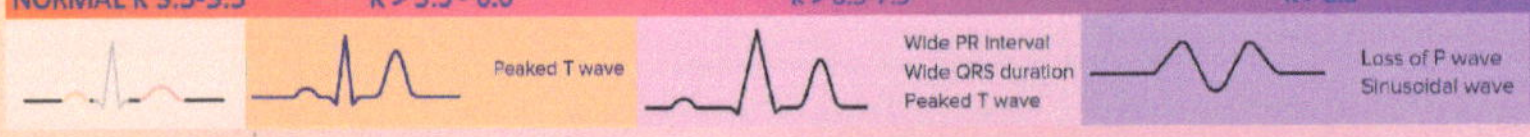

↑K — Rule out pseudohyperkalemia →

PSEUDOHYPERKALEMIA

- Hemolysis
- Small needle size/excessive aspiration
- Centrifuging before clot formation
- Excercising muscles/fist clenching before sampling/Excessively tight tourniquet
- Leucocytosis >70,000/cm³
- Thrombocytosis >1000000/cm³

CAUSES

EXCESSIVE POTASSIUM INTAKE/RELEASE

K supplements, Drugs, Salt substitues, Dates, Peanuts, Cashews, Dried figs

Spinach, Avocadoes, Tomatoes, Potatoes, Carrots, Cauliflower, Broccoli

Bananas, Kiwis, Mangos, Oranges, Enteral Nutrition supplements

Tissue necrosis

- Rhabdomyolysis
  - crush injury, seizures, electric shock, cocaine, sepssi, blunt or penetrating trauma
- Ischemia
- Hemorrhage

REDISTRIBUTION

- METABOLIC ACIDOSIS
- HYPEROSMOLALITY
- HYPERGLYCEMIA/TYPE 4 RTA
- HYPOALDOSTERONISM- Addison's disease
- DRUGS
  - Drugs inhibiting the RAAS
  - Decrease renin secretion-Beta adrenergic agonists, ANP
  - Block renin-Direct renin inhibitors
  - RAAS inhibitors ACE inhibitors, ARBs
  - Decrease adrenal aldosterone synthesis-Heparin
  - Inhibit alosterone action-Spironlactone, Eplerenone

DECREASE RENAL POTASSIUM EXCRETION

- DRUGS
  - Potassium Sparing Diuretics
  - SulfamethaoxazoleTrimethoprim
  - Lithium therapy
  - NSAIDS
  - Digoxin
  - Calcineurin Inhibitors-Tacrolimus, Cyclosporine
- OBSTRUCTIVE UROPATHY
- KIDNEY DISEASE
- GENETIC HYPERKALEMIC SYNDROMES
  - Pseudohypoaldosteronism type 1
    - Hypotension, dehydration, metabolic acidosis, hyperkalemia, Normal/high aldosterone levels, present in infancy
  - Pseudohypoaldosteronism type 2/Gordon's syndrome
    - Hypertensions, hyperkalemia, low renin and aldosterone levels, present in adolescence or young adults.

TREATMENT

MECHANISM	THERAPY	DOSE	ONSET
MEMBRANE STABILIZATION	Calcium Gluconate	Calcium Gluconate 10%, 10ml iv, over 10 minutes	1-3 minutes
	Insulin	10 units IV in 50ml 50% dextrose solution	30 minutes
	Albuterol	10-20mg, nebulized over 10 minutes	30 minutes
SHIFT POTASSIUM INTRACELLULAR	Furosemide	40-80mg IV	15 minutes
	Sodium bicarbonate	150mmol/L IV infusion	Hours
	Sodium polystyrene sulfonate	15-30g in 15ml sorbitol orally	1-2 hours
	Patiromer	8.4-25.2g daily	7 hours
REMOVE POTASSIUM	Hemodialysis	------	Immediate

ACE : Angiotension converting enzyme, ***ANP :*** Atrial natriuretic peptide, ***ARB :***Angiotensin receptor blockers, ***K :*** Potassium, ***NSAIDS :*** Non-steroidal anti-inflammatory drugs, ***RAAS :*** renin-angiotensin-aldosterone system, ***RTA :*** Renal tubular acidosis

METABOLIC ACIDOSIS

Paromita Das, Priti Meena

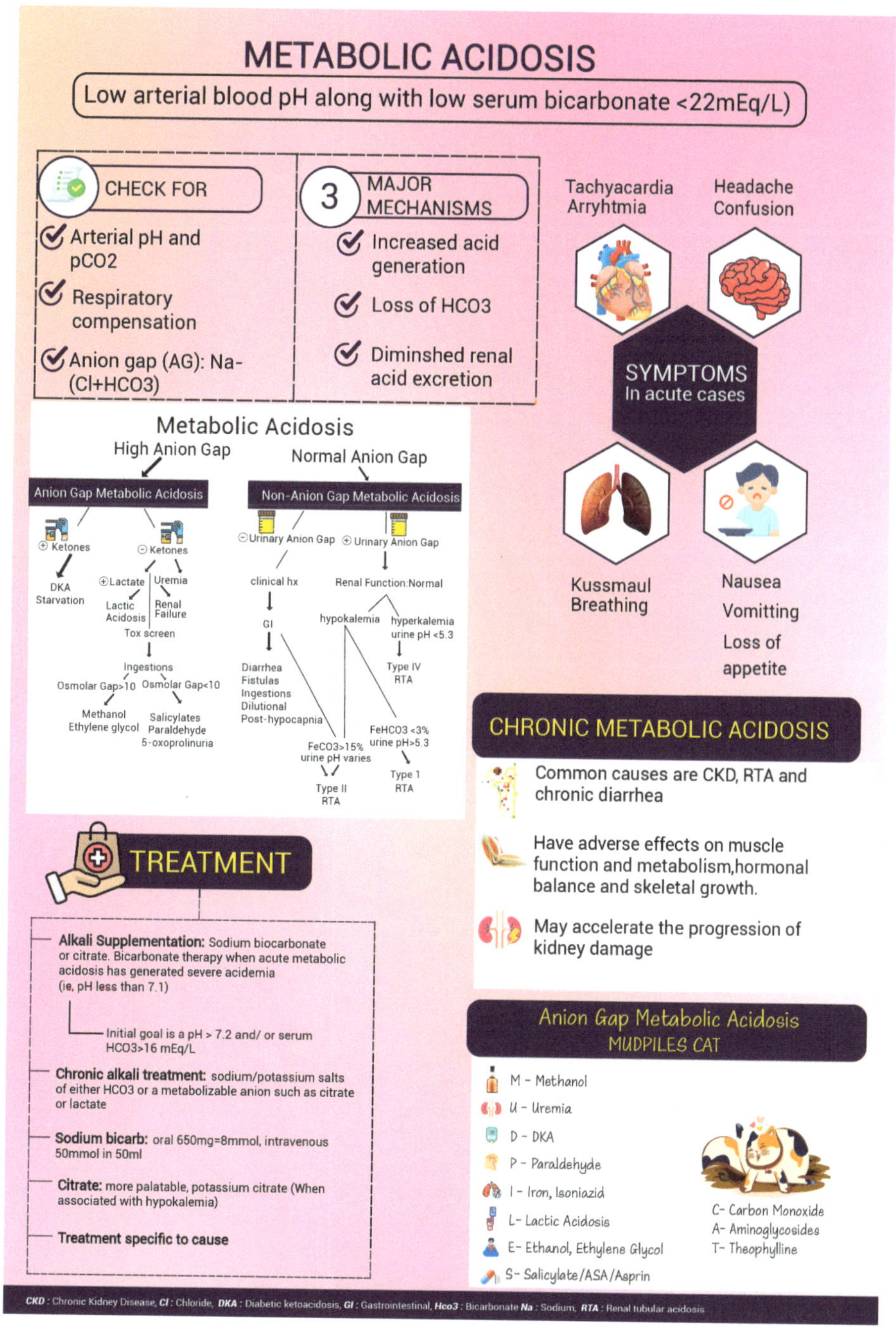

METABOLIC ALKALOSIS

Garima Aggarwal

PATHOPHYSIOLOGY

Generation of Metabolic Alkalosis

- Loss of acid in urine
- Loss of acid in GI tract (vomitting/GI suctioning)
- Excessive intake of bicarb/ equivalents (acetate/citrate/ lactate)
- Volume depletion

Maintenance of Metabolic Alkalosis

- ↓GFR -> reduced bicarbonate filtrate
- ↑Reabsorption of Hco3 <- increased Aldosterone/ Volume depletion
- Impaired secretion of Hco3 in urine -> decreased chloride delivery to distal tubule<- Volume depletion
- Hypokalemia
- Increased distal Na delivery->Increased K+/H+ secretion <- diuretic use

Disorder	Metabolic Alkalosis
Arterial Blood Gas	↑pH > 7.45 ↑Hco3 > 27 ↓H+
Respiratory Compensation	Hypoventilation ↑paCo2
Renal Compensation	Excrete Hco3 Conserve H+

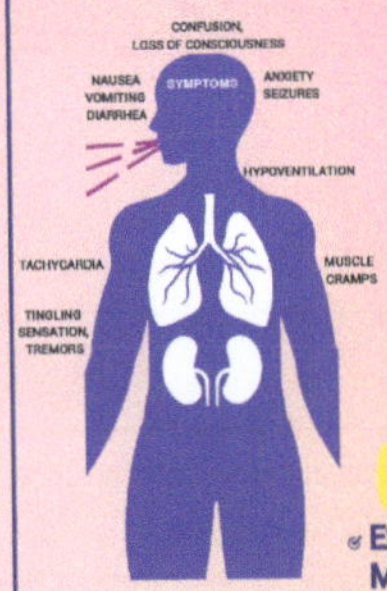

METABOLIC ALKALOSIS

Urine Chloride

<10 meq/L — Appropriate Renal Response
- **Vomiting**
- **NG suction**
- **Chloride Diarrhea**
- **Post Hypercapnoeic compensation**
- Previous diuretics use

>20 meq/L → **Hypertension**

- **Yes** → **Renin & Adolsterone Levels**
  - **Low**
    - **Exogenous Mineralocorticold excess (Licorice)**
    - Ectopic ACTH (Cushing's)
    - Liddle Syndrome
    - Congential Adrenal Hyperplasia
    - Apparent Mineralocorticold excess
  - **High**
    - Primary hyperaldosteronism (low renin, high aldosterone)
    - Renin secreting tumor
    - **Diuretic use**
    - Renovascular Hypertension
- **No**
  - **Diuretics**
  - Bartter's Syndrome
  - Gitelman Syndrome

TREATMENT OF METABOLIC ALKALOSIS

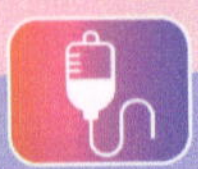

VOLUME REPLACEMENT

SALINE REPLACEMENT

Potassium Chloride

IF EDEMATOUS

Continue Diuretics

Consider Acetazolamide

MINERALOCORTICOID EXCESS

Spironolactone

Amiloride

Surgical removal

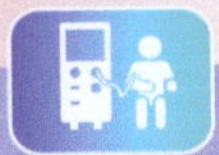

KIDNEY DYSFUNCTION

Dialysis with low bicarbonate

ACTH : Adrenocorticotropic hormone, ***GI :*** Gastrointestinal, ***GFR :*** Glomerular filtration rate, ***Hco3 :*** Bicarbonate, ***H + :*** Hydrogen ion, ***K :*** Potassium, ***Na :*** Sodium, ***NG :*** Nasogastric, PaCO2 : Partial pressure of carbon dioxide

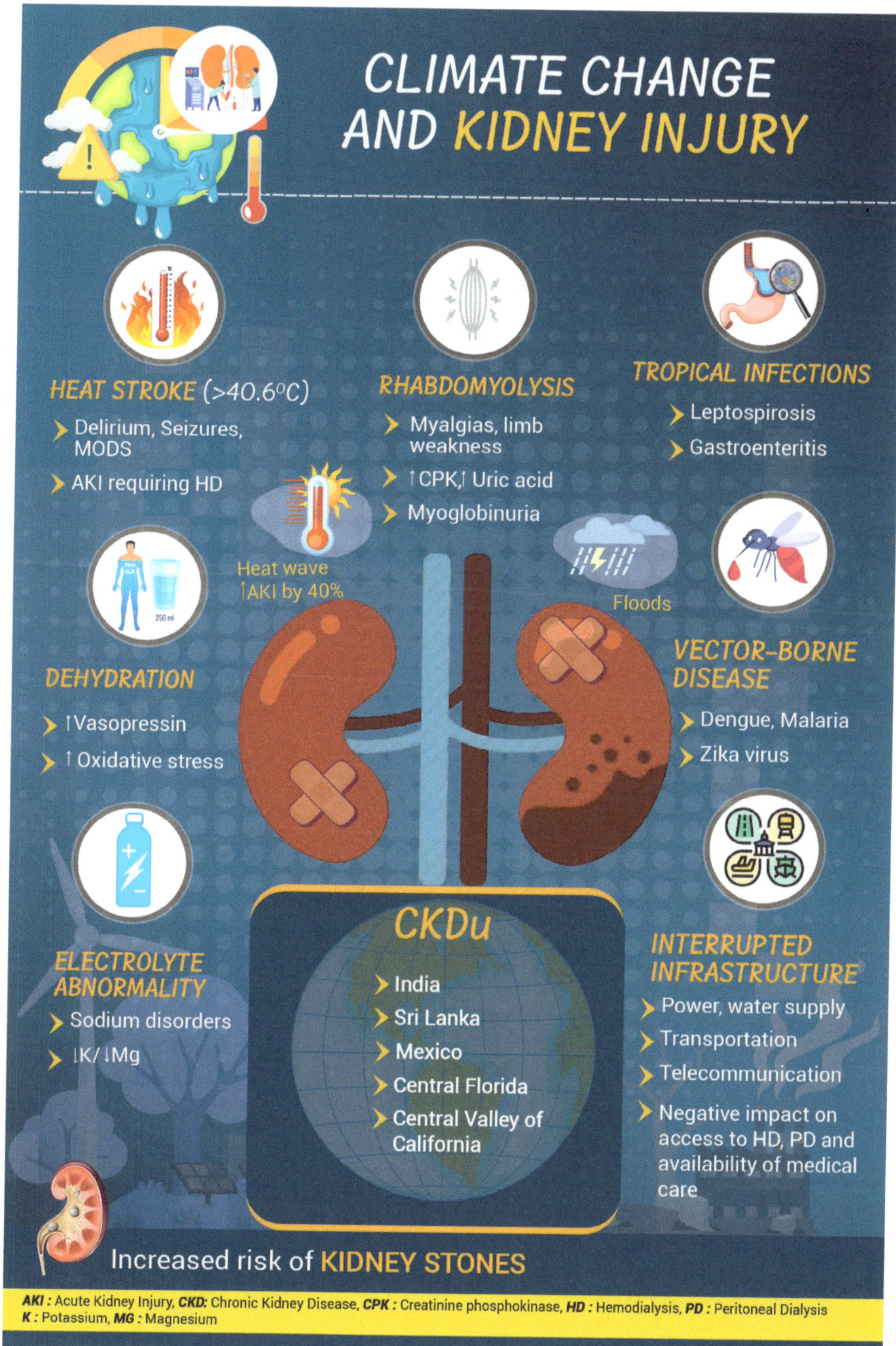
CLIMATE CHANGE AND KIDNEY INJURY
HEAT STROKE (>40.6°C)
Delirium, Seizures, MODS
AKI requiring HD
RHABDOMYOLYSIS
Myalgias, limb weakness
↑CPK,↑ Uric acid
Myoglobinuria
TROPICAL INFECTIONS
Leptospirosis
Gastroenteritis
Heat wave ↑AKI by 40%
Floods
DEHYDRATION
↑Vasopressin
↑ Oxidative stress
VECTOR-BORNE DISEASE
Dengue, Malaria
Zika virus
CKDu
India
Sri Lanka
Mexico
Central Florida
Central Valley of California
ELECTROLYTE ABNORMALITY
Sodium disorders
↓K/↓Mg
INTERRUPTED INFRASTRUCTURE
Power, water supply
Transportation
Telecommunication
Negative impact on access to HD, PD and availability of medical care
Increased risk of KIDNEY STONES
AKI : Acute Kidney Injury, CKD: Chronic Kidney Disease, CPK : Creatinine phosphokinase, HD : Hemodialysis, PD : Peritoneal Dialysis
K : Potassium, MG : Magnesium

www.ingramcontent.com/pod-product-compliance
Ingram Content Group UK Ltd.
Pitfield, Milton Keynes, MK11 3LW, UK
UKHW062019030826
14089UKWH00029B/168
* 9 7 9 8 8 9 6 7 3 4 5 2 9 *